9-26-11

THE
PALEO
DIET
FOR
ATHLETES

THE ANCIENT NUTRITIONAL FORMULA FOR
PEAK ATHLETIC PERFORMANCE

LOREN CORDAIN, PhD
AUTHOR OF *THE PALEO DIET*

AND ## JOE FRIEL, MS
AUTHOR OF THE TRAINING BIBLE BOOK SERIES

RODALE.

Revised edition published by Rodale Inc. in September 2012.

© 2005, 2012 by Loren Cordain and Joe Friel

Rodale books may be purchased for business or promotional use or for special sales. For information, please write to:
Special Markets Department, Rodale Inc., 733 Third Avenue, New York, NY 10017
Printed in the United States of America

Rodale Inc. makes every effort to use acid-free ∞, recycled paper ♻.

Book design by Chris Rhoads

Library of Congress Cataloging-in-Publication Data is on file with the publisher.
ISBN 978–1–60961–935–0 direct hardcover
ISBN 978–1–60961–917–6 trade paperback

Distributed to the trade by Macmillan
4   6   8   10   9   7   5   3   direct hardcover
                10   9   trade paperback

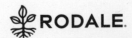

We inspire and enable people to improve their lives and the world around them.
rodalebooks.com

CONTENTS

ACKNOWLEDGMENTS

FROM JOE FRIEL:

First, I want to thank my coauthor, Dr. Loren Cordain, for introducing me to the Paleo Diet in 1995. In doing so, he forever changed the way I train athletes and improved the health and well-being not only of me but also of my family and friends. What I have learned from Loren has done more to improve my ongoing athletic performance than anything else I've done with my training in the last 20 years. I still view our chance meeting and subsequent conversations as we became good friends as turning points in my life.

Second, I want to thank the scores of athletes I have coached—from novice to Olympian—who allowed me to change their diets in order to refine the concepts you will read about here. Chief among them is Dirk Friel, my son, who continues to offer valuable feedback on the relationship between his high-level training for bike racing and his diet. And, finally, I want to thank Joyce, my wife of 46 years, for her assistance with many of the recipes included here and for allowing me the freedom to tinker in her kitchen and to get up at 4:00 a.m. to research and write about things that fascinate me.

FROM LOREN CORDAIN:

On a beautiful spring morning about 20 years ago, I went out for an early-morning run on the deserted roads and trails above Fort Collins, Colorado. About 2 miles into my 7-mile run, I noticed a lean silhouette following me about a half mile behind. Being somewhat competitive in those days, I picked up the tempo and expected to shake this lone runner. Nothing doing; he picked up the pace as well. After another mile, I put it into high gear, expecting to bury this upstart. Unbelievably, this unknown figure had managed to close the distance to less than 200 yards. By the end of the run, we were both in full sprint. As I was totally spent at the end of my run, Joe passed me and said, "Good morning!" I want to thank my coauthor for encouraging me to write this book in a slightly gentler manner than he pushed me on that Colorado spring morning. Finally, I want to thank my wife, Lorrie, and my three sons, Kyle, Kevin, and Kenny, for putting up with all of the lost weekends and late evenings needed to make this book happen.

INTRODUCTION

Information on the topic of nutrition for athletes has been on the market for the better part of the past century. It's interesting to note the changes that have occurred in such advice. For example, in 1945, Coach Willie Honeman offered the following dietary suggestions for bike racers:

> The question of food and what to eat is one that would take much space to cover. A good rule of thumb is to eat whatever foods appeal to you, but be sure they are of good quality and fresh. Avoid too many starchy foods, such as bread, potatoes, pies, pastries, etc. Eat plenty of green and cooked vegetables.
>
> —Willie Honeman, in *American Bicyclist,* 1945

Contrast Honeman's suggestions with what two modern cycling authorities proposed to athletes.

> Carbohydrate supplementation is essential to meet the needs of heavy training. Greater portions of pasta, potatoes, and breads can help, but many athletes may prefer the concentrated carbohydrate found in "high-carbohydrate drinks." Such products as Ultra Fuel, Exceed High-Carbohydrate Source, and Gatorlode are used to generate additional carbohydrate intake without the bulk of solid food.
>
> —Edmund Burke, PhD, and Jacqueline Berning, PhD, RD,
> in *Training Nutrition,* 1996

These selections illustrate what has happened to the logic of coaches, athletes, and even sports scientists since the 1970s. The current thinking is that athletes should load up on carbohydrate continuously, even to the extent of supplementing their diets with commercial products while avoiding "real" foods. The shift away from "good quality and fresh" foods, especially fruits, vegetables, and animal proteins, is widespread in the athletic world. Such a shift, while beneficial in terms of glycogen stores, which are necessary for performance—especially in endurance events—overlooks the necessity of eating foods that are also rich in other nutrients. This conventional viewpoint not only has negative consequences for health but also compromises an athlete's capacity for recovery and subsequent quality of training.

In *The Paleo Diet for Athletes,* we propose that this trend must be reversed and that the optimal model for the athlete is the same one that we as *Homo sapiens* have thrived on for nearly all of our existence on the planet—a Paleolithic, or Old Stone Age, diet, albeit one slightly modified to meet the unique demands of athletes.

The Paleo Diet is somewhat higher in protein and fat and lower in carbohydrate, relative to what sports nutritionists encourage American athletes to eat. But the greatest differences in what we propose here may be found in the timing of carbohydrate and protein ingestion, especially branched-chain amino acids; selecting foods based on glycemic load at certain times relative to training; the base-enhancing effects of our diet on blood and other body fluids; and periodization of diet in parallel with training. All of this means that you will recover faster and perform better by following our program: the Paleo Diet for Athletes. We've seen it happen in athlete after athlete for the past 15 years.

What we propose here is not intended as a quick-fix weight-loss diet, although many of the athletes who have converted to it have reduced their excess fat stores. The dietary strategies we offer are intended for health and performance enhancement.

Performance is obvious, but why health enhancement? Unfortunately, many athletes are not truly healthy, despite being magnificently fit. Health and fitness do not always go hand in hand.

High volumes of training, often exceeding 2 hours per day, play havoc on the human immune system when it is not given adequate nutrients for renewal in the hours following training. A daily diet top-heavy in starch, especially from a single source such as grains, is bound to leave the athlete's body starved for protein and many trace nutrients. The Paleo Diet for Athletes satisfies those demands daily.

Although heavily based upon science and thoroughly tested and honed in the real world of athletics, the value of eating much as our prehistoric ancestors ate is not generally accepted at face value by some scientists or athletes, as it flies in the face of much that we have been taught to believe about diet. When one suggests eating in this manner, many arguments against it are proposed. You may also be experiencing some healthy skepticism at this point—and some skepticism is a good thing. In order for you to continue reading this book in a more open manner, we need to address the most common of these concerns.

COMMON COUNTERARGUMENTS

Some of the most widespread, intuitive counterarguments against the Paleo Diet are that "they [hunter-gatherers] died at an early age" and thus "didn't live long enough to develop heart disease, cancer, and other chronic illnesses." Consequently, "they really were not healthier or fitter than modern people."

If you have bought into the first statement, then you are absolutely correct. There is no doubt that the average life span of hunter-gatherers and Stone Age people was quite short, compared with our own. Case in point: The average age of Neanderthals has been estimated at 12 to 15 years; pre-European-contact American Indians, 20 to 25 years. Today, US women live to age 79; men to 72. It should be pointed out, though, that "average life span" is a misleading term. In reality, average life span is nothing more than the average age at death for an entire population; it tells us zilch about the age and health characteristics of individual, living people. For example, if two parents lived to the ages of 79 and 72, were healthy for most of their adult lives, and had two children who died at birth, the average life span of this group of four people ([79 + 72 + 0 + 0]/4) would be 37.7 years. On the surface, based upon the low average life span, it would appear that all people in this group were not very healthy.

In order to more accurately portray a population's age and health characteristics, scientists have devised what are called life tables—charts that show the entire living population by age group, not just the people who have died. In a study of more than 450 !Kung hunter-gatherers in Botswana, life tables revealed that 10 percent of the population was age 60 and older. But more important, the aged populations in hunter-gatherer societies are virtually free of obesity, hypertension, high cholesterol, diabetes, and other chronic diseases that are near-universal afflictions of the elderly in Western societies. Hunter-gatherers died not from chronic, degenerative disease but from the accidents and trauma of a hazardous life spent in a perilous environment.

Think about camping out for your entire life, and you can get an appreciation for how harsh and dangerous their lifestyle was. While most of us really need not worry about death until middle or old age, hunter-gatherers commonly suffered early death from causes that claim comparatively few of us. They had no modern medicine, no advanced surgical procedures, no antibiotics, and no understanding of the germs that cause infection and disease. Civil war, strife, and regional conflict were a fact of life that continually raged throughout most of their lifetimes, and infanticide (the deliberate killing of infants) was commonly practiced. Because they lived outdoors their entire lives and were constantly challenged by the elements and the physical environment, the risk of injury from accidents was quite high over the course of their lifetimes. Hunting of big game, then as now, would have been a risky business, increasing the likelihood of accident or injury. The net result of living an entire life in a perilous environment produced a high death rate from trauma and accident in these people. It is rather remarkable that 10 to 20 percent of the population lived to 60 and beyond.

However, again, the take-home message is that the living, regardless of their age, were universally lean, fit, and free of the chronic degenerative diseases that are epidemic in our world. Figure I.1 shows that the aerobic fitness levels of young men, age 20 to 30 years, from hunter-gatherer and non-Westernized populations are far superior to that of the average Western couch potato, while Figure I.2 on page xii shows that their body fat levels are much lower.

It may surprise you, but despite diets rich in animal foods, these people have healthful blood cholesterol levels that leave the average Westerner in the dust (see Table I.1 on page xii). Further, high blood pressure—the most prevalent risk factor for coronary heart disease in the United States, affecting at least 50 million Americans—is rare or not present in non-Westernized societies.

The Yanomamo Indians of South America, to whom salt was unknown in the late 1960s and early 1970s, were completely free of high blood pressure. Table I.2 on page xiii shows the remarkable results of their salt-free diet in conjunction with their non-Westernized lifestyle on blood pressure. Not only is their average population blood pressure

FIGURE I-1

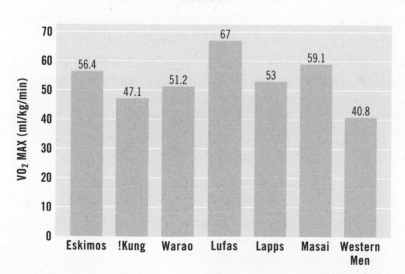

FIGURE I-2

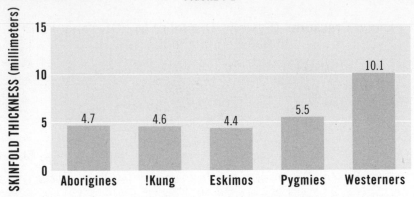

(102/64) lower than values considered to be normal (120/80) in the United States, but also there is no age-associated rise in blood pressure. In the United States, by the ages of 65 to 74, 65 percent of all Americans have high blood pressure (140/90 or greater).

The superb health and fitness levels of hunter-gatherers were recorded not only in the medical literature but also in historical accounts by early explorers, adventurers, and frontiersmen. Cabeza de Vaca, the Spanish explorer, saw Native Americans in Florida in 1527 and described them as "wonderfully well built, spare, very strong, and very swift." Similar obser-

TABLE I.1

Blood Cholesterol Levels in Non-Westernized Populations

SOCIETY	LOCATION	MEAN SERUM CHOLESTEROL (MG/DL)
Aborigines	Australia	139
Eskimos	Canada	141
Hadza	Tanzania	110
!Kung	Botswana	120
Pygmies	Zaire	106
Yanomamo (men)	Brazil	123
Yanomamo (women)	Brazil	142
Westerners	United States	210

TABLE I.2

Blood Pressures (Systolic/Diastolic) in 506 Yanomamo Indians Throughout Life

Males		Females	
AGE	BLOOD PRESSURE	AGE	BLOOD PRESSURE
0–9	93/59	0–9	96/62
10–19	108/67	10–19	105/65
20–29	108/69	20–29	100/63
30–39	106/69	30–39	100/63
40–49	107/67	40–49	98/62
50+	100/64	50+	106/64

vations of these Indians were made in 1564 by the French explorer Rene de Laudonniere, who noted, "The agility of the women is so great that they can swim over great rivers, bearing their children upon one of their arms. They climb up, also, very nimbly upon the highest trees in the country . . . even the most ancient women of the country dance with the others."

In his 1773 account of California Native Americans, Jacob Baegert noted that "the Californians are seldom sick. They are in general strong, hardy, and much healthier than the many thousands who live daily in abundance and on the choicest fare that the skill of Parisian cooks can prepare." In his book *Across Unknown South America*, Henry Savage Landor describes the Borono Indians of the Amazon in 1913.

They displayed powerful chests, with ribs well covered with flesh and muscle. With their dark yellow skins they were not unlike beautiful bronze torsi. The abdominal region was never unduly enlarged, perhaps owing to the fact that their digestion was good, and also because they took a considerable amount of daily exercise. . . . The anatomical detail of the body was perfectly balanced. The arms were powerful, but with fine, well-formed wrists—exquisitely chiseled, as were all attachments of their limbs. Great refinement of the race was also to be noticed in the shape of their legs—marvelously modeled, without an ounce of extra flesh, and with small ankles.

Captain Cook, who visited New Zealand in 1772, was particularly impressed by the good health of the native Maori.

It cannot be thought strange that these people enjoy perfect and uninterrupted health. In all our visits to their towns, where young and old, men and women, crowd about us, prompted by the same curiosity that carried us to look at them, we never saw a single person who appeared to have any bodily complaint, nor among the numbers that we have seen naked did we perceive the slightest eruption upon the skin, or any marks that an eruption had been left behind. . . . A further proof that human nature is here untainted with disease is the great number of old men that we saw . . . appeared to be very ancient, yet none of them were decrepit; and though not equal to the young in muscular strength, were not a whit behind them in cheerfulness and vivacity.

Another common counterargument proposed by doubting Thomases is this: "We don't really know what they, our Stone Age ancestors, ate." In Chapter 8, we will delve into all the archaeological, anthropological, physiological, and fossil evidence showing us exactly what Stone Age hunter-gatherers ate. But for now, let us challenge you with a simple question that most of you could intuitively work out with little or zero knowledge of the fossil record or archaeology.

What foods could not have been consumed by Stone Age people?

This is no trick question; just do a little bit of reasoning with what you know about how some of the foods on your daily platter got there. Let's tackle some of the easy ones first. How about the cup of milk you had with your breakfast cereal—where did it come from? Well, of course, a farmer milked a cow, and the milk was processed, pasteurized, homogenized, and bottled at a dairy, then eventually made its way to your local supermarket. Bingo—as simple as that, right?

Now stop and think a moment about where that docile, milkable cow came from. Were these peaceful, domesticated beasts always with us? Of course not! Modern-day milk cows were domesticated from wild, unruly beasts bearing enormous horns, called aurochs. Julius Caesar, who encountered these fierce brutes in Europe before they became extinct, remarked, "They are a little below the elephant in size, and of the appearance, color, and shape of a bull. Their strength and speed are extraordinary; they spare neither man nor wild beast which they have espied." Prior to domestication, aurochs, like all wild mammals, would not let humans approach them, much less milk them. So, you can see that all of the milk and dairy products we consume today simply would not have been on the menu of our hunter-gatherer ancestors. In the average US diet, milk and dairy represent 10.6 percent of total daily energy intake.

How about refined sugars? The annual per capita consumption of all sugars in the United States is a staggering 152 pounds, or 18.6 percent of our total daily calories from all foods combined! Do you think it would have been possible for your Stone Age ancestors to have consumed that much refined sugar? Absolutely not! Table sugar (sucrose) comes from either the sugarcane plant or sugar beets. Hunter-gatherers simply did not possess either the tools or knowledge to make refined sugars. In fact, sugar from sugarcane was first manufactured in northern India about 500 BC, whereas sugar extracted from sugar beets dates back to only 1747, in Germany. The ubiquitous high-fructose corn syrup, the preferred sweetener in soft drinks and many processed foods, was introduced into the US food supply as recently as the late 1970s. We now consume almost as much high-fructose corn syrup (63.6 pounds per capita) as we do sucrose (65.6 pounds per capita). There is no doubt that hunter-gatherers would have relished refined sugars, just as we do. However, except for honey, which was rare and only seasonally available, they simply had no readily available source of refined sugar.

Now that you are getting the drift of which foods could and could not have been on hunter-gatherers' menus, it becomes apparent that no highly processed foods were ever eaten. This isn't rocket science by any means—just simple, deductive logic that almost anyone can work out with a few basic facts.

However, here's a fact that may surprise you. Although bread, grains, and cereals symbolize "the staff of life" in virtually all Westernized societies and now represent almost 25 percent of the calories in the typical US diet, they were rarely or never consumed by our Stone Age ancestors. How do we know this? Have you ever tried to pop down a handful of uncooked whole wheat berries? How about some uncooked corn kernels or brown rice grains? If you perform these little experiments, you will see that the hard morsels come out of your body just like they went in— fully intact and undigested! Whole grains are tough as old boots unless their cell walls are first broken down by milling and their starch made digestible by cooking. Although our Stone Age ancestors had controlled fire by about 250,000 years ago, we know that grains did not become staple foods until the very recent appearance of crude stone grinding tools 13,000 years ago in the Middle East, according to fossil records. The bottom line is that grains, like dairy products and refined sugars, were not part of the native human diet.

While a cheese puff may look quite a bit different from a tortilla chip or a frozen waffle or even a bagel, all of these processed foods are almost indistinguishable from one another when you look at their individual food components. Think about it. They are really nothing more than mixtures of the same old three to six major ingredients—refined grains, refined sugars, some kind of processed vegetable oil, salt, artificial flavoring, and, perhaps, some kind of processed dairy product. Processed vegetable oils and salt, just like dairy food, refined sugars, and grains, are Johnny-come-latelies into the human diet. These ubiquitous foods and processed food mixtures made with them now compose 70 percent of all the food consumed in the US diet. By default, their inclusion into our diets displaces more healthful fruits, veggies, lean meats, and seafood—the staples of our Stone Age ancestors. As the next 12 chapters unfold, we will show you how you can improve your diet and thereby maximize your potential to improve your performance by increasing your intake of lean meats, seafood, fruits, and vegetables, along with careful and judicious consumption of certain "non-Paleo" modern foods.

CHAPTER 1

THE DIET REVOLUTION

When Joe and I began writing *The Paleo Diet for Athletes* in 2004, books on low-carbohydrate diets such as Dr. Atkins's New Diet Revolution, Protein Power, the Zone, and the South Beach Diet had ruled the bestselling book lists for at least a decade. At the time, millions of Americans lost weight with diets that flew directly in the face of conventional medical and nutritional wisdom, which advocated low-fat, high-carbohydrate diets. If we fast-forward to 2012, most (but not all) things have remained the same. The USDA replaced its "Food Pyramid" with the "MyPlate" in June 2011; however, the change was only cosmetic in nature, as the same old low-fat, high-carbohydrate recommendations remained firmly in place. *The Zone* and *Protein Power* have disappeared from the bestseller lists, only to be replaced by the latest reincarnation of *Atkins* and *The South Beach Diet*. In the ensuing 7 years since our book was first published, a new concept has arrived on the dietary scene that threatens to displace not only the low-carb diets but also government- and institution-recommended low-fat, high-carbohydrate diets.

In the past 2 years, Paleo diets have become internationally known, and books such as *The Paleo Diet, The Paleo Solution, The Paleo Diet Cookbook, The Paleo Diet for Athletes, Paleo Comfort Foods, Everyday Paleo, The Paleo Answer, Make It Paleo, The Primal Blueprint,*

Well Fed: Paleo Recipes for People Who Love to Eat, and others have dominated the bestseller lists. In Figure 1.1 from Google Trends from a search of "Paleo Diet" (www.google.com/trends?q=the+paleo+diet), it is apparent that, except for a small group of dedicated followers, the Paleo Diet concept was virtually unknown to the world in the 4 years following the publication of our book in 2005. In contrast, during the past 2 years, "Paleo" has literally become a household word and is perhaps the hottest new concept in diet, health, nutrition, and lifestyle. More important, as we will show you, the fundamental science behind contemporary diets based upon Stone Age food groups underlies their acceptance in both the scientific and popular literature.

A similar revolution in dietary thinking has made waves in the sports world by athletes worldwide who happen to be privy to this way of eating that has dramatically improved their athletic performances. Their dietary formula for success was not accidentally stumbled upon by trial and error but resulted from a chance conversation between two old friends, Joe Friel and myself, in the spring of 1995.

Fast-forward 17 years. Joe has become an internationally recognized coach of world-class athletes, has written 11 bestselling books on ath-

FIGURE 1.1

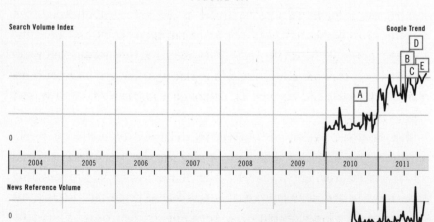

letic training, and is a worldwide authority on endurance training. Meanwhile, Loren, a university professor, has become a leading international scientific authority on Stone Age (Paleolithic) diets, and has written more than 50 scientific papers on the topic as well as five popular diet books. Had Joe and I not had that conversation in the spring of 1995, the small ripple that eventually became a tidal wave concerning diet and athletic performance likely never would have surfaced.

LOREN'S CHALLENGE:
THE PALEO DIET IN A NUTSHELL

In 1995, I challenged Joe to give the Paleo Diet a try. Joe had been a longtime adherent to the standard very high-carbohydrate diet for athletes and was skeptical of my claim that eating less starch would benefit performance. Nearly every successful endurance athlete that Joe had known ate as he did, with a heavy emphasis on cereals, bagels, bread, rice, pasta, pancakes, and potatoes. In fact, Joe had done quite well on this diet as an All-American duathlete (run-bike-run) in his age group, winning national races and finishing in the top 10 at World Championships. Joe had also coached many successful athletes, both professional and amateur, who ate the same way he did.

I suggested Joe try eating a diet more in line with the Paleo Diet for 1 month. Joe took the challenge, determined to show me that eating as he had for years was the way to go. He started by simply cutting back significantly on starches and dairy and replacing those lost calories with fruits, vegetables, and lean meats. Although a simple formula, it wasn't easy at first.

For the first 2 weeks, Joe felt miserable. His recovery following workouts was slow, and his workouts were sluggish. He figured he was well on his way to proving that I was wrong. But in week 3, a curious thing happened. He noticed not only that he was feeling better but also that his recovery following workouts was speeding up significantly, and he decided to experiment to see how many hours he could train. Since his early forties (he was 51 at the time), he had not been able to train more than about 12 hours per week; whenever he exceeded that weekly volume, upper respiratory infections would soon set him back. In week 4, he trained 16 hours without a sign of a cold, sore throat, or ear infection. He was amazed—he hadn't done that many hours in nearly 15 years. He decided to keep the experiment going. That year Joe finished third at the US National Championship with an excellent race and qualified for the US team for the World Championships. He had a stellar season, one of his best in years.

Joe's little experiment proved to have far-reaching effects. After making certain refinements to my basic Paleo Diet, Joe found this way of eating to be "ergogenic," a term exercise physiologists use to describe nutritional supplements that can enhance athletic performance. By the late 1990s, Joe was recommending the Paleo Diet to the athletes he coached, including Ryan Bolton, a member of the US Olympic Triathlon team in the 2000 Sydney Olympics and a winner of the Ironman USA Triathlon. Increasingly, by word of mouth and the Internet, athletes worldwide were becoming aware of the competitive edge they could gain by adopting a diet based upon my dietary principles and fine-tuned by Joe's practical experience with it.

The Paleo Diet for Athletes is not just for world-class performers like Ryan Bolton and Gordo Bryn (an ardent devotee of the Paleo Diet and past winner of the Ultraman Triathlon and the World's Toughest Half-Ironman Triathlon) but also for everyday fitness enthusiasts like Don Moffat. Here's Don's story.

> I wish I had known about the Paleo Diet 5 years ago, when I was a sub-3-hour marathoner before my health started breaking down due to insulin resistance-related issues. Following a high-protein, low-carb diet for the last 2 months has created startling results in my fitness. I've lost 3 inches from my waist (down to 32), and I can't believe how, at 38, I'm putting on muscle. My run times have

dropped by 25 percent. (I'm still not fast again, but I'm seeing steady, week-to-week progress.) I find the increase in muscle strength particularly gratifying, as this was always a problem for me before, even in my early twenties. It's sort of like getting some youth back.

WHY IS THE PALEO DIET FOR ATHLETES ERGOGENIC?

There is indeed a method to this madness, and I have uncovered the scientific basis for the effectiveness of the modification of the original Paleo Diet. In a nutshell, there are four basic reasons the Paleo Diet enhances athletic performance.

1. Branched-chain amino acids. First, the diet is high in animal protein, which is the richest source of the branched-chain amino acids— valine, leucine, and isoleucine. Branched-chain amino acids (BCAA) are different from other amino acids that collectively make up protein in that they are potent stimulants for building and repairing muscle. This information is new and has been reported in the scientific literature only in the past decade. But the dig is this: These amino acids work best when consumed in the postexercise window.

Lean meats and fish are far and away the greatest sources of BCAA. A 1,000-calorie serving of lean beef provides 33.7 grams of BCAA, whereas the same serving of whole grains supplies a paltry 6 grams. Because most endurance athletes focus on starches (breads, cereals, pasta, rice, and potatoes) and sugars at the expense of lean meats, particularly following a hard workout, they get precious little muscle-building BCAA in their diets. By consuming high amounts of animal protein (and hence BCAA) along with sufficient carbohydrate, athletes can rapidly reverse the natural breakdown of muscle that occurs following a workout and thereby reduce recovery time and train at a greater intensity at the next session. Joe's advice for athletes to increase fresh meats along with plenty of fruits and vegetables now makes perfect sense and explains the athletes' near-universal report of improved recovery with these dietary recommendations.

2. Blood acidity versus alkalinity. In addition to stimulating muscle growth via BCAA, the Paleo Diet for Athletes simultaneously prevents muscle protein breakdown because it produces a net metabolic alkalosis. All foods, upon digestion, report to the kidney as either acid or alkali (base). The typical American diet is net acid producing because of its high reliance upon acid-yielding grains, cheeses, and salty processed foods at the expense of base-producing fruits and veggies. The athlete's body is even more prone to blood acidosis due to the by-products of exercise. One way the body neutralizes a net acid-producing diet is by breaking down muscle tissue. Because the Paleo Diet for Athletes is rich in fruits and veggies, it reverses the metabolic acidosis produced from the typical grain- and starch-laden diet that many athletes consume, thereby preventing muscle loss.

3. Trace nutrients. Fruits and vegetables are also rich sources of anti-oxidant vitamins, minerals, and phytochemicals and, together with fresh meats (excellent sources of zinc and B vitamins), promote optimal immune-system functioning. The refined grains, oils, sugars, and processed foods that represent the typical staples for most athletes are nearly devoid of these trace nutrients. From examining the training logs of numerous people he has coached, Joe found that the frequency and duration of colds, flu, and upper respiratory illnesses are reduced when athletes adopt the Paleo Diet. A healthy athlete, free of colds and illness, can train more consistently and intensely and thereby improve performance.

4. Glycogen stores. One of the most important goals of any athletic diet is to maintain high muscle stores of glycogen, a body fuel absolutely essential for high-level performance. Dietary starches and sugars are the body's number one source for making muscle glycogen. Protein won't do, and neither will fat. Athletes and sports scientists have known this truth for decades. Regrettably, they took this concept to extremes; high-starch, cereal-based, carbohydrate-rich diets were followed with near-fanatical zeal 24 hours a day, 7 days a week.

It is a little-known fact, but, similar to the situation with branched-chain amino acids, glycogen synthesis by muscles occurs most effectively in the immediate postexercise window. Muscles can build all the glycogen they need when they get starch and sugar in the narrow time frame following exercise. Eating carbs all day long is overkill and actually serves to displace the muscle-building animal proteins and alkalinity-enhancing, nutrient-dense fruits and veggies that are needed to promote muscle growth and boost the immune system. Perhaps the most important refinement made to my original Paleo Diet was Joe's recognition that consumption of starches and simple sugars was necessary and useful only during exercise and in the immediate postexercise period. Joe has also found that certain carbohydrates are more effective than others in restoring muscle glycogen, particularly specific types of sugar, such as glucose and net alkaline-producing starches found in bananas, sweet potatoes, and yams.

NOTHING NEW IN 40 YEARS

The standard dietary advice given to athletes by sports physiologists, nutritionists, and physicians hasn't changed much in 40 years. It is similar to the USDA's Food Pyramid (recently renamed the MyPlate)—high in grain-based carbohydrates and low in fat—the same diet that many scientists believe is partially responsible for the obesity epidemic in this country. The world now is aware that an alternative exists to the Food Pyramid/MyPlate. Low-carbohydrate, high-protein diets have proven to be more effective in promoting weight loss than are conventional high-carbohydrate, low-fat diets. Unfortunately, many people in the athletic world are little aware that these same types of diets (higher in protein and lower in carbohydrate) can be extremely effective in enhancing performance. Except for the athletes privy to my research and Joe's practical implementation of it, athletes in general are unaware that an alternative diet exists—a diet that can maximize performance in a range of sports, from bodybuilding and tennis to running and the triathlon.

The Paleo Diet for Athletes was and is revolutionary and is creating an upheaval in the sports world, similar to the commotion set in play by the therapeutic and health effects of the Paleo Diet. The information contained in this book is thoroughly supported by scientific literature, to which Loren continues to make cutting-edge contributions. More important, Joe has shown that the Stone Age diet of our ancient ancestors, with slight modifications, works extremely well for recreational athletes all the way up to Olympians. The Paleo Diet for Athletes has passed the most important test by the most critical audience of all: the athletes themselves.

THE PALEO DIET FOR ATHLETES: NUTRITIONAL CHARACTERISTICS IN A NUTSHELL

The essential dietary principles of the Paleo Diet for Athletes are straight-forward: You can eat as much fresh meat, poultry, seafood, fruit, and veggies as you like. Foods that are not part of modern-day Paleolithic fare include cereal grains, dairy products, legumes, alcohol, salty foods, processed meats, refined sugars, and nearly all processed foods.

There are a number of crucial exceptions to these fundamental rules that will be completely explained in coming chapters. Case in point: Immediately before, during, and after a workout or competition, certain non-Paleo foods should be eaten to promote a quick recovery. During all other times, meals that closely follow the 21st-century Paleolithic diet, described in Chapter 9, will encourage comprehensive long-term recovery and allow you to attain your maximal performance potential.

At first glance, you might think it counterproductive or even foolish to reduce or eliminate two entire food groups (cereal grains and dairy),

TABLE 1.1

Sample 1-Day Menu from a Modern Diet Based on Paleolithic Food Groups for a Woman
(25 years old; 2,200-calorie daily intake)

FOOD	QUANTITY (g)	ENERGY (kcal)
Breakfast		
Cantaloupe	276	97
Atlantic salmon (broiled)	333	605
Lunch		
Vegetable salad with walnuts		
Shredded romaine lettuce	68	10
Sliced carrot	61	26
Sliced cucumber	78	10
Quartered tomatoes	246	52
Lemon-juice dressing	31	8
Walnuts	11	70
Broiled lean pork loin	86	205
Dinner		
Vegetable, avocado, and almond salad		
Shredded mixed greens	112	16
Tomato	123	26
Avocado	85	150
Slivered almonds	45	260
Sliced red onion	29	11
Lemon-juice dressing	31	8
Steamed broccoli	468	131
Lean beef sirloin tip roast	235	400
Dessert		
Strawberries	130	39
Snacks		
Orange	66	30
Carrot sticks	81	35
Celery sticks	90	14

along with most of the processed foods in your diet. One way of looking at our Paleo dietary recommendations is to compare them with the USDA Food Pyramid/MyPlate, the diet officially recommended by the US government and specifically designed to improve our health and reduce our risk of chronic disease. The USDA has published an extensive handbook, *Using the Food Guide Pyramid: A Resource for Nutrition Educators* (available on the Web at www.nal.usda.gov/fnic/Fpyr/guide.pdf), in which government dietitians have outlined sample 5-day menus that conform to Food Pyramid guidelines. The USDA has also been gracious enough to provide us with the vitamins, minerals, and nutrient values in its example menus. Consequently, it is a relatively simple exercise to compare modern-day Paleo diets with those officially sanctioned by the USDA.

Remember the ground rules of modern-day Stone Age diets: The diets contain no grains, dairy products, salt, processed foods, or processed meats; they consist almost entirely of fresh fruits, veggies, meats, and seafood. Table 1.1 on page 9 outlines a typical menu for a 25-year-old woman whose daily caloric intake is 2,200 calories.

Now let's see how this representative day's worth of modern Paleo food stacks up against the USDA Food Pyramid/MyPlate. First, take a look at the major dietary components, which are listed in Table 1.2. You immediately see that the Paleo Diet is much higher in protein and lower in carbohydrate than the Food Pyramid/MyPlate diet. Notice that a little more than half of the calories in the Paleo Diet come from meat and seafood, and that almost 40 percent of the daily energy comes from fat. The fats you will be getting in this diet are just plain good for you! Observe that the good fats (monounsaturated and polyunsaturated fats) that lower blood cholesterol levels are considerably higher than what you would get by following the Food Pyramid/MyPlate diet.

Many people have heard that omega-3 fatty acids found in fish like salmon are healthful, but fewer are aware that a family of fats called omega-6 fatty acids, found in vegetable oils, margarine, and processed foods, can be harmful when consumed at the expense of omega-3s. In the standard American diet, the ratio of omega-6 to omega-3 fatty acids

TABLE 1.2

Dietary Characteristics of a Contemporary Diet Based on Paleolithic Food Groups and in a Recommended USDA Food Pyramid Diet for a Woman (25 years old; 2,200-calorie daily intake)

NUTRIENT	FOOD PYRAMID	MODERN PALEO DIET
Protein (g)	113	217
Protein (% energy)	20	38
Carbohydrate (g)	302	129
Carbohydrate (% energy)	53	23
Total sugars (g)	96.6	76.5
Fiber (g)	30	42.5
Fat (grams)	67	100.3
Fat (% total energy)	27	39
Saturated fat (g)	19.6	18
Saturated fat (% total energy)	7	6.4
Monounsaturated fat (g)	22.8	44.3
Polyunsaturated fat (g)	19	26.7
Omega-3 fatty acids (g)	1	9.6
Omega-6 fatty acids (g)	14.3	14.2
Cholesterol (mg)	219	461
Sodium (mg)	2,626	726
Potassium (mg)	3,450	9,062

is an unhealthy 10:1. Contrast this ratio to the wholesome 1:1 to 3:1 in the native human diet. Now take a look at the Food Pyramid/MyPlate: The recommendation is an appalling 14:1 and is actually worse than what the average American is currently eating! The Food Pyramid was originally conceived and thrust upon a trusting US public in 1992, prior to the widespread knowledge that an imbalance in omega-6 and omega-3 fatty acids had much to do with health and well-being. Unfortunately, we are still saddled with this botched bit of advice even after the Pyramid was revised in June 2011 to the current MyPlate recommendations.

But just wait—there are troubles with the Food Pyramid/MyPlate beyond its improper fat balance. In 1992, the concept of a glycemic load and its impact on health were unknown to the dietitians who designed the Pyramid. Should we be concerned about the glycemic load of a food? Absolutely! Does the Food Pyramid/MyPlate differentiate between high and low glycemic foods? Absolutely not! There is little doubt that even the recently revised MyPlate is badly in need of repair. It's high time that nutritionists consider the evolutionary basis for the optimal human diet rather than relying upon human foibles and biases in developing healthful, performance-enhancing diets.

As an athlete, you want to maximize your performance by maximizing your diet. This includes the amount of vitamins and minerals that you get from your food. Let's contrast the nutrient density of our sample

TABLE 1.3

Trace Nutrients in a Modern Diet Based on Paleolithic Food Groups and in a Recommended USDA Food Pyramid Diet for Women (25 years old; 2,200-calorie daily intake)

	FOOD PYRAMID		MODERN PALEOLITHIC DIET	
Nutrient	Amount	% RDA	Amount	% RDA
Vitamin A	1,659 mcg RE	207	6,386 mcg RE	798
Vitamin B$_1$	2.3 mg	209	3.4 mg	309
Vitamin B$_2$	2.6 mg	236	4.2 mg	355
Vitamin B$_3$	30 mg	214	60 mg	428
Vitamin B$_6$	2.6 mg	200	6.7 mg	515
Folate	453 mcg	113	891 mcg	223
Vitamin B$_{12}$	4.7 mcg	196	17.6 mcg	733
Vitamin C	233 mg	388	748 mg	1,247
Vitamin E	10 IU	125	19.5 IU	244
Calcium	1,215 mg	122	691 mg	69
Phosphorus	808 mg	258	2,546 mg	364
Magnesium	427 mg	138	643 mg	207
Iron	19 mg	127	24.3 mg	162
Zinc	14 mg	116	27.4 mg	228

Paleo Diet to the USDA Food Pyramid/MyPlate. Take a quick look at the values in Table 1.3, and you will see that there is really no comparison. Except for calcium, the Paleo Diet simply blows away the Food Pyramid/MyPlate. In Chapters 5 and 9, we fully explain why a reduced calcium intake does not represent a problem, particularly if you eat ample fruits and vegetables.

An essential part of making this diet work for endurance athletes like you is to maintain an adequate carbohydrate intake so that your muscle glycogen levels will be fully restored before your next workout. Consequently, you will need to include additional carbohydrates in your diet, particularly during and following long workouts. In Chapters 2, 3, and 4, we fully explain the ins and outs of carbohydrate ingestion relative to your workout, your training schedule, and your personal needs.

PART I

THE ROAD MAP TO PEAK PERFORMANCE AND HEALTH

CHAPTER 2

STAGE I:
EATING BEFORE
EXERCISE

What should an athlete eat before, during, and after exercise? This is a question to which athletes have sought the answer for as long as there have been competitive sports. In the days of the Roman Empire, gladiators ate the heart and muscle of lions before the contest, believing this would give them the ferocious qualities of the animal. As late as the 1960s, athletes were still eating prodigious quantities of red meat before engaging in "battle." In the 1970s, there was a swing toward consuming carbohydrates on race day. That trend still continues, but recently there has been an increased interest in protein and fat in the athlete's race-day diet. And so the pendulum swings the other way once again.

While the role of carbohydrate ingestion before, during, and after exercise has been studied extensively over the past 40 years, only recently has there been much research into the role and timing of dietary protein and fat relative to exercise. Since such research is still in its infancy, there is a great deal not fully understood, and, further complicating the matter, there are contradictions in the limited research available.

THE DEMANDS OF ENDURANCE TRAINING

Training for endurance sports such as running, cycling, triathlon, rowing, swimming, and cross-country skiing places great demands on the body, putting the athlete in some stage of recovery almost continuously during periods of heavy training. The keys to optimum recovery are sleep and diet. Even though we recommend that everyone eat a diet similar to what our Stone Age ancestors ate, we realize that nutritional concessions must be made for the athlete who is training at a high volume in the range of 10 to 35 or more hours per week of rigorous exercise. Rapid recovery is the biggest issue facing such an athlete. While it's not impossible to recover from such training loads on a strict Paleo Diet, it is somewhat more difficult to recover quickly. If it is modified before, during, and immediately following challenging workouts, the Paleo Diet provides two benefits sought by all athletes— quick recovery for the next workout and superior health for the rest of your life.

Such high training loads require a great intake of carbohydrate for short-term replenishment of expended glycogen stores, perhaps as much as 1,200 to 1,500 calories. Eating low to moderate glycemic index foods in the Paleo-approved categories of fruits and vegetables may certainly replace such deficiencies, but will be accompanied by several pounds of fiber. Such a diet will also be slow to replace expended glycogen stores in the muscles following hard workouts or races, thus delaying or substantially affecting a subsequent workout or race in the next few hours and days. This is when modification of a strict Paleo Diet is beneficial to the serious athlete.

While highly fit and athletic, our Stone Age ancestors never ran 26.2 miles at the fastest pace possible or willingly took on any of the other racing challenges of 21st-century athletes. Evolutionarily, today's athletes are pushing the limits of physiology. Their diets must be adjusted to meet these demands.

In this and the next two chapters, we will examine the times when eating in ways other than the more conventional Paleo Diet is appropriate for the serious endurance athlete. But we can't emphasize strongly enough that these are exceptions to the standards discussed in Chapter 9 and are limited to specific time windows relative to training sessions and races. In Chapters 2, 3, and 4, we discuss the five recovery stages through which the athlete passes on most days that include exercise. By dividing the day into the following stages and eating appropriate foods in adequate amounts in each, you can enhance your recovery and maximize performance.

Stage I: Immediately before exercise

Stage II: During exercise

Stage III: 30 minutes immediately following exercise

Stage IV: A period equal to the duration of the preceding exercise session

Stage V: Long-term, postexercise recovery preceding the next Stage I

Before getting into the details of these stages, let's take a look at diet during a time when most athletes seem to be unsure of what to eat—the week of the race. To differentiate the importance of all of the race events on your schedule, we classify them as priority A, B, or C. Priority A events are the most important on your schedule. Normally an athlete will have only two or three of these planned for a given season since each involves cutting back on the training load for several days to a few weeks prior. Such reductions, while allowing the athlete to fully realize race readiness, may well lead to diminished fitness if done more frequently than a few times per season. Priority C races are the least important events on your schedule. There may be many of these because they are considered little more than challenging workouts done, for example, to test fitness or to make final preparations for a higher-priority race. As you might expect, priority B events fall between A and C in terms of importance. You want to do well at these races, so you may rest for a few days before them, but you won't taper your training over the longer period as is done for the highest-priority events.

EATING DURING RACE WEEK

This is not a time to make wholesale changes in your diet. Stick with the foods you've been eating, but be aware that if this is a priority A event, you will probably need to reduce the amount of food that you eat this week, as your training volume is reduced, so you may avoid excessive weight gain. You might still put on as much as 2 or 3 pounds, but most of that is water. For every gram of glycogen your body stores away in the muscles, it also packs away 2.6 grams of water. Having extra water on board may well be an advantage, especially if you'll be racing in hot or humid conditions.

The day before the race, if you've been carefully following a Paleo Diet, shift your food choices by taking in slightly more carbohydrate than usual to ensure that your carbohydrate storage sites are full. With the reduced volume this week, your body is primed to store glycogen, so this last day of shifting your diet to increased carbohydrate should be adequate.

Now is a good time to eat more fruits such as bananas, peaches, cantaloupe, watermelon, and honeydew melon, along with vegetables such as potatoes, sweet potatoes, and yams. Snack on dried fruit today. To moderate the glycemic index of these foods, include protein and fat with each meal. Examples of good fats to select today are olive and flaxseed oils as salad dressing along with cold-water fish such as salmon, halibut, haddock, herring, and mackerel. Such fish, as always, will satisfy both the protein and fat needs the evening before the race. Skip the pasta party.

In addition, reduce dietary fiber to allow for easier digestion of foods in preparation for the next day's race. Otherwise, eat at usual times and keep food types as normal as possible.

STAGE I: EATING BEFORE EXERCISE

It happens all too often: An athlete prepares meticulously for weeks and months for an important event. There is no workout that is too demanding, no sacrifice too great. Then comes race day, and an error is made in the prerace meal: choosing food that takes too long to digest or digests too quickly; eating too much too close to the race start; taking in too little fluid; or eating nothing at all. The result is a disastrous performance—all that preparation for naught. We've seen it happen too many times. In fact, we've experienced it ourselves. Live and learn.

How could this have been prevented? How, indeed, could the athletic performance have been enhanced by the foods eaten before a demanding race or training session? The purpose of this section is to help you establish a dietary routine that serves you well, whether for a workout starting at your back door or a race a thousand miles away. Of course, it's easier if you're at home than on the road. Our goal here is to establish a select menu of foods that you can find whether you're in Hometown, USA, or traveling to Hobart, Australia, for a race.

Preexercise Eating Goals

Let's start by examining the goals for preexercise foods and fluids. There are five major objectives we are trying to accomplish with nutrient intake just before the race or workout.

Satisfy hunger. This is pretty basic, so it's a wonder that some athletes ignore food first thing in the morning. If it's race day, you may be too preoccupied to be aware of telltale signs at first, but your body will soon cry out for food. The longer you put it off, the greater the risk of starting exercise underfueled. The biggest downside of such a mistake is what cyclists call "bonking" and runners call "hitting the wall." You simply run very low on muscle and liver glycogen—the body's storage form of carbohydrate. When that happens, you're forced to slow down or completely stop.

Realizing that you're hungry in the last hour before exercise may well be too late. Eating so close to starting is likely to do more harm than good. Don't start hungry and don't put off eating. If possible, eat at least an hour in advance of exercise. The higher the intensity of the workout or race, the more time is necessary for digestion. At first you may find it difficult to eat right out of bed, but this aversion is mostly mental. Get used to taking in food of some sort early every day and it will be much easier on race day. You may find that a liquid meal is the best option if you dislike eating early in the morning.

Restock carbohydrate stores depleted by the overnight fast. During the night, as you slept, your body was busy repairing and replacing tissues in an ongoing maintenance routine it has been engaged in since your conception. And, of course, there were energy demands throughout the night simply related to being alive—breathing, cardiac activity, movement, digestion, and other life-sustaining functions. All of this takes energy, and one of the most available fuel sources for this activity is the carbohydrate stored in your muscles as glycogen. So when you awake after several hours of sleep, your carbohydrate stores may be depleted by as much as 140 to 260 calories, depending on your body size and fat-free mass (muscles, bones, hair, fingernails, organs—everything other than fat). Replacing these expended calories, roughly 10 percent of your carbohydrate stores, is important to your immediate athletic performance, and the longer the race or workout session, the more critical this becomes.

Reestablish normal body fluid levels. Besides expending energy as you slept, your body also lost water in your breath, through your pores, and during any bathroom visits. First thing in the morning, your body may be down several ounces from normal hydration levels. Failing to replenish fluids prior to exercise could set you up for a substandard race or workout.

Optimize performance. This is a big one. Other than simply restoring your fuel and fluid levels, proper preexercise nutrition has a lot to do with how you perform. Certain nutrients have been shown to boost performance for some types of events. We'll examine these possibilities later in this chapter.

Prepare the body to recover quickly postexercise. The better your hydration and fuel levels are going into the race or workout, the faster you'll recover, assuming you refuel and rehydrate adequately during exercise. But if you start with a low tank, even if you eat and drink as you should during activity, recovery may well be delayed. This means it will take you longer to return to a high level of training in subsequent days. It's even more critical if you are working out two or three times a day or if you are stage racing, as road cyclists often do.

Preexercise Eating

There is little doubt that preexercise nutrient intake can help your athletic performance. The big question has to do with what you should eat and drink. We can offer several guidelines that come not only from the research but also from our personal experiences as athletes and from coaching hundreds of others in several sports over the past 30 years. In a nutshell, here are the guidelines that will help you make decisions about what to take in before starting a race or workout.

Consume 200 to 300 calories per hour prior to exercise. The amount you need is determined by your body size, how much you ate the night before, what time that meal was eaten, and your experience with eating before exercise. We recommend eating no less than 2 hours before the race or workout when possible. Three hours is usually better, especially if you tend to have a nervous stomach on race days. If you eat 2 hours before, take in 400 to 600 calories. If eating 3 hours before, you could eat 600 to 900 calories. Your body size and experience should help you narrow the range.

Take in mostly carbohydrate. As was explained in the previous section, during the multihour fast of your night's sleep, your body's stores of glycogen were reduced. The fastest, most efficient way to restore this vital fuel source is by eating carbohydrate. If chosen wisely, carbohydrate also has the advantage of digesting fairly quickly so that you won't be carrying a load of undigested foodstuffs early in the training session or race. The type of foods to eat will be addressed shortly.

The more time before the start of the race or workout, the more you should reduce the glycemic index of the meal. The glycemic index of a food indicates how quickly a carbohydrate's sugar gets into the blood. A quick release of sugar from the meal triggers the release of the hormone insulin by the pancreas. This results in a rapid decrease in the blood sugar level, followed quickly by increased hunger shortly before the race begins. That's not what you want to happen. But by eating a lower glycemic index food 2 or more hours before starting, your gut will have time to digest it and slowly replenish glycogen stores. Fruit, for example, is a good choice because its sugar, fructose, is slow to digest, lowering the glycemic index.

Keep the meal low in fiber. There are several ways to reduce the glycemic index of a food. One of the most effective is the addition of fiber. But this may be too effective for a preexercise meal; the fiber in some foods, such as coarse, whole-grain cereals, is so dense that it could well sit in your gut for several hours, soaking up fluids and swelling. That's not a good feeling to have at the start of a race or hard workout.

Include protein, especially the branched-chain amino acids. Amino acids are the building blocks of protein. Certain amino acids, the "essential" ones, are critical for your health and fitness and must be in the foods you eat because the body can't produce them. Research out of the lab of Peter Lemon, PhD, at the University of Western Ontario reveals that three of these essential amino acids, those called branched-chain amino acids (BCAA), have benefits for performance when taken before aerobic exercise. (If you study protein for athletes, you're sure to come across Dr. Lemon's name often, as he is considered one of the leading authorities in the world on this topic.) In this study, cyclists were given 6 grams of BCAA or 6 grams of gelatin 1 hour before an exhaustive session on a bicycle. Compared with the gelatin feeding, the BCAA significantly improved time to exhaustion and maximum power output, while lowering heart rate at submaximum efforts. Blood sugar and lactate levels did not differ between the two trials.

Other research has revealed that a mixture of the essential amino acids and carbohydrate taken before strenuous exercise not only improves endurance performance but also effectively stimulates protein synthesis after exercise. This is great news for the serious endurance athlete, as time to recovery is critical for performance. The faster you recover, the sooner you can do another quality workout; the more quality workouts in a given period of training, the better your subsequent performances in races.

Finally, an additional benefit of adding protein to a preexercise meal is that this lowers the glycemic index of the carbohydrate ingested along with it. A lowered glycemic index means a longer, slower release of sugar into the bloodstream during the subsequent exercise session, thus delaying the onset of fatigue.

Drink to satisfy thirst. You can prevent dehydration during exercise by making sure that you are well hydrated before starting. Furthermore, research has shown that consuming adequate fluids relative to thirst reduces protein breakdown during exercise. Anything you can do to spare protein or prevent its use as a fuel during a race or workout benefits both performance and recovery. You don't want to use muscle tissue to fuel exercise. Drinking to satisfy thirst before exercise is one simple way to help ensure this doesn't happen.

Take in water only in the last hour. The purpose here is to prevent a rapid influx of sugar to the blood, followed by the release of insulin to control it. Such a sugar-insulin (hypoglycemic) reaction is likely to leave you low on blood sugar at the start—just the opposite of what you intended—so you feel slightly dizzy and light-headed within a few minutes of starting exercise.

The exception to this guideline is that in the last 10 minutes prior to exercise, high glycemic index fluids may be consumed. This is explained in greater detail below.

Preexercise Food Choices

Foods to eat before exercise should be those that can be found in grocery stores, no matter where you are racing, or easily be carried during travel. The following are examples of such food sources to eat prior to the last hour before starting exercise. You should select those that appeal to you in the morning and are well tolerated by your body. Try them on the days of race-simulation workouts and priority C races, well before the targeted priority A event for which you intend to use them. You may want to combine two or more of these to create some variety in your preexercise meal.

Fruit with eggs. Eggs are loaded with protein and easily digested by most people. Boiled eggs may be taken to a race venue if they are kept chilled, or you can order scrambled eggs at a restaurant. One large, whole egg contains about 6 grams of protein and 1.5 grams of BCAA. Combine this with fresh fruit, especially fruit that is low in fiber, such as bananas, peaches, cantaloupe, honeydew, and watermelon. Fibrous fruits to avoid include apples, berries, dates, figs, grapes, pears, mango, papaya, and pineapple.

Applesauce mixed with protein powder. Look for unsweetened applesauce. This is low in fiber and has a low glycemic index primarily due to its fructose content, and it's well tolerated by most people. Stir in 2 or 3 tablespoons of powdered egg or whey protein to further slow the glycemic reaction and to add BCAA. The BCAA content of protein powders varies with source and manufacturer, but they contain roughly 2.2 grams per tablespoon. Carry protein powder in a plastic bag when traveling to races and purchase applesauce at your destination. While this doesn't exactly sound like a gourmet meal, realize that you are eating before the race only to provide fuel for your body. Be sure to try this in training or before a priority C race.

Baby food, including animal products. This may sound strange, but it works well. Chopped and pureed baby food can be found anywhere and is easily digested by the human gut at any age. Good choices are fruits or vegetables, along with chopped meats such as turkey, fish, or chicken.

Liquid meals. If you tend to have a very nervous stomach prior to races, blending foods may produce a liquid you can more easily digest. Blend low-fiber fruit, such as those listed above, with fruit juice and 2 or 3 tablespoons of powdered egg or whey protein.

Commercial meal-replacement drinks, although not optimal, are an option when you are away from home and don't have any other options for real food. Look for products with added protein, such as Ensure High Protein. It's best to avoid those drinks that use milk as a base. Whey protein as an ingredient, however, will meet your protein needs for the prerace meal. Be aware that these drinks are becoming so popular with endurance athletes that stores in the vicinity of races often sell out days in advance. Bring your own or shop early.

Sports bar with protein. This is the least attractive of the options, but it'll work in a pinch. Protein bars, sometimes called meal-replacement bars, are easily carried and available almost everywhere. While primarily a carbohydrate-based food source, they contain just enough protein to slow the glycemic reaction and add some BCAA to the meal.

Fluids, especially water. You may also use coffee or tea, which have known benefits associated with caffeine. As little as 1 or 2 cups (depending on body size) of strongly brewed coffee, which has about 3 times as much caffeine as tea, before exercise has been shown to improve endurance performance in athletes who are not chronic users. However, be aware that there are potential downsides with caffeine, such as upset stomach and increased nervousness. Most studies have found that caffeine is not a diuretic. The need to urinate after drinking caffeinated drinks probably has to do with drinking beyond thirst. The World Anti-Doping Association (WADA) does not consider caffeine to be a prohibited substance, while the International Olympic Committee (IOC) as of 2008 enforces a limit of 12 mg per liter of urine. It would take most athletes 6 to 8 cups of strong coffee to reach this level.

Fruit and vegetables juices may also be taken in before exercise, but not in the last hour prior. Be sure to experiment with these during training sessions. Good choices are tomato, apple, and orange. Tomato juice often has added sodium, which may increase your thirst and need for fluids (there is more on sodium in Chapter 3).

10 Minutes Before Start

Taking in carbohydrate within the last hour or so of starting exercise, not including the final 10 minutes before, may cause hypoglycemia (low blood sugar) during the first several minutes of exercise in some people who are especially sensitive to sugar. For them, carbohydrate, especially a high glycemic load source, causes an almost immediate increase in blood insulin levels to reduce the blood's sugar level, resulting in hypoglycemia.

Many athletes may well experience light-headedness or dizziness in the ensuing exercise because of this reaction. Why doesn't this happen when high glycemic index carbohydrate is taken in during the final 10 minutes before starting? The answer is that there just isn't enough time for the body to respond by pumping out insulin. By the time exercise occurs, the body immediately begins to down-regulate its need for insulin. During exercise, sugar intake produces smaller increases of this hormone because the muscles become more sensitive to insulin and permeable to glucose, reducing the need for large amounts of insulin that normally are required to escort the sugar into the muscle.

Taking in 100 to 200 calories from a few ounces of sports drink or gel, followed by 6 to 8 ounces of water, may well give you the energy boost needed right before starting, without any negative effects. This is especially beneficial for those early-morning workouts when you get out of bed within an hour of heading out the door. It may also prove helpful to the athlete who just can't eat first thing in the morning.

Just as with the preexercise meal examples offered above, the purpose of this 10-minute topping off is to replenish glycogen stores while ensuring adequate hydration levels.

CHAPTER 3

Stage II: Eating During Exercise

Eating during exercise is a learned skill that requires considerable planning and testing and includes discovering tasty nutrient sources along with the amounts and timing that work best for you. This demands careful trial and error and meticulous attention to detail. Don't assume that just because certain sources work well for someone else, they will also work well for you. Tolerance for food during exercise is an individual matter.

FOOD TOLERANCE DURING EXERCISE

The workouts that are the best indicators of what you can or cannot eat are the ones that most closely simulate the event for which you are training, including the expected race duration, intensity, terrain, and weather. You will find that your body's tolerances for food and fluid change as conditions vary. The least important priority C races on your schedule that mimic the conditions of the priority A events serve as even better tests for nutrition because these also place psychological demands on you. The ultimate test is the goal race. From this experience, you can draw even better conclusions for future races.

The intensity of exercise has a great deal to do with how well the stomach tolerates food and drink. At very high intensities, such as above 85 percent max VO$_2$ (approximately at anaerobic threshold), the gastro-intestinal system essentially stops functioning as blood is shunted to the hardworking muscles and to the skin for cooling. Conversely, at low intensities, such as when racing in an ultra-marathon event that takes many hours to complete, many athletes experience an as-yet-unexplained mechanism that produces nausea. Fortunately, if the event for which you are training is short and intense, such as a 5-K run or bicycle criterium, there is no need to take in additional fuel. You have plenty on board already.

If, on the other hand, your event is long and not a steady effort but, rather, punctuated by high-intensity efforts that determine the outcome, such as a bicycle road race, then eating and drinking must occur at times when the intensity is low. The nausea associated with very long events, such as Ironman triathlons or ultra-marathons, isn't as simple. Among the possible reasons for the queasiness:

Poor pacing. This is the most common cause of nausea early in a long, steady race. Going too fast in the early stages—perhaps because of nervous energy and a poor pacing strategy while simultaneously taking in food, whether solid or liquid—causes the digestive tract to fill excessively. Due to the high intensity, the gut doesn't process what's taken in. Continuing to consume calories even after the intensity has settled at a more conservative level just exacerbates the problem. Slowing down dramatically and temporarily stopping food intake are the only solutions.

Excessive fluids. Another possible cause of nausea in long-duration events is overdrinking. The stomach can hold roughly 32 ounces and empties at a rate of approximately 30 to 42 ounces per hour, depending on body size and exercise intensity. If the stomach's reservoir capacity is exceeded, as can be the case with poor race-nutrition planning and a lack of refueling rehearsal, it has no choice but to remove the excess by vomiting.

Excessive nutrients. Related to the last cause is another: taking in food or drink that is excessively concentrated with nutrients. The greater the fuel's nutrient content, the slower the stomach processes it. While physiology textbooks say that, on average, the stomach empties about 6 calories per minute, or 360 calories per hour, most long-distance athletes know it is possible to handle far more than that—perhaps as much as 600 calories per hour (and maybe even more in some large athletes). There seems to be a lot of variation in individual tolerance for food volume. Whatever your limit, slightly exceeding it for several hours will eventually lead to the stomach overfilling, with but one solution—puking.

Dehydration. Excessive dehydration in the heat may also contribute to nausea. If fluid intake is well below one's sweat rate for a long period of time, body fluids are shunted away from the digestive system to the skin (for cooling) and muscles (for work production). When that happens, the processing of fuel and fluids is reduced. In other words, the stomach's emptying rate falls and whatever is taken in accumulates until the excess triggers nausea.

Saltwater ingestion. In ocean-swim events, such as Ironman-distance triathlons or long-distance swimming, swallowing seawater may set up the athlete for nausea later in the event. "Seawater poisoning" occurs when the high sodium content of ocean water causes the stomach to shut down until the gut's sodium content is diluted, preferably by drinking plain water. If the athlete does not gradually take in water to dilute the sodium, or if he or she takes in fuel in any form (including liquid), the body will make its own adjustments by pulling water from the blood and intracellular space into the stomach or by vomiting.

None of the above. Your gut's displeasure during a given event could be due to several of the above scenarios—or it could be caused by something altogether different, such as nervous excitement, food poisoning, exhaustion, or extreme heat. It may also be that your body, while in good shape, is not yet fully prepared for a long-distance event. An extreme event relative to your fitness level may simply overwhelm your body's ability to cope.

The good news is that once you vomit, it's likely that you'll start feeling better. But don't get carried away by the newfound relief—the problem could soon come back to haunt you. At this point, slow down if you haven't already, and begin sipping water to see how that is accepted. If your stomach seems to handle that for 10 to 20 minutes or so, progress to a diluted drink by mixing water and a sports beverage. Take in only 2 to 3 ounces over 10 to 20 minutes. Again, if that stays down, try a normally concentrated sports drink. At some point, you will know that the conservative approach is working and you can resume a greater intensity, but be cautious; your stomach may still be upset. Even though this may cost you time, it is better to finish than to make the DNF (did not finish) list.

HYDRATION DURING EXERCISE

Athletes are generally greatly concerned by dehydration. After a poor race performance, especially on a hot day, they are likely to blame the less-than-stellar experience on excessive loss of body fluids. Recent research is showing, however, that the level of dehydration necessary to affect performance is greater than formerly believed. The trend is toward accepting dehydration at some level as a normal condition of exercise. For example, the American College of Sports Medicine in 1996 concluded that athletes should prevent any level of dehydration by continually replacing all water lost during exercise. By 2007 the ACSM's position had changed due to concerns about excessive drinking resulting in hyponatremia (discussed later in this chapter), a far worse problem than dehydration. They now advise athletes to restrict water losses during exercise to less than 2 percent. But even that is questionable.

The clinical evidence is not overwhelming that losing 2 percent of body weight due to sweat is harmful to your health or to endurance performance. In fact, field studies conducted on athletes at long-distance races in hot and humid conditions, such as the Ironman Triathlon World Championship in Kailua-Kona, Hawaii, find that athletes continue to perform at very high levels with body-weight losses of 3 percent or even greater. Some exercise scientists point out that the most dehydrated athletes in a race are typically the first to finish. They certainly were not slowed down by body-weight losses of greater than 2 percent.

Body weight is not recommended as a way to determine your fluid needs. For, after all, while racing or training you don't have the opportunity to weigh yourself to gauge fluid replacement needs. Nor can you use past experiences when you've weighed before and after exercise. There are many variable conditions when you are training and racing that impact fluid levels. Small changes in air temperature, humidity, wind speed, exercise intensity, exercise duration, altitude, hydration status at the start line, glycogen storage levels, and other factors affect how much fluid your body loses through sweat and breathing. Knowing that one set of such conditions caused a loss of a certain amount of body weight does not mean that all exercise will result in the same or even similar losses. So how should you gauge fluid losses to prevent what could be excessive dehydration?

The answer is simple: thirst. Somehow, athletes have come to believe that thirst is not a good predictor of their body's fluid needs. It's likely due to effective marketing by sports drink companies, which has been shown to have a great influence on what athletes believe about hydration. If thirst does not work for humans, then we would be the only species in the animal world to have such a condition. And it's unlikely that as a species we would have flourished and spread around the world to so many extreme environments.

Early humans evolved while running and walking long distances in the heat of the dry African savannah while hunting and gathering. Water was not readily available. There were no aid stations. They drank just enough to maintain healthy fluid levels, but not necessarily body weight. The key to this delicate balance, now as much as 10,000 years ago, is the sensation of thirst. If you learn to pay attention to how thirsty you are and drink enough to satisfy it, you will no longer need to be concerned with body weight. Nor will you need a "drinking schedule," which is, at best, based on flimsy conclusions about what the many conditions will be during exercise. It's actually quite simple: If you are thirsty, drink; stop drinking when you are no longer thirsty.

SODIUM AND EXERCISE

Let's address another rehydration issue common in endurance sport— the need for sodium intake to maintain or even improve performance.

During exercise, as fluid is lost through sweating and breathing, the concentration of sodium in the body actually increases. The reason is because much more fluid than sodium is lost through sweating. One might sweat off around a liter of water during intense exercise on a warm day, but lose only a tiny amount of sodium. Normal body sodium levels are about 140 millimoles per liter (mmol/l) of water while the level of sweat is about 20 to 60 mmol/l.

So let's say an average-size human body contains 40 liters of water when at rest and normally hydrated. That means it has stored away something like 5,600 mmol of sodium (40 x 140 = 5,600). If 1 liter of fluid is lost during exercise and with that 60 mmol of sodium is excreted (the high end or "salty" sweater), then the new sodium concentration is about 142 mmol/l (5,600 – 60 = 5,540 / 39 = 142.05). The concentration of sodium has risen, not declined. Guess what happens next after a sufficiently large rise in sodium concentration occurs? Your thirst mechanism kicks in and you drink water to dilute the sodium, bringing it back down to something closer to 140 mmol/l. A study by Hubbard and associates found that a rise of about 2 or 3 percent of plasma sodium concentration evoked a strong desire to drink.

So your sodium content becomes more concentrated during exercise as you sweat, not less, as we've been led to believe. In other words, you don't need to replace lost sodium during exercise because the loss is inconsequential, while the volume of water lost is significant. But even if you did, the sodium content of most sports drinks is only 10 to 25 mmol/l, not enough to replace the loss. More than that makes the drink unpalatable. The extracellular fluid in your body, where much of the sodium is stored, has about the concentration of seawater. If you've ever swallowed seawater, you know how nasty that would be as a sports drink.

Would *not* taking in sodium during a long race or workout impact your performance? Not according to the research. For example, a study by Merson and associates found that adding sodium to a sports drink did not improve performance in a time trial effort after 4 hours of exercise at a moderate intensity. Similarly, a study by Barr and associates found that sodium in a sports drink did not impact the ability to complete 6 hours of moderate-intensity exercise.

Should you take in sodium at all during a race or workout? There is no known downside to doing so. In fact, there may be a slight advantage, but not for the reasons we've been led to believe. A bit of sodium may improve the rate of absorption of both water and carbohydrate in the upper part of the small intestine. Sodium during exercise also is known to expand blood plasma volume, increasing the amount of blood pumped by the heart for each stroke. That's a good thing. And after exercise, extra sodium may be needed to prevent dilution in the cells as water is taken in to recover from the slight dehydration that occurred. So the bottom line is that it's okay to take in sodium during and after a race or workout.

HYPONATREMIA

The greater issue for the long-duration athlete is hyponatremia—low sodium concentrations in the body fluids. This can lead to not only poor performance but also acute health problems and even death. In recent years there have been two reported deaths in marathons related to over-hydration-induced hyponatremia. Both were back-of-the-pack runners who had been on the road for several hours. Studies of Ironman-distance triathletes have shown that many competitors experience mild levels of hyponatremia.

This condition is considered to be a sodium concentration level of less than 135 mmol/l by some experts. The most common way this occurs is through dilution of sodium stores caused by overdrinking during exercise. So the main issue is not replacing sodium, but rather not drinking too much fluid. Thirst is the key to this balance. If you drink only when thirsty and to a level that satisfies thirst, then you will not drink too much. Drinking as much as possible, which used to be a common tip for athletes, or drinking to a predetermined schedule during events lasting longer than about 4 hours, has the potential to cause hyponatremia.

Hyponatremia occurs when the sodium concentration of the blood is reduced to dangerous levels. It can result from prolonged vomiting or diarrhea or from taking diuretics; but in endurance athletics, it's most commonly seen with excessive intake of fluid during long events. And the fluid doesn't have to be water. The death of one of the two marathoners mentioned above occurred from overdrinking a commercial sports beverage. Even though these drinks have sodium as an ingredient, they do not maintain a healthy concentration if you drink to excess. Hyponatremia is extremely rare in events lasting less than 4 hours, but it's common in competitions taking 8 or more hours to complete. In studies at the New Zealand and Hawaii Ironman Triathlons, events that take 8 to 17 hours to complete, researchers found that up to 30 percent of finishers experienced mild to severe hyponatremia.

How does this happen? In a mistaken belief that one cannot take in too much water during exercise, the athlete overhydrates and may even gain weight during the event. The problem is most common with slower participants because they have greater opportunity and more time to drink. (The fastest athletes are more prone to dehydration than to hyponatremia; they find it more difficult to take in fluids at their level of competitiveness, plus they spend less time on the course.)

It can be difficult to determine if you are experiencing hyponatremia because the signs come on slowly. Early symptoms include headache in the forehead, nausea, muscle cramps, lethargy, confusion, disorientation, reduced coordination, and tunnel vision. One sure sign of hyponatremia is bloating. Look for puffiness and tightness around rings, watches, sock bands, and elastic waistbands. In extreme cases, the athlete may experience convulsions, unconsciousness, respiratory distress, or cardiac arrest. Because urination is greatly reduced or stops altogether when blood sodium concentrations are low, hyponatremia is often misdiagnosed as dehydration—and that can be a fatal error. If water intake is increased in a mistaken attempt to rehydrate the athlete, the condition worsens.

Let's now examine the unique nutritional characteristics of workouts and races of various duration ranges.

EATING DURING 2- TO 90-MINUTE EVENTS

These are the shortest exercise sessions that qualify as endurance activities and include 800-meter through about half-marathon runs, sprint-distance triathlons, bicycle criteriums and time trials, some mountain bike races, 5-K to about 30-K cross-country ski races, and most rowing events.

What sets such events apart from longer-distance racing is the high intensity. At the pace the athlete is traveling, taking in solid food is out of the question and, thankfully, not necessary. The focus of nutrition during training or racing for these events, regardless of one's speed, is on hydration, which is resolved by drinking enough to satisfy thirst.

Assuming adequate nutrition in the days and hours preceding a 2- to 90-minute session, the athlete's body is well prepared with glycogen stores. The risk of bonking is quite low for experienced athletes. Novices and weekend warriors may need to assume their starting point for taking in carbohydrate is 60 minutes, because they don't store as much glycogen in their muscles. There is no harm in novices or advanced athletes using a sports drink, regardless of the duration. Some research has even found performance benefits from the intake of a sugar-based fuel source in events lasting less than an hour. Interestingly, one study found that rinsing one's mouth with a sports drink and spitting it out improved performance in relatively short events. The mechanism for this isn't understood and the research is contradictory.

With this in mind, however, the greatest nutritional need at this duration is water. As explained above, it's best to drink enough to satisfy your thirst. In such a short race, that may not be possible, especially for the fastest athletes, who find it difficult to move at high speed and drink at the same time. There should be little cause for concern if that is the case. With such a short event, dehydration is unlikely to be sufficient to harm your health or even to result in a poor performance.

EATING DURING 90-MINUTE TO 4-HOUR EVENTS

Examples of race events in this range are half- to full-marathon runs, Olympic to half-Ironman-distance multisport races, bicycle criteriums and road races, mountain bike races, and 30-K to 100-K cross-country ski events. Longer workouts at a more leisurely effort are also included here.

At this duration, inadequate nutrition and environmental stresses on the body begin to take a toll on performance. All athletes are at risk for depleted muscle glycogen stores, and very fast athletes face the possibility of dehydration, so nutritional goals must begin with taking in adequate fluids and carbohydrate. It is best to use a sports drink or gel with water to maintain carbohydrate stores. Take in 200 to 300 calories per hour, depending on your body size and experience. The longer the event, the more important it is to replenish fuel stores.

From the outset of the exercise session, replace some of the expended glycogen to delay the onset of fatigue while maintaining power. Do not wait until the latter stages of the workout or race to take in carbohydrate, as that may well set you up for a poor performance or even a bonk. The carbohydrate at this duration is best in a liquid form. There is little reason to use solid foods. Assuming a good nutritional intake before the event and the consumption of carbohydrate throughout, food in solid form will have no marked advantage, but the potential for nausea at race intensity is significant.

Especially for longer events in this range, using sports drinks and gels instead of only water has the added advantage of limiting muscle damage. For high-intensity exercise sessions, the body will turn to protein for a fuel source as glycogen stores run low. Much of that protein will come from muscle. Failing to get adequate carbohydrate during intense exercise at the longer end of this duration range can result in muscle wasting.

In studies comparing the effects of carbohydrate and water on perceived exertion during intense exercise at this duration, carbohydrate was the clear winner. This means that even though your heart rate and blood acidosis levels may be the same whether you drink water or a sports drink, the effort will feel lower with the sports drink. The combination of carbohydrate and protein (primarily the branched-chain amino acids, described in Chapter 4) may enhance performance and post-exercise recovery, while helping to prevent the transport of excessive amounts of serotonin to the brain. Serotonin is a chemical that can cause the onset of central nervous system fatigue, accompanied by increased sensations of exertion and even sleepiness. The research on sports drinks that combine carbohydrate and protein is not conclusive. When carb-only and carb-plus-protein drinks with equal amounts of calories are compared in such studies, there is generally no significant performance improvement. For some athletes, the consumption of protein during exercise seems to contribute to nausea.

For the shorter end of this duration range many athletes will get by with minimum fuel intake. When exercising at maximum intensity for the longer end of this duration, take in up to 200 to 300 calories per hour in an equal distribution every 10 to 20 minutes, primarily from liquid sources. The minimum intake is 1 calorie of carbohydrate per pound of body weight per hour.

As always, drink enough to satisfy your thirst. Doing this is a skill that must be developed in training and priority C races, as some athletes

(continued on page 42)

LACTIC ACID'S BAD RAP

For the better part of a century, athletes and physiologists alike have considered lactic acid a primary cause of fatigue during high-intensity exercise and referred to it as a "waste product" of muscle metabolism. But now this way of thinking has changed, as scientists have learned that this substance we produce in large quantities during exercise, especially highly intense exercise, is not a cause of fatigue and actually helps to prevent it.

The former misrepresentation started with British physiologist and Nobel laureate Archibald V. Hill, who in 1929 flexed frog muscles to fatigue in his lab and noted that lactic acid accumulated when muscular failure occurred. He concluded that the lactic acid caused the fatigue associated with repeated muscle contractions. What he didn't know is that when the muscle is examined as part of a complete biological system instead of in isolation from the rest of the body,

we can see that lactic acid is processed and converted to fuel to help keep the muscles going. It does not cause fatigue.

Nor does lactic acid cause muscle soreness the day after hard exercise. This myth has been around for decades and refuses to go away, despite evidence to the contrary over the past 30 years. Soreness is more likely the result of damaged muscle cells resulting from excessive usage.

So if lactic acid is not the villain we've made it out to be, what does cause fatigue and the burning sensation in the muscles during short, intense exercise bouts, such as intervals or races lasting just a few minutes? To get at the answer, it's necessary to understand the pH scale, which tells us how acidic or alkaline (base) the body's fluids are in a range of 1 to 14, as hydrogen ions increase or decrease. On this scale, hydrogen readings dropping below neutral 7 indicate increasing acidity, while those rising above 7 indicate escalating alkalinity. Examples of acidic fluids are hydrochloric acid (pH = 1) and vinegar (pH = 3), while milk of magnesia (pH = 10.5) and ammonia (pH = 11.7) are alkaline.

At rest, the pH of your blood is around 7.4—slightly alkaline. In terms of your blood, small absolute changes in acid-base balance have major consequences. For example, during a 2- to 3-minute all-out effort, your blood's pH may drop as low as 6.8 to 7.0. In biochemical terms, this is a huge acidic swing, producing a burning sensation in the working muscles and an inability for them to continue contracting. Fatigue has set in.

If lactic acid didn't cause the drop in pH, what did? The answer has to do with our sources of fuel during such short exercise bouts— glycogen and glucose. Both are carbohydrates, but they have slightly different chemical compositions. Glycogen is stored inside the muscle, where it can be quickly broken down to produce energy. Glucose, a form of this carbohydrate-based fuel that is stored in the liver and floats around in the bloodstream, is called on to produce energy for exercise when muscle glycogen stores can no longer keep up with the demand or are running low. As glycogen is broken down to produce energy, it releases one unit of hydrogen. But if glucose must be used for fuel, such as when the intensity of the exercise exceeds glycogen's ability to keep up, two units of hydrogen are released. This rapid doubling of hydrogen ions in the system lowers the blood's pH, causing the burning and fatigue associated with acidosis. The same amount of lactic acid is released no matter which fuel is used.

Far from being an evildoer, lactic acid is an ally during intense exercise. It does a great deal to keep the body going when the going gets hard. Besides being converted back into a fuel source, when hydrogen begins to accumulate, lactate transports it out of the working muscle cells and helps to buffer or offset its negative consequences.

After 80 years, lactic acid's bad boy reputation has been lifted.

become so focused on performance that they forget to pay attention to their thirst. High glycemic index drinks with much greater maltodextrin or glucose than fructose content are preferred, as some athletes experience gastrointestinal distress from even a moderate amount of fructose. Most commercial drinks include at least some fructose. Let experience be your guide.

Consider using a caffeinated sports drink or gel; this has been shown to enhance the utilization of the glucose in sports drinks. The mechanism here is not fully understood, and research in this area is limited. Could using caffeine result in an upset stomach? In the only study on this topic, conducted at University Hospital, Maastricht, Netherlands, there was no difference in the stomach-acid levels of the people using drinks with caffeine and those who didn't use caffeine. But as always, it's best to experiment with caffeinated drinks in training and priority C races than to try them for the first time in an important event.

EATING DURING 4- TO 12-HOUR EVENTS

At this duration we are moving into events in which the athlete's health and well-being during exercise cannot be taken for granted. Hyponatremia, as described earlier, is now a real threat, and nutritional planning is critical in ways other than simply performance.

Races in this range include marathon and ultra-marathon running, half-Ironman- to Ironman-distance events, bicycle road races and century rides, and ultra-marathon cross-country ski and rowing events.

At such durations the intensity of exercise is quite low, with the effort seldom, if ever, approaching the anaerobic threshold in most sports. The exception is bicycle road racing, in which episodes lasting about 2 minutes during breakaways occur at a highly anaerobic level. With this exception, the fuel source for long, steady events is now very heavily weighted in favor of fat, with carbohydrate playing a smaller, but no less important, role. There is an old saying in exercise science that "fat burns in a carbohydrate fire." In the real world of endurance athletics, this means that if carbohydrate stored as muscle glycogen runs low, the body will gradually lose its capacity to produce energy from fat. In other words, a bonk is highly likely during events in this category if carbohydrate ingestion is neglected for even a little while. Once an athlete is well behind the carbohydrate intake versus expenditure curve, catching up is difficult and may be accomplished only by slowing dramatically or stopping exercise altogether. This is the dreaded "death march" so commonly found late in these events.

Carbohydrate must be taken in right from the beginning of these sessions in order to stay close to the expenditure rate, delaying the onset of fatigue while maintaining power. Although replacing most of the expended glycogen is the goal for this duration, it's doubtful you will be able to restock all of it. At the highest intensities, the fastest athletes expend about 1,000 calories per hour, with perhaps up to 60 percent of that coming from carbohydrate-based glycogen. It's unlikely that all but the largest athletes consume that much carbohydrate. In fact, you don't need to replace it at all if you did a good job of eating quality carbohydrate in the 24 hours leading up to the race or workout. If you did, you have probably stored 1,500 to 2,000 calories as carbohydrate in your muscles and liver, depending on your body size. By keeping the hourly deficit (exercise expenditure minus intake) at less than 100 calories, even the elite athletes in the longest of these events—those who are likely to burn the most calories—can avoid bonking. Slower athletes can keep the deficit even smaller, but that isn't particularly a problem because their burn rate is lower.

In such events, get about 200 to 400 calories per hour in an equal distribution every 10 to 20 minutes, primarily from liquid sources with a minimum of 1 calorie of carbohydrate per pound of body weight per hour. At the upper end of this race-duration range, around 12 hours, sports bars or even solid foods may be used as desired. Solid foods must be of moderate to high glycemic index, low in fiber, and easily digested.

Some athletes have success when using commercial meal-replacement drinks at durations of about 8 hours or more. If you decide to experiment

(continued on page 46)

WHAT CAUSES MUSCLE CRAMPS?

We've all had it happen. The race is going great—then all of a sudden, from out of nowhere, a muscle begins to feel "twitchy" and seizes up. You slow down, hoping it will go away. It does, but as soon as you start pouring on the power, it comes back. The promise of a stellar race is gone.

There is no more perplexing problem for athletes than cramps. Muscles seem to knot up at the worst possible times—seldom in training, but frequently in races.

The real problem is that no one knows what causes cramps. There are theories, the most popular being that muscle cramps result from dehydration or electrolyte imbalances. These arguments seem to make sense—at least on the surface. Cramps are most common in the heat of summer, when low body-fluid levels and decreases in body salts due to sweating are likely to occur.

But the research doesn't always support these explanations. For example, in the mid-1980s, 82 male runners were tested before and after a marathon for certain blood parameters considered to be likely causes of muscle cramps. Fifteen of the runners experienced cramps after 18 miles. There was no difference, either before or after the race, in blood levels of sodium, potassium, bicarbonate, hemoglobin, or hematocrit. There was also no difference in blood volume between the crampers and the noncrampers, nor were there significant differences in the way the two groups trained.

Note that we are talking about exercise-induced cramps here. In such cases of cramping, the knotted muscle is almost always one that is involved in movement in the sport. If depletion of electrolytes was a cause of cramping during exercise, why wouldn't the entire body cramp up? Why just the working muscles? Electrolytes are lost throughout the body, not just in working muscles. We know that people who become clinically hyponatremic by losing a great deal of body salts (not exercise-induced) cramp in *all* of their muscles. It's generalized, not localized.

It should also be pointed out that when someone cramps, the "fix" is not hurriedly drinking a solution of electrolytes, but rather stretching the offending muscle. For example, a runner with a calf cramp will stop and stretch the calf muscle by leaning against a wall or other object while dorsiflexing the ankle against resistance—the standard "runners stretch."

In fact, what is known is that sweat, with regard to electrolytes, is hypotonic. That means the concentration of sodium, potassium, magnesium, chloride, and calcium is weaker than it is in the body. This indicates that more water is lost in the sweat than electrolytes. So if the body lost more of its stored water but not as much of its electrolytes, what would happen to electrolyte concentration in the body? The concentration would increase. So during exercise when you dehydrate and lose electrolytes, their concentration in the body is greater than it was before you started to exercise. The body functions based on concentrations, not on absolute amounts. That alone presents a great problem for the argument that the cause of cramping is the loss of electrolytes that must be replaced.

So if dehydration or electrolyte loss through sweat doesn't cause cramping, what does? No one knows for sure, but theories are emerging. Some researchers blame poor posture or inefficient biomechanics. Poor movement patterns may cause a disturbance in the activity of the Golgi tendon organs—"strain gauges" built into the tendon to prevent muscle tears. When activated, these organs cause the threatened muscle to relax while stimulating the antagonistic muscle—the one that moves the joint in the opposite way—to fire. There may be some quirk of body mechanics that upsets a Golgi device and sets off the cramping pattern. If that is the cause, prevention may involve improving biomechanics and regularly stretching and strengthening muscles that seem to cramp, along with stretching and strengthening their antagonistic muscles.

Another theory is that cramps result from the burning of protein for fuel in the absence of readily available carbohydrate. In fact, one study supports such a notion: Muscle cramps occurred in exercising subjects who reached the highest levels of ammonia release, indicating that protein was being used to fuel the muscles during exercise. This suggests a need for greater carbohydrate stores before, and replacement of those stores during, intense and long-lasting exercise.

When you feel a cramp coming on, there are two ways to deal with it. One is to reduce your intensity and slow down—not a popular option in an important race. Another is to alternately stretch and relax the affected muscle group while continuing to move. This is difficult if not impossible to do in some sports, such as running, and with certain muscles.

There is a third option that some athletes swear by: pinching the upper lip. Who knows—it may work for you the next time a cramp strikes.

with these, it's best to avoid those that use dairy products as the primary source. Unfortunately, most drinks in this category are largely cow's milk. One exception is Ensure.

Otherwise, the guidelines for carbohydrate fuel replacement are the same as in the previous section, including the possible use of a caffeinated drink with added protein. As with the 90-minute to 4-hour events, taking in some protein may help prevent the onset of central nervous system fatigue, which is marked by general malaise and even yawning—even though you're consuming adequate carbohydrate and aren't particularly bored. But once again you must consider the possible downside of nausea. Experiment in training and low-priority events to see if the addition of protein to your sports drink can be managed by your gut.

The elite athlete's greatest concern at this distance is dehydration. Slower athletes should be able to easily avoid this calamity by drinking when thirsty, but they need to be aware of overdrinking resulting in hyponatremia, as described above. Overhydrating with water by as little as 2 percent can bring on this dreaded condition.

Solid food is more likely to be needed only during the longest events in this range, although some athletes continue to use only liquid sources of fuel even when approaching 12 hours.

EATING DURING 12- TO 18-HOUR EVENTS

Events in this duration include the Ironman-distance triathlon, double-century bike ride, and ultra-marathons in such sports as running, mountain biking, cross-country skiing, swimming, and kayaking. The stresses placed on the athlete can be extreme, with fatigue, heat, humidity, hills, wind, and currents taking their toll and gradually reducing performance. Nutrition is critical for these events.

Much of what was said in the previous section remains true here. The caveats are that solid foods now become a necessity, and hunger may well dictate what you decide to use for fuel. This might include bananas, cookies, jelly sandwiches, fruit juices, and soup. All of the foods selected should be toward the high end of the glycemic index. Otherwise, intake of carbohydrate, protein (especially branched-chain amino acids), and caffeine, as described above, may be continued.

EATING DURING EVENTS LONGER THAN 18 HOURS

These are the true "ultra" events of the world of endurance sports: the Race Across America (RAAM) and Paris-Brest-Paris bike races, double-Ironman-distance triathlon, Western States 100-mile run, and multiday bicycle racing tours such as the grueling Tour de France, the Vuelta a España, and the Giro d'Italia. It can be very difficult to take in adequate food and water, but for events done in daily stages, such as the Tour de France, daily nutritional intake between stages is often the difference between finishing and dropping out.

The longer the event, the more crucial it is that caloric needs be met by balancing nutrient intake with expenditure. Unsupported events require the athlete to carry nutrients or purchase them along the route, which makes planning all the more critical—the preferred sources must be light or generally available at convenience stores. Plan on taking in at least 6,000 calories daily—and that's conservative. RAAM riders who spend at least 5 days riding across the United States, from the West to the East Coast, typically report 10,000-calorie days.

The longer the event, the lower the intensity, diminishing the relative amount of carbohydrate used as fuel. Whereas carbohydrate may account for 80 percent of the expended calories in events that last less than 90 minutes, it may contribute only about 50 percent of the total energy used in ultra-events. This means that the carbohydrate content of your fuel need not be as carbohydrate-rich as for shorter events. Conversely, protein intake becomes more important and should make up 5 to 15 percent of your fuel, so your nutritional source should reflect this demand. Not getting enough protein may well result in muscle wasting. That's not conducive to good performance.

Fat also becomes more important in events of this duration. You'll burn a lot of it, so it's okay to take in a considerable amount—a fifth to a third of your fuel source—during the activity. In fact, ultra-marathoners often report a craving for fat during their events. Fat tends to present fewer gut problems during exercise than carbohydrate does, but that doesn't mean it won't affect your stomach at all. Before the event, be sure to experiment to discover the mix and types of fuels that work best for you.

Nutritional Goals for 18+ Hour Events

Given the importance of refueling in events of this duration, it's a good idea to closely examine all aspects of nutrition in great detail. Let's start by considering the nutritional goals for the ultra-marathon athlete.

Replace all of the expended carbohydrate. Even at relatively slow velocities, a considerable amount of dietary carbohydrate is needed to delay the onset of fatigue while maintaining power. Carbohydrate should be taken in from the outset of exercise, using predominantly high glycemic index sources. It's generally best that the sports drinks you choose have greater maltodextrin or glucose sources than fructose.

What changes from the previous discussions, however, is that the demand for carbohydrate relative to time is reduced. You'll be using less fuel per hour while burning fewer calories from carbohydrate sources and more from fat than for short events, so the total replacement of carbohydrate is not as difficult as in shorter, faster events.

Prevent excessive dehydration while avoiding hyponatremia. Staying adequately hydrated for such events is critical. Once you are excessively dehydrated, it is difficult to get fluid levels back to normal. As always, use thirst as your guide to drinking. Hyponatremia is a threat to all athletes, including the faster ones, in events of this duration. The key, again, is drinking to satisfy thirst and not on a schedule. There will be a significant loss of body weight due to dehydration in each day's activity in multiday events even while you are drinking to thirst. During rest and recovery times fluids should be consumed as desired.

Prevent central nervous system fatigue. Low levels of branched-chain amino acids in the blood during these long events can allow serotonin to enter the brain, causing the central nervous system to fatigue even though the other systems of the body are doing well. (See "What Is Fatigue?" on page 124.)

Prevent muscle wasting. It is not unusual for athletes in ultra-distance events, such as the Tour de France, to lose several pounds, mostly from muscle. A study of trekkers in the Andes found that those who supplemented their diet with branched-chain amino acids gained muscle mass over 21 days, while their placebo-supplemented companions who otherwise ate the same diet lost muscle. Without adequate protein intake, the trekkers' bodies were "cannibalizing" themselves. This helps us understand why, after ultra-marathon events, athletes look so gaunt. To prevent muscle catabolism, it is critical that the athlete take in protein along with carbohydrate during the race.

Prevent hunger. You will become quite hungry if you go 18 hours or longer with nothing more than sports drinks and gels. Foods including solid sources are a necessity, as they are more energy-dense than liquid sources. You'll also find that after several hours, you become very tired of sweets and crave fat. Follow your desires and eat what sounds appealing, but consider these treats rather than main sources of fuel. The typical warnings still stand: Keep these foods low in fiber, and try them in workouts before using them in races.

Nutritional Guidelines for 18+ Hour Events

The guidelines for including fat and protein (primarily branched-chain amino acids) now shift toward fat and protein and slightly away from carbohydrate. Your 300 to 600 calories hourly from carbohydrate, fat, and protein should be broken down, respectively, as 60 to 70 percent, 20 to 30 percent, and 10 to 15 percent. This proportion may enhance performance and recovery, while helping to prevent the serotonin buildup that can cause central nervous system fatigue and greater exertion.

Races of this distance often provide or allow support in the form of aid stations, feed zones, or even following support vehicles. This makes the replacement of huge energy needs throughout the event possible. For multiday events such as bicycle stage races, rest and recovery breaks are the times when the day's caloric expenditures must be made up. During these times, which are essentially Stages IV and V of daily recovery, an assortment of foods such as potatoes, sweet potatoes, yams, vegetables, turkey sandwiches, fresh fruits, and soup will provide carbohydrate, fat, and protein.

CHAPTER 4

STAGES III, IV, AND V: EATING AFTER EXERCISE

Immediately after a race or workout ends, it's time to start focusing on recovery. This should be your highest priority. The higher your athletic goals, the more important quick recovery becomes. If you aspire to achieve at your peak levels, then both the quantity and quality of training are crucial for success. The sooner you can do another key workout, the faster you will get into race shape and the better your results will be.

If everything is done right nutritionally, both before and during the exercise session, then you're well on your way to accomplishing this result. Following exercise, your objective must be to return your body to its preexercise levels of hydration, glycogen storage, and muscle protein status as quickly as possible. Diet is the critical component in this process.

There are three stages in this process: 30 minutes postexercise (Stage III); short-term postexercise (Stage IV), lasting as long as the exercise session; and long-term postexercise (Stage V), lasting until the next Stage I. Generally these stages will occur in sequential order from I through V. But on days when multiple workouts are done with only a few hours between sessions, Stages III and IV may be completed followed by a return to Stage 1, repeating the entire process. Stage V would then be very late in the day. This is quite common for serious athletes who train and race at a high level. Stages III and IV may also be modified based on the total stress of the workout. Let's examine the details of each stage of postexercise recovery.

STAGE III: EATING 30 MINUTES POSTEXERCISE

Following a highly stressful workout or race, this is the most critical phase. During the first 30 minutes after exercise stops, your body is better prepared to receive and store carbohydrate than at any other time during the day. If the preceding session was challenging, your body's glycogen stores have been significantly diminished and there may be damage to muscles as well. Get nutrition right now, and you are well on your way to the next key workout. Blow it, and you're certain to delay recovery.

Timing is a critical component for this stage. At no other time in the day is your body as receptive as it is now to macronutrient intake. Research shows that the restocking of the muscles' carbohydrate stores is two to three times as rapid immediately after exercise as it is a few hours later. In the same way, other research reveals that the repair of muscles damaged during exercise is more effective if protein is consumed immediately after exercise. Don't delay. Begin refueling as soon as possible after your cooldown.

There are five goals for this brief but critical window of opportunity.

Goal #1: Replace expended carbohydrate stores. During highly intense exercise, especially if it lasted longer than about 1 hour, you used up much of your carbohydrate-based energy sources. Even though you may have taken in fuel during the session, you were unable to replace all that was expended. Muscle glycogen stores are now at a low level. These can best be restored by taking in carbohydrates that are high on the glycemic load scale for quick replenishment, along with sources that are lower on the scale to provide for a steady release of carbohydrates into the blood. Glucose, the sugar in starchy foods such as potatoes, rice, and grains, is a good source for quick recovery, while fructose, the sugar in fruit and fruit juices, provides a steady, slowly released level of sugar into the bloodstream. Take in at least three-fourths of a gram (3 calories) of carbohydrate per pound of body weight from such sources. This recovery "meal" is generally best taken in liquid rather than solid form, partly because solid foods often aren't very appealing at this time. A liquid meal also is absorbed more quickly and contributes to the rehydration process. Good sources are commercially produced recovery drinks. Or you can make your own "homebrew" recovery drink, which is much cheaper and exactly designed to suit your tastes. (See Table 4.5 on page 60.)

One of the highest glycemic load carbohydrates is glucose. By adding glucose to the homebrew, you replace the body's expended carbohydrate stores more quickly than by eating fruit and drinking fruit juice alone, because these foods are rich in fructose, which the body takes somewhat longer to digest. Pure glucose, sometimes referred to as "dextrose," is difficult to find, although it is typically in commercial sports and recovery drinks. You can purchase glucose from various sources on the Internet, such as amazon.com, bulkfoods.com, carbopro.com, honeyvillegrain.com, iherb.com, and nuts.com. As of this writing it cost about $3 per pound.

Goal #2: Rehydrate. Chances are good that you are experiencing some level of dehydration following a long or hard workout or race. Losing a quart of fluids an hour—about 2 pounds—is fairly common, especially on hot days. At the greatest sweat rates, an athlete may lose around a half gallon (1,800 milliliters) of sweat per hour. That's about 4 pounds. Among the highest sweat rates ever reported in the research literature was about 1 gallon per hour in one of America's best all-time marathoners, 147-pound Alberto Salazar. That would be about 8 pounds— roughly 5 percent of his body weight. Replacing such high rates of fluid loss during exercise is difficult, if not impossible, potentially leaving the athlete in a dehydrated state as the postexercise stage of recovery begins.

To replenish fluid levels, begin taking in 16 ounces (500 milliliters) of liquid for every pound lost during exercise. You probably won't accomplish this in 30 minutes, especially after a long session on a hot day, so plan on continuing throughout the next few hours into Stage IV. You may need to take in 150 percent of what your weight indicates you lost just to keep up with your body's ongoing need for fluids in the hours following the workout or race. Thirst also plays a role here just as it did during exercise. When it is quenched, whether you have replaced all lost body weight or not, reduce or stop your intake of fluids. Forcing down fluids when you are not thirsty is never a good idea.

Goal #3: Provide amino acids for resynthesis of protein that may have been damaged during exercise. In an intense 1-hour workout, it's possible to use 30 grams (1 ounce) of muscle protein for fuel. With even longer exercise sessions, the protein cost of fueling the body is likely to rise. As carbohydrate is depleted in the working muscles, the body begins to break down protein structures within the muscle cells to create more glycogen. In addition, cells may have been damaged during exercise, and consuming protein immediately after will hasten their repair while diminishing or even preventing the delayed onset of muscle soreness.

Protein, particularly sources that are rich in the branched-chain amino acids (leucine, isoleucine, and valine), should be taken in at a carb-to-protein ratio of about 4:1 or 5:1 over the 30-minute recovery period. The research is clear on the need for protein after stressful sessions; the exact amount is not clear, however. We've found that 4 or 5 parts carbohydrate to 1 part protein seems to be palatable and effective. If you are using a protein powder to mix a recovery drink, the best sources of protein are egg or whey products, which contain all of the essential amino acids and a healthy dose of branched-chain amino acids, as can be seen in Table 4.1.

Table 4.2 on page 56 provides a breakdown by body weight of the caloric components of a recovery drink with a 4:1 or 5:1 ratio of carbohydrate to protein. You may feel the need to take in more or fewer calories depending on how intense or long the workout was, your nutritional

STAGES III, IV, AND V: EATING AFTER EXERCISE

status prior to the session, what and how much you took in during exercise, and how good eating sounds to you at this time. Even if you don't feel up to taking in this much immediately after your workout, at least begin to sip the recovery drink, and spread its intake over a longer period. The research on recovery meals isn't conclusive as to how long the window is open. But 30 minutes is known to be an effective duration. The workout or race conditions may also influence how much you take in. For example, as it does with fluids, heat increases the need for both carbohydrate and protein.

Goal #4: Begin replacing electrolytes. Electrolytes are the salts sodium, chloride, potassium, calcium, and magnesium, which are found either within the body's cells or in extracellular fluids, including blood. Dissolved in the body fluids as ions, they conduct an electric current and

TABLE 4.1

Branched-Chain Amino Acid Content of Selected Foods

SOURCE (100-Calorie Sample)	ISOLEUCINE (mg)	LEUCINE (mg)	VALINE (mg)	TOTAL BCAA (mg)
Egg white, powder	1,200	1,791	1,352	4,343
Egg white, raw	1,188	1,774	1,340	4,302
Whey protein	922	1,719	896	3,537
Meats	928	1,474	967	3,369
Soy protein	886	1,481	923	3,290
Seafood	744	1,285	803	2,832
Hard-boiled egg	389	442	494	1,325
Milk	323	524	358	1,205
Beans	319	524	349	1,192
Vegetables	238	287	245	770
Grains	130	303	172	605
Nuts and seeds	111	198	149	458
Starchy root vegetables	45	66	58	169
Fruits	20	31	29	80

TABLE 4.2

Recovery Drink Calories by Body Weight

WEIGHT (lbs)	CARBOHYDRATE CALORIES (Minimum)	PROTEIN CALORIES	TOTAL CALORIES
100	300	60–75	360–375
110	330	66–83	396–413
120	360	72–90	432–450
130	390	78–98	468–488
140	420	84–105	504–525
150	450	90–113	540–563
160	480	96–120	576–600
170	510	102–128	612–638
180	540	108–135	648–675
190	570	114–143	684–713
200	600	120–150	720–750
210	630	126–158	756–788

are critical for muscle contraction and relaxation and for maintaining fluid levels. During exercise, the body loses a small portion of these salts, primarily through sweat. So an imbalance between electrolytes and fluids occurs while sweating, with their concentrations increasing. Following exercise, as you begin to drink, you will gradually return body fluids levels to a more normal level. This will result in a low concentration of electrolytes if they aren't taken in now.

Most of the electrolytes are found in abundance in natural food, which makes their replacement fairly easy. Drinking juice or eating fruit will easily replace nearly all of the electrolytes expended during exercise—with the exception of sodium, which is not naturally abundant in fruits and juices. Two or three pinches of table salt may be added to a postexercise recovery drink for sodium replenishment. Table 4.3 lists good juice and fruit sources to use in a Stage III postworkout drink for the replenishment of sodium, magnesium, calcium, and potassium. Chloride is not included, as there is limited research on its availability in these foods.

TABLE 4.3

Electrolytes in Juices and Fruits Used during Recovery

	SODIUM (mg)	MAGNESIUM (mg)	CALCIUM (mg)	POTASSIUM (mg)
Juice (12 oz)				
Apple, frozen	26	18	21	450
Grape, frozen	7	16	12	80
Grapefruit, frozen	3	45	33	505
Orange, fresh	3	41	41	744
Pineapple, frozen	4	35	42	510
Fruit				
Apple, 1 medium, raw	1	6	10	159
Banana, 1 medium, raw	1	33	7	451
Blackberries, 1 cup, frozen	2	33	44	211
Blueberries, 1 cup, raw	9	7	9	129
Cantaloupe, 1½ cups, raw	21	25	25	741
Grapes, 1½ cups, raw	3	8	20	264
Orange, 1 large, raw	2	22	84	375
Papaya, 1 medium, raw	8	31	72	780
Peaches, 3 medium, raw	0	18	15	513
Pineapple, 1½ cups, raw	2	32	17	262
Raspberries, 1½ cups, raw	0	33	40	280
Strawberries, 2 cups, raw	4	32	42	494
Watermelon, 2 cups, raw	6	34	26	372

Goal #5: Reduce the acidity of body fluids. During exercise, body fluids trend increasingly toward acidity. There is also evidence indicating that as we age, our blood and other body fluids also have a tendency toward acidity. The cumulative effect is a slight lowering of pH (increased acidity), which the body offsets by drawing on its alkaline sources. Regardless of your age, if this acidic trend following exercise is allowed to persist for some period of time, the risk of nitrogen and calcium loss is greatly increased. The body reduces the acidity by releasing minerals into the blood as well as other body fluids that have a net alkaline-enhancing effect, thus counteracting the acid. Calcium from the bones and nitrogen from the muscles meet this need. The trend toward greater acidosis is stopped. This prevents a health catastrophe, but at a great cost.

The problem is that in neutralizing the acid this way, we give up valuable structural resources. You're essentially peeing off bone and muscle as the acidity of your blood stays high. While cannibalizing tissue is necessary from a strictly biological perspective, this is an expensive solution from an athletic and a long-term health perspective. While body fluids may be chemically balanced by the process, future performance and health may well be jeopardized as muscle and bone are compromised.

Research has shown that fruits and vegetables have a net alkaline-enhancing effect. Table 4.4 demonstrates the acid- and alkaline-enhancing effects of various foods. The foods with a plus sign (+) indicate increased acidity; the greater the plus value, the higher the acid effect. Those foods with a minus sign (-) decrease the acid of the body fluids in direct proportion to their magnitude. So, by preparing a recovery drink with fruits and juices that have a net alkaline-enhancing effect (they reduce acidity), you are doing more than merely replacing carbohydrate stores; you're also potentially sparing bone and muscle. Interestingly, a recent study by Cao and associates at the US Department of Agriculture found that although animal protein increased the urinary excretion of calcium, it did not have any negative consequences for bone health.

HOMEBREW RECIPES

Based on all of the above, then, here's what you want in a homemade recovery drink: fruits and juices (to provide fluids and slow-releasing

TABLE 4.4

Acid/Base Values of Food
(100 g portions)

ACID FOODS (+)		ALKALINE FOODS (-)	
Grains		**Fruits**	
Brown rice	+12.5	Raisins	-21.0
Rolled oats	+10.7	Black currants	-6.5
Whole wheat bread	+8.2	Bananas	-5.5
Spaghetti	+7.3	Apricots	-4.8
Corn flakes	+6.0	Kiwifruit	-4.1
White rice	+4.6	Cherries	-3.6
Rye bread	+4.1	Pears	-2.9
White bread	+3.7	Pineapple	-2.7
		Peaches	-2.4
Dairy		Apples	-2.2
Parmesan cheese	+34.2	Watermelon	-1.9
Processed cheese	+28.7		
Hard cheese	+19.2	**Vegetables**	
Gouda cheese	+18.6	Spinach	-14.0
Cottage cheese	+8.7	Celery	-5.2
Whole milk	+0.7	Carrots	-4.9
		Zucchini	-4.6
Legumes		Cauliflower	-4.0
Peanuts	+8.3	Potatoes	-4.0
Lentils	+3.5	Radishes	-3.7
Peas	+1.2	Eggplant	-3.4
		Tomatoes	-3.1
Meats, Eggs, Fish		Lettuce	-2.5
Trout	+10.8	Chicory	-2.0
Turkey	+9.9	Leeks	-1.8
Chicken	+8.7	Onions	-1.5
Eggs	+8.1	Mushrooms	-1.4
Pork	+7.9	Green peppers	-1.4
Beef	+7.8	Broccoli	-1.2
Cod	+7.1	Cucumber	-0.8
Herring	+7.0		

Reprinted from the Journal of the American Dietetic Association, *V95(7), Thomas Remer and Friedrich Manz, "Potential renal acid load of foods and its influence on urine pH," pp. 791–97, 1995, with permission from the American Dietetic Association.*

carbohydrate with electrolytes while reducing blood acidity), glucose (a quickly absorbed energy source), protein (to replace what was used in exercise and hasten muscle recovery from breakdown occurring during exercise), and sodium (because fruits and juices are low in this electrolyte). Using ingredients that are mostly found in your own kitchen, you can make a smoothie that fulfills all those requirements.

Start by filling a blender with about 12 to 24 ounces of fruit juice, based on your body weight (see Table 4.5). Apple, grape, grapefruit, orange, and pineapple are good choices due to their relatively high glycemic loads and electrolyte contents. Next, add a fruit from the list in Table 4.3 (see page 57) and glucose, also sometimes called dextrose (see Table 4.5). Then, with the blender still running, add protein powder from either egg or whey sources (see Table 4.1 on page 55). Sprinkle in two or three pinches of table salt. If you didn't use frozen berries, add a handful of ice. There you have it—a fairly inexpensive drink that has all of the ingredients needed for immediate recovery.

TABLE 4.5

Ingredients for Homebrew Recovery Drink (by body weight)

BODY WEIGHT IN POUNDS (kg)	FRUIT JUICE (oz)	GLUCOSE (tbsp)	PROTEIN POWDER (tbsp)	TOTAL CALORIES (approx.)
100 (45.5)	12	2	1½–2	390–415
110 (50)	12	2	1½–2	390–415
120 (54.5)	12	3	2	445
130 (59.1)	12	4	2–2½	470–495
140 (63.6)	16	4	2½–3	550–575
150 (68.2)	16	4	2½–3	550–575
160 (72.7)	16	5	2½–3	580–605
170 (77.3)	20	5	3–3½	660–685
180 (81.8)	20	5	3–3½	660–685
190 (86.4)	24	5	3–3½	720–740
200 (90.9)	24	5	3–3½	720–740
210 (95.5)	24	6	3–4	750–790

Each smoothie also includes one fruit and two or three pinches of table salt.

You don't need to use this type of recovery drink after every workout, just those that include a significant amount of intensity or last at least 60 to 90 minutes. In fact, avoid using this drink when you don't need it, as the high glycemic load is likely to add unwanted pounds of body fat. After short and low-intensity workouts, you can make a smaller version of the homebrew without the glucose.

STAGE IV: SHORT-TERM POSTEXERCISE

For very intense, short workouts or those longer than about 60 to 90 minutes, recovery needs to continue beyond the initial 30-minute window. Although there is no research supporting this, we have had success in coaching athletes who eat a Paleo diet in Stage V in continuing to focus on recovery for the same amount of time that the workout or race took. Stage III is unlikely to fully meet all of your recovery needs following a workout that lasted longer than about 90 minutes. Recovery needs to continue into Stage IV following such lengthy sessions. And the longer the workout was, the more critical Stage IV becomes. When athletes tell me they don't recover well as Paleo dieters, I usually discover through questioning that they go straight to Stage V without inserting a Stage IV. Stage IV is critical to your recovery. Don't omit it.

So how does Stage IV work? Let's say you exercised for 2 hours and it was a challenging workout. The initial 30-minute recovery period (Stage III) should be followed by an additional 90 minutes in Stage IV. In the same way, a 4-hour workout or race should be followed by the standard 30 minutes in Stage III and then by 3½ hours in Stage IV. This critical stage continues the focus on "macrolevel" recovery, meaning the emphasis is still primarily on the intake of carbohydrate and protein.

As your body returns to a resting state following exercise, sensations of hunger will emerge. After not taking in any substantial food sources for perhaps several hours, the body begins to cry out for complete nutrition. How long it takes for hunger to appear depends on how long and intense the preceding exercise was, how well stocked your carbohydrate stores were before starting the session, how much carbohydrate you took in during the session, and even how efficient your body is in using fat for fuel while sparing glycogen. The foods you eat now should emphasize moderate to high glycemic load carbohydrates.

Stage IV Recovery Guidelines

The focus of this period is similar to that of the 30-minute window preceding it. The difference is that now there is a shift toward taking in more solid foods, although continued fluid consumption is also important. Here are guidelines for eating during this extended recovery period.

Carbohydrate remains very important at this stage of recovery, but the difference is inclusion of more solid foods, especially starchy vegetables that are high on the glycemic load scale while having a net alkaline-enhancing effect on body fluids. Good choices include potatoes, yams, and sweet potatoes, as well as dried fruits, especially raisins. These are excellent to snack on or even make a meal of during Stage IV recovery because they have the greatest alkaline-enhancing effect of any food studied while also having a high glycemic load. That means a great amount of carbohydrate is delivered to the muscles quickly, which is more valuable at this time than having a high glycemic index. Table 4.6 lists the glycemic loads of various alkaline-enhancing fruits, juices, and vegetables. Notice that while some foods, such as watermelon, have a high glycemic index, their glycemic loads are low; the lower the load, the more of the food you will need to eat. Glycemic load is a measure of not only how quickly a food's sugar gets into your blood but also how much sugar is delivered. The foods listed first are preferred, but all are good choices. You may also select grains such as corn, bread, a bagel, rice, and cereal to continue the rapid replacement of carbohydrate stores. Grains are not optimal, for while most have a high glycemic load, they have a net acid-enhancing effect, so be certain to include plenty of vegetables, fruits, and fruit juices to counteract the negative consequence.

During this extended recovery stage, continue taking in carbohydrate at the rate of at least 0.75 gram (3 calories) per pound of body weight per hour. Otherwise, your appetite may serve as a guide as to how much to eat. After especially long or intense exercise, you may find liquids more appealing than solids. If so, continue using a recovery drink, just as in the first 30 minutes postexercise.

At this time you must also maintain your lean protein intake, using the same 4:1 or 5:1 ratio with carbohydrate. The purpose, as before, is to continue providing amino acids for the resynthesis of muscle protein and maintenance of other physiological structures that rely on amino acids, such as the nervous system. Animal products are the best sources

TABLE 4.6

Glycemic Load and Index of Selected Alkaline-Enhancing Foods (100 g serving)

FOOD	GLYCEMIC LOAD	GLYCEMIC INDEX
Raisins	48.8	64
Potato, plain	18.4	85
Sweet potato	13.1	54
Banana	2.1	53
Yam	11.5	51
Pineapple	8.2	66
Grapes	7.7	43
Kiwifruit	7.4	52
Carrots	7.2	71
Apple	6.0	39
Pineapple juice	5.9	46
Pear	5.4	36
Cantaloupe	5.4	65
Watermelon	5.2	72
Orange juice	5.1	50
Orange	5.1	43
Apple juice	4.9	40
Peach	3.1	28
Strawberries	2.8	40

of this protein because they're rich in essential amino acids, including the branched-chain amino acids that we now know to be critical to the recovery process. Fish, shellfish, egg whites, and turkey breast are excellent choices. It is best to avoid farm-bred fish and feedlot-raised animals, and not just at this time but throughout the day. The physical composition of their meat, especially the oils, is dramatically different from that of wild game and free-ranging animals. It's common for Paleo athletes to keep a stock of boiled eggs, deli-sliced turkey breast, tuna salad, and other such protein sources easily available in their refrigerators just for this purpose.

If you continue eating fruits and vegetables now, you will also restock electrolytes that may be necessary for recovery, depending on how long the exercise session was and how hot the weather.

It's still important to drink adequate amounts to satisfy your thirst. This may vary greatly depending on how long the session lasted, its intensity, and the weather. Thirst will tell you when to drink and when to stop. Fruit juices are an excellent choice because they also bolster carbohydrate stores and are rich in most electrolytes. If you've otherwise met your carbohydrate-restocking needs by late in Stage IV, then drink water to quench thirst.

Again, we want to emphasize how critical it is to follow these Stage IV recovery guidelines, especially after very long and stressful sessions. If you rush into Stage V directly from Stage III after a long and hard workout or race, then your full recovery may well be delayed.

STAGE V: LONG-TERM POSTEXERCISE

You've gotten yourself through a grueling workout and refueled as you should in Stages I through IV of recovery. You're back at work or in class, spending time with the family, maintaining your house and landscaping—whatever it is you do when you're not training or racing. This part of your day may look ordinary to the rest of the world, but it really isn't. You're still focused on nutrition for long-term recovery.

This is the time when many athletes get sloppy with their diets. The most common mistake is to continue eating a high glycemic load diet that is low in micronutrient value and marked by the high starch and sugar intake prescribed for Stages III and IV. Eating in this way compromises your development as an athlete. It's a shame to spend hours training only to squander a portion of the potential fitness gains by eating less-than-optimal foods.

What are optimal foods? These are the categories of foods that have been eaten by our Paleolithic ancestors for millions of years; the ones to which we are fully adapted through an inheritance of genes from the many generations that preceded us here on Earth: fruits, vegetables, and lean protein from animal sources. Optimal foods also include nuts, seeds, and berries. These are also the most micronutrient-dense foods available to us—they're rich in vitamins, minerals, and other trace elements necessary for health, growth, and recovery. Table 4.7 on page 66 compares the vitamin and mineral density of several foods. Those with the highest content are in boldface. Notice that vegetables especially provide an abundant level of vitamins and minerals; most other foods pale by comparison.

Stage V Recovery Guidelines

In terms of athletic performance, the nutritional goals and guidelines for this stage of recovery are as follows.

Maintain glycogen stores. For some time prior to this stage of recovery, you intently focused your diet around carbohydrate, especially high glycemic load sources such as the sugars in starchy foods. While these foods are excellent for restocking the body's glycogen stores, they are not nutrient dense (see Table 4.7 on page 66). There is no longer a need to eat large quantities of such foods; in fact, they will diminish your potential for recovery. Every calorie eaten from a less-than-optimal food means a lost opportunity to take in much larger amounts of health- and fitness-enhancing vitamins and minerals from vegetables,

(continued on page 68)

TABLE 4.7

Comparison of Vitamin and Mineral Density of Selected Foods (standard units)

FOOD	A	C	B$_1$	B$_2$	Nia	B$_6$	B$_{12}$	Fol
Vegetables								
Broccoli	**478**	213	**0.3**	**0.7**	0.3	**0.7**	0	234
Cauliflower	6	**226**	**0.3**	0.2	2	**0.9**	0	213
Spinach	**3,509**	43	**0.4**	**1**	5	0.5	0	**624**
Asparagus	341	**82**	**0.4**	**0.5**	4	**0.6**	0	**400**
Fruits								
Apple	9	10	0.02	0.02	0.1	0.1	0	5
Banana	9	10	0.04	0.1	0.6	0.6	0	21
Peach	127	16	0.1	0.1	2	0.1	0	8
Pear	3	7	0.03	0.1	0.2	0.03	0	12
Meats								
Tuna	**1,364**	*	0.2	0.2	**6**	0.3	**6**	*
Salmon	214	*	0.2	0.2	**7**	0.2	**6**	*
Turkey	0	0	**0.4**	0.08	4	0.3	0.2	4
T-bone steak	*	0	0.04	0.1	2	0.2	1	3
Grains								
Bagel	*	0	0.1	0.1	1	0.01	0	8
Whole-wheat bread	*	0	0.1	0.08	2	0.08	0	23
Long-grain rice	*	0.7	0.1	0.01	2	0.01	0.01	2
Yellow corn	20	6	0.2	0.07	1	0.06	0	43
Dairy								
Skim milk	173	2	0.1	0.4	0.02	0.1	**1**	15
Low-fat yogurt	25	1	0.07	0.3	0.2	0.08	0.9	17
American cheese	*	0	0.01	0.1	0	0.04	0.4	2
Swiss cheese	*	0	0	0.1	0	*	0.7	*
Legumes								
Soybeans	0.7	1	0.1	0.2	0.2	0.1	0	31
Baked beans	18	*	0.2	0.06	0.5	0.1	0	26
Broad beans	2	0.5	0.1	0.1	0.6	0.1	0	95
Peanuts	0	0	0.1	0.02	2	0.04	0	25
Nuts								
Almonds	0	0	0.04	0.1	0.6	0.2	0	10
Cashews	0	0	0.04	0.04	0.2	0.04	0	12
Macadamia	*	0	0.04	0.02	0.4	0.03	0	36
Walnuts	2	1	0.06	0.02	0.2	0.09	0	10

The highest vitamin and mineral contents in each column are indicated by a bold listing.

* No information available

Pant	Na	K	Ca	P	Mg	Fe	Zn	Cu	Mn
Vegetables									
1	34	552	**386**	160	**204**	**3**	0.5	0.2	**0.8**
0.5	26	**1,333**	113	147	47	2	1	0.04	0.7
0.6	**300**	**1,995**	**581**	238	**376**	**15**	**3**	**0.7**	**4**
0.7	18	**1,268**	100	**245**	**77**	3	2	**0.4**	**0.8**
Fruits									
0.1	1	196	12	12	7	0.3	0.06	0.07	0.08
0.3	1	430	7	21	31	0.3	0.2	0.1	0.2
0.4	0	462	14	30	16	0.3	0.3	0.2	0.1
0.1	1	208	19	18	9	0.4	0.2	0.2	0.1
Meats									
*	27	175	*	*	*	0.7	0.4	0.05	*
*	67	384	7	**282**	31	0.6	0.5	0.07	*
0.4	41	194	12	139	18	0.9	1	0.03	0.01
0.1	28	158	4	83	11	1	**2**	0.06	0.006
Grains									
0.1	121	25	14	23	7	1	0.2	0.03	*
0.3	261	72	30	107	38	1	0.7	0.1	1
0.09	0	27	9	17	7	1	0.2	0.03	*
0.8	16	229	2	94	29	0.6	0.4	0.05	0.2
Dairy									
1	147	472	**351**	**287**	33	0.1	1	*	*
0.9	110	369	288	226	28	0.1	1	*	*
0.3	291	110	150	120	9	0.3	1	*	*
0.2	**478**	88	223	162	9	0.2	1	*	*
Legumes									
0.1	0.3	297	59	141	50	**3**	0.7	0.2	0.5
0.1	**429**	320	54	112	35	0.3	1	0.2	0.4
0.1	4	245	33	114	39	1	1	0.2	0.4
0.2	139	112	9	61	30	0.4	0.6	0.1	0.4
Nuts									
0.1	2	125	45	89	50	0.6	0.5	0.2	0.4
0.2	2	98	8	85	45	1	1	**0.4**	*
0.04	61	39	11	63	15	0.4	0.3	0.2	*
0.1	2	78	15	49	26	0.4	0.4	0.2	0.5

fruits, and lean animal protein. The more serious you are about your athletic performance, the more important this is.

Furthermore, one of the beauties of the human body is that, regardless of which system or function we are talking about, it takes less concentrated effort to maintain than to rebuild. This means that by eating prodigious quantities of high glycemic load carbohydrates in the previous stages, you've rebuilt your body's glycogen stores, and now less carbohydrate is required to maintain that level. Low glycemic load fruits and vegetables will accomplish that while also providing the micronutrients needed for this last stage of recovery.

Rebuild muscle tissues. Despite your best efforts to take in amino acids in recovery, if the workout was sufficiently difficult, you will have suffered some muscle cell damage. If you could use an electron microscope to look into the muscles used in an intensely hard training today, it would look like a war zone, albeit a very tiny one. You would see tattered cell membranes and leaking fluids. The body would be mobilizing its "triage services" to repair the damage as quickly as possible. To do this, the body needs amino acids in rather large quantities. Most needed are the branched-chain amino acids (BCAA) you read about earlier. Without them, the body is forced to cannibalize other protein cells to find sufficient amounts of the right amino acids to complete the job. Also needed are the essential amino acids, those that the body cannot produce and that must come from food.

BCAA and essential amino acids are most abundant in animal products. If you're hesitant to eat red meat from feedlot-raised animals, we don't blame you. The common beef products you buy in supermarkets are a poor source of food. While certainly rich in BCAA, meats from feedlot-raised animals are also packed with omega-6 polyunsaturated fats and other questionable chemical additives and are best avoided.

So what should you eat to provide BCAA and the essential amino acids for your rebuilding muscles? The best possible source would be meat from game animals such as deer, elk, and buffalo. Of course, chances are that you don't have the time to go hunting, given your workout and career choices. (For our ancestors, hunting was exercise and

TABLE 4.8

Suggested Daily Protein Intake per Pound of Body Weight

TRAINING VOLUME IN HOURS/WEEK	PROTEIN/DAY/POUND OF BODY WEIGHT IN GRAMS (calories)
< 5	0.6–0.7 (2.4–2.8)
5–10	0.7–0.8 (2.8–3.2)
10–15	0.8–0.9 (3.2–3.6)
16–20	0.9–1.0 (3.6–4.0)
> 20	1.0 (4.0)

career all rolled into one activity.) No, it's unlikely that you will find game meat outside your back door, and it can't be sold in supermarkets, either. But there are other readily available choices that are almost as good.

Ocean- or stream-caught fish and shellfish are among the best protein sources; they are, after all, wild game. It's best, however, to avoid farm-raised fish, which is essentially the same as feedlot-raised cattle. Another good choice is turkey breast. It comes as close to providing the lean protein and fat makeup of game animals as any domestic meat available. It's still a good idea to seek out meat from turkeys that were allowed to range freely in search of food. The same goes for any meat you may choose. Free-ranging animals have not only exercised but have also more likely eaten foods that are optimal for their health. This means that omega-6 and omega-3 polyunsaturated fats are in better balance. You'll find that such meats are more expensive than the more common meat of penned-up animals. It's just like so much in life: Quality costs more. You get what you pay for.

In Stage V, continue to take in 0.6 gram to 1 gram (2.4 to 4 calories) of protein per pound of body weight relative to your training load. The longer or more intense your exercise was, the more protein you should take in, as shown in Table 4.8.

Maintain a healthy pH. In our discussion of Stage III, we told you about the acid- and base-enhancing properties of foods, illustrated by

Table 4.4 on page 59. The need to maintain a healthy pH continues in this stage in order to reduce the risk of losing nitrogen and calcium. This is especially critical for older athletes whose bodies tend toward acidity more so than young athletes'. As explained earlier, nitrogen is an essential component of muscle, and calcium is crucial for bone health. Fortunately, the very foods that are the most nutrient-dense are also the ones—the only ones—that reduce blood acidity: fruits and vegetables. Any fruit will do now, so eat whichever appeal to you. As for vegetables, it's best to choose those of vibrant colors—red, yellow, green, and orange—while avoiding white ones. Be aware that beans, although often categorized as vegetables, are net acid-enhancing and best avoided. This includes peanuts, which are legumes.

Prevent or reduce inflammation. All athletes are susceptible to inflammation of muscles and tendons—it comes with the territory. You may have a tendon that is a persistent problem for you following high-effort workouts and sometimes flares up, causing pain or discomfort. Muscle tissue damaged during an intense workout may also result in inflammation. If allowed to go unchecked, nagging inflammation can become a full-blown injury, causing you to miss training and lose fitness. Omega-3 polyunsaturated fat supplements have been shown to reduce inflammation by lowering the ratio of omega-6 to omega-3 fatty acids, which should be approximately two parts omega-6 to one part omega-3 or less. Due to the high intake of omega-6 from snacks and other packaged foods that are abundant in our society, the average American diet has a 10:1 ratio of omega-6 to omega-3. In fact, avoiding omega-6 is quite a challenge in Western society. By consuming foods that are rich in omega-3—cold-water fish, leafy vegetables, macadamia nuts and walnuts, eggs enriched with omega-3, and liver—you can lower this ratio and reduce your inflammation risk. We recommend that to improve the odds of accomplishing this, you take an omega-3 supplement, such as fish oil or flaxseed oil.

Optimize body weight. For most endurance sports, maintaining a low body mass translates into better performances (see Chapter 6 for more details on this). Yet, even with a lot of daily exercise to burn calories, avoiding weight gain can be a struggle for many endurance athletes. We think you will find that by eating a Stage V diet made up primarily of fruits, vegetables, and animal protein, weight control will not be a problem. It's when you eat less-than-optimal foods that you tend to add body fat.

STAGE V AND CARBOHYDRATE

On a conventional Stone Age nutrition plan, such as the one described in *The Paleo Diet,* a person would be eating much more protein and less carbohydrate than the diet we suggest here for athletes. The shift toward more carbohydrate is due to the need to quickly recover from strenuous exercise, a need that the average, sedentary person does not have—and that our Stone Age ancestors did not have. For the athlete who trains more than once per day or has exceptionally long workouts, as is common with many serious athletes, the absolute carbohydrate intake is even higher because the need to recover increases as the number of training hours rises.

For example, an athlete training once a day for 90 minutes may burn 600 calories from carbohydrate during exercise and needs to take in at least that much during Stages I, II, III, and IV of recovery. This athlete may be eating around 3,000 total calories daily. If he gets 50 percent of his daily calories from carbohydrate, he would take in an additional 900 calories in carbs that day in Stage V, above and beyond the carbohydrate consumed in the earlier stages of the day. Of course, this carbohydrate should primarily come from fruits and especially vegetables, so calories aren't wasted by eating foods lacking in micronutrients.

The high-volume athlete may do two of these 90-minute exercise sessions a day, thus doubling the total requirement for carbohydrate to 1,200 calories during the first four stages that day. This shift toward greater volume of training also should be accompanied by an increase in total calories consumed daily. Say 3,600 calories are taken in on such a day; if the athlete is also eating a half-carbohydrate diet, he will need another 600 calories from carbohydrate sources this day in Stage V. This illustrates how the absolute carbohydrate intake varies with the training load of the athlete, despite the percentage of intake being the same.

STAGE V AND PROTEIN

Getting too little carbohydrate in the diet is seldom a problem for athletes; it's abundant in grocery stores, inexpensive, and enjoyable to eat. No, the real stumbling block is protein intake. When we do dietary assessments of athletes, we typically find that they aren't eating enough protein. Why? Because protein is not abundant in stores, it's relatively expensive, and it's not as enjoyable to eat as a sweet or starchy food. Protein in the form of meat has also gotten a bad rap in the last few decades. We've been taught that animal meat is bad for us, as it contributes to heart disease, cancer, and assorted other evils. The problem with this conclusion is that it doesn't isolate the true causes of these diseases. It's not protein that is to blame for Western society's health woes but, largely, the omega-6 fats and other additives that often accompany it. And combining saturated fat with high glycemic load foods (think mashed potatoes and gravy or bread and butter) is a double whammy. Protein from free-ranging animals and fish does not cause heart disease. And, in fact, is quite healthy.

Let's not throw the baby out with the bathwater. Feedlot-produced animal protein should be eliminated from your diet, but not the protein from free-ranging animals. Fish, shellfish, and turkey breast are excellent sources of healthy protein and rich in essential and branched-chain amino acids. For now, the take-home message is that athletes need an abundance of amino acids daily, and these are best found in free-ranging animal sources.

Since protein is so important to your total recovery, this is a good place to begin deciding what to eat at meals in Stage V. The first concept to understand is that the amount of protein you need is related to how much you train. For the average person on the street who does little or no exercise, the level of protein intake stays much the same from day to day, as physical activity is usually quite limited. It's different for the athlete who often pushes his or her body to near its limits and, in the process, potentially damages a lot of muscle tissue while perhaps using some protein as fuel. The greater your training volume or intensity, the greater the likelihood such cellular harm will occur. A considerable amount of amino acids from animal protein sources is needed in the hours of Stage V recovery to repair this tissue and prevent the body from seeking amino acids from internal sources, such as other muscles or the immune system. Without adequate protein, the risk of a compromised immune system increases and the possibility of muscle wasting rises.

Table 4.8 on page 69 provides general guidelines for how much protein to eat with regard to your weekly training volume. Intensity of training is much harder to quantify, but you may also assume that when doing a lot of interval training, hill work, resistance training, or other high-effort exercise, you probably need to increase your protein intake to the next level in the table.

The next matter is deciding where you will get this lean protein. You may be aware that you can obtain all of the essential amino acids by mixing grains and legumes in a meal. Each of those food categories is lacking in one or more of the essential amino acids, but when you eat them in combination, the meal becomes more balanced (although plant-based diets will always be lacking in the essential amino acids lysine and tryptophan). What is not generally explained, however, is that the volume of plant-based foods one has to eat to get adequate daily protein (see Table 4.9 on page 74) requires eating considerable amounts of grains and beans because these foods are nutritionally poor. In addition, they contribute to body acidity and the loss of nitrogen and calcium (see Table 4.4 on page 59). A serious athlete attempting to get nearly a gram of protein per pound of body weight from a combination of grains and legumes would need to eat all day long—and have a gut that can process a significant amount of fiber. Even if he or she could do this, blood

TABLE 4.9

Protein and Essential Amino Acid Content of Common Foods

FOOD (100-calorie serving size)	PROTEIN CONTENT (grams)	ESSENTIAL AMINO ACID CONTENT (grams)
Animal		
Cod (3.4 oz)	22	8.7
Shrimp (3.6 oz)	21	8.2
Lobster (3.6 oz)	21	8.1
Halibut (2.5 oz)	19	7.5
Chicken (2 oz)	18	6.8
Turkey breast (2 oz)	17	6.9
Tuna (1.9 oz)	16	6.3
Tenderloin steak (1.75 oz)	14	5.1
Eggs, whole (1¼)	7.7	3.4
Legumes		
Tofu (½ cup)	10	3.6
Kidney beans (½ cup)	7	2.8
Navy beans (⅓ cup)	6	1.9
Red beans (½ cup)	5	2.5
Peanut butter (1 tbsp)	4.6	1.4
Grains		
Brown rice (½ cup)	2.1	0.7
Whole-wheat bread (1½ slices)	3	0.8
Corn (¾ cup)	3.7	1.4
Bagel (½ bagel)	3.8	1.1

acidity levels would stay high, and anti-nutrients would prevent the absorption of much of the limited micronutrients these foods have.

A 150-pound athlete training 15 hours a week would need to take in about 135 grams of protein a day (150 x 0.9), according to Table 4.8 on page 69. Assuming 20 percent of that comes from assorted vegetables, fruits, fruit juices, sports bars, and sports drinks consumed throughout the day, including during the workout, another 108 grams of protein would be needed that day. To get that from animal sources, he could eat:

4 ounces of cod

6 ounces of turkey breast

4 ounces of chicken

Those foods would provide all of the additional protein and contain 44.5 grams of the all-important essential amino acids for our theoretical athlete. The total energy eaten to get these nutrients would be 454 calories. To get the same amount of protein by combining grains and beans, he would have to eat all of the following in one day:

1 cup of tofu

1 cup of kidney beans

6 slices of whole wheat bread

1 cup of navy beans

1½ cups of corn

1 cup of red beans

1 cup of brown rice

2 bagels

2 tablespoons of peanut butter

Our athlete had better like beans and have a huge appetite! The above requires eating an additional 2,300 calories that day—more than five times as much as when eating animal products—just to get 108 grams of protein. Eating grains and legumes to get daily protein is not only very inefficient, but, far worse, the vegetarian athlete will come up short on essential amino acids—even if he or she can stomach all those beans and grains.

STAGE V AND FAT

Just as there are good and bad sources of carbohydrate and protein, there are fats and oils you should pursue in your daily diet and certain others to avoid. The desirables include omega-3 polyunsaturated and monounsaturated types. As described earlier in this chapter, lowering the ratio of omega-6 to omega-3 has positive implications for reducing the likelihood of inflammation, a persistent problem for athletes. Omega-6s, while necessary for health, are more than abundant in our modern diet. This fat is common in vegetable oils such as soybean, peanut, cottonseed, safflower, sunflower, sesame, and corn. Most snack foods and many grain products, including breads and bagels, rely heavily on vegetable oils due to their low cost.

Monounsaturated fats should also be included in the athlete's diet because of their health benefits, including lowering cholesterol and triglyceride levels, thinning the blood, preventing fatal heartbeat irregularities, and reducing the risk of breast cancer. Remember that health always comes before fitness. Good sources of monounsaturated fat are avocados, nuts, and olive oil.

Avoid the fats found in abundance in whole dairy foods and feedlot-raised animals, especially beef, and trans fat found in many of the foods in our grocery stores—not only snack foods but also many bread products, peanut butter, margarine, and packaged meals. Steer clear of trans fat, referred to as "partially hydrogenated" oil on food labels, whenever possible. Trans fat increases LDL (the "bad" cholesterol associated with heart disease) and also decreases your body's production of HDL (the "good" cholesterol linked with a low incidence of heart disease). That's a double whammy best avoided.

PART II

NUTRITION 101: UNDERSTANDING BASIC CONCEPTS

CHAPTER 5

Food as Fuel During Exercise

DIETARY ORIGINS

Upon introduction to the Paleo Diet concept, many people assume that there was a single universal diet that all Stone Age people ate. Nothing could be further from the truth. In the 5 million to 7 million years since the evolutionary split between apes and hominins (primates who walk upright on two feet), as many as 20 or more different species of hominins may have existed. Their diets varied by latitude, season, climate, and food availability. But there was one universal characteristic: They all ate minimally processed wild plant and animal foods. In the Introduction, we told you all about the foods they couldn't have consumed; in Chapter 8, we will show you the evidence for the food that they ate. But in the meantime, it's important to understand how the current Western diet differs from theirs and how these differences may affect exercise performance.

If you contrast the average American diet to hunter-gatherer diets (even at their most extreme deviations), the standard American diet falls outside the hunter-gatherer range for certain crucial nutritional characteristics. By examining the diets of more than 200 hunter-gatherer societies, we have found that the typical Western diet varies from ancestral hunter-gatherer diets in these seven key features:

1. Macronutrient balance

2. Glycemic load

3. Fatty acid balance

4. Potassium/sodium balance

5. Acid/base balance

6. Fiber intake

7. Trace nutrient density

MACRONUTRIENT BALANCE
AND GLYCEMIC LOAD

Figure 5.1 compares the macronutrient composition (protein, fat, carbo-hydrate) of hunter-gatherer and typical US diets. Note that in hunter-gatherer diets, protein is universally elevated at the expense of carbohydrate, while the diets usually contained more fat than what we

FIGURE 5.1

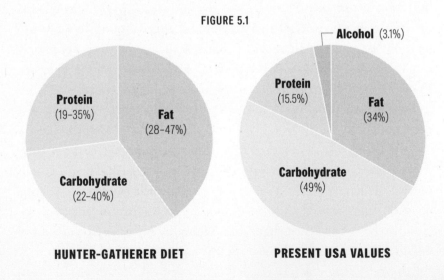

Alcohol (3.1%)

HUNTER-GATHERER DIET   **PRESENT USA VALUES**

get. However, the types of fat they consumed were healthful omega-3 and monounsaturated fats, and certain polyunsaturated and saturated fats. But the important issue here for the athlete is the carbohydrate story. Not only was the carbohydrate content of their diet lower, but the quality of their carbs was worlds apart from what most of us eat.

Glycemic Index and Glycemic Load

One quality of any carbohydrate food is its glycemic index. The glycemic index, a scale that rates how much certain foods raise blood sugar levels compared with glucose, was developed by Dr. David Jenkins at the University of Toronto in 1981. Sometimes white bread, which has a glycemic index of 100, is used as the reference food rather than glucose. One of the shortcomings of the original glycemic index is that it only compares equal quantities of carbohydrate (usually 50 grams) among foods to evaluate the blood glucose response. It doesn't take into account the total amount of carbohydrate in a typical serving. This limitation has created quite a bit of confusion. For instance, watermelon has a glycemic index (GI) of 72, while a milk chocolate candy bar tops out with a GI of only 43. Does that mean we should eat candy bars rather than fruit? Of course not! The candy bar is a much more concentrated source of carbohydrate (sugar) than watermelon is. You would have to eat only 3 ounces of the chocolate to get 50 grams of carbohydrate, whereas you would have to eat a half pound of watermelon to get 50 grams of carbs. To overcome this limitation, scientists at Harvard University in 1997 proposed using a new scale called the glycemic load, defined as the GI multiplied by the carbohydrate content in a typical serving. The glycemic load effectively equalized the playing field and made real-world food comparisons possible.

Almost all processed foods made from refined grains and sugars have quite high glycemic loads, whereas virtually all fresh fruits and veggies have very low glycemic loads (see Table 5.1 on page 82). The Web site www.glycemicindex.com helps you determine the GI and glycemic load of almost any food.

TABLE 5.1

Comparison of Glycemic Index and Load of Refined and Unrefined Foods (100 g portions)

WESTERN REFINED FOODS			UNREFINED TRADITIONAL FOODS		
Food	Glycemic Index	Glycemic Load	Food	Glycemic Index	Glycemic Load
Crisped rice cereal	88	77.3	Parsnips	97	19.5
Jelly beans	80	74.5	Baked potato	85	18.4
Cornflakes	84	72.7	Boiled millet	71	16.8
Life Savers	70	67.9	Boiled broad beans	79	15.5
Rice cakes	82	66.9	Boiled couscous	65	15.1
Table sugar (sucrose)	65	64.9	Boiled sweet potato	54	13.1
Shredded wheat cereal	69	57.0	Boiled brown rice	55	12.6
Graham crackers	74	56.8	Banana	53	12.1
Grape-Nuts cereal	67	54.3	Boiled yam	51	11.5
Cheerios cereal	74	54.2	Boiled garbanzo beans	33	9
Rye crisp bread	65	53.4	Pineapple	66	8.2
Vanilla wafers	77	49.7	Grapes	43	7.7
Corn chips	73	46.3	Kiwifruit	52	7.4
Mars bar	68	42.2	Carrots	71	7.2
Shortbread cookies	64	41.9	Boiled beets	64	6.3
Granola bar	61	39.3	Boiled kidney beans	27	6.2
Angel food cake	67	38.7	Apple	39	6.0
Bagel	72	38.4	Boiled lentils	29	5.8
Doughnut	76	37.8	Pear	36	5.4
White bread	70	34.7	Watermelon	72	5.2
Waffles	76	34.2	Orange	43	5.1
100% bran cereal	42	32.5	Cherries	22	3.7
Whole wheat bread	69	31.8	Peach	28	3.1
Croissant	67	31.2	Peanuts	14	2.6

TABLE 5.2

Blood Glucose and Insulin Responses (239-kcal sample)

FOOD	GLUCOSE	INSULIN
White bread	100	100
Eggs	42	31
Beef	21	51
Fish	28	59

The glycemic reference is white bread with a glucose and insulin response of 100.

Meat and seafood generally don't contain any carbohydrate and cause minimal rises in blood sugar and insulin levels (see Table 5.2).

Surprising—and somewhat alarming—is the paradoxically high insulin response of milk (90) and fermented milk (98) compared with their low glycemic responses (30 and 15, respectively). A similar dissociation of the blood insulin and glucose response occurs in yogurt. Generally, however, the GI of most foods nicely parallels the insulin response or insulin index (II). Hence, high GI foods are almost always high II foods.

Because the carbohydrates in Paleolithic diets came from minimally processed wild plants, and because hunter-gatherers ate no refined grains or sugars (except for seasonal honey), the glycemic loads of their diets would have been very low by modern standards. But remember, the fat and protein intake would have been higher. What are the implications of these dietary macronutrient patterns upon endurance performance?

Muscle Fuel Sources

When you are at rest and not exercising, about 60 percent of the energy needed to fuel your body is provided by fats. The balance is provided by carbohydrate because protein is a relatively minor source of energy. When you are at rest, free fatty acids (FFA) circulating in the bloodstream provide the major source of fat to fuel metabolism. FFA in the blood comes from fat stored in cells in your belly, thighs, and any other place where you accumulate fat. At low exercise levels (25 percent of your aerobic capacity or max VO_2), fat provides 80 percent of the muscle's fuel, and the balance (about 20 percent) comes from carbohydrate. At 25 percent max VO_2, most of the fat fueling muscle contraction still comes from FFA in the blood, although a small amount is derived from stored fat droplets inside muscle cells—the intramuscular triglycerides (IMT). Twenty to 30 years ago, exercise scientists didn't pay much attention to IMT when it came to endurance performance; their sights were narrowly focused upon glycogen. Glycogen is made up of chains of glucose molecules, which is how carbs are stored inside muscle cells.

Let's continue with the tutorial on muscle fuel sources so you can eventually see how Paleolithic macronutrient patterns weren't necessarily a liability for performance. As exercise intensity increases, so does IMT usage by the muscles. At approximately 65 percent max VO_2, IMT stores are being maximally drawn on, so that energy contribution from fats and carbs is about 50:50. When exercise intensity increases to 85 percent max VO_2, IMT supplies only 25 percent of the energy needed for muscle contraction. Finally, as you continue to 100 percent of your aerobic capacity, glucose from muscle glycogen stores becomes the preferred and necessary fuel source. Why is that? Why isn't fat used to fuel very intense and high-level exercise?

If you look at the caloric density of fat, it has 9 calories per gram—more than twice as much as carbohydrate's 4 calories per gram. So, at least on the surface, it looks like fat would be the preferred fuel for high-level exercise because it's such a concentrated energy source. But there's another side to the story, and it's called fuel efficiency—a concept you know better as "miles per gallon." When you look at body fuel efficiency in terms of oxygen rather than energy density, the picture changes. It takes considerably more oxygen for muscles to burn fat than to burn carbohydrate. Carbohydrate yields 5.05 calories per liter of oxygen, whereas fat gives only 4.69—a difference of 7 percent. During aerobic metabolism, this 7 percent caloric advantage for carbs translates into a threefold faster energy production in the muscles. The take-home message: Muscle stores of glycogen are absolutely essential in performing endurance exercise at or above 85 percent max VO_2 for any extended period.

But here's the problem: There is a limit to how much glycogen the muscles can store. Trained endurance athletes can store twice as much muscle glycogen as couch potatoes can. However, it's important to know that muscle glycogen stockpiles cannot be shifted from one muscle to another during exercise: Any glycogen in your arms will not help your legs and vice versa. The values for muscle glycogen in Table 5.3 represent whole-body muscle stores and obviously will be considerably lower for specific muscle groups.

Because the muscle glycogen stores are limited, high-intensity endurance activity (> 85 percent max VO_2) can last only as long as the glycogen lasts. But there's a catch here, and if you are an experienced endurance athlete, you know it: You can drink athletic beverages containing glucose to slow the muscle's glycogen loss during exercise but, unfortunately, you cannot drink them fast enough. The maximum rate that ingested glucose can be metabolized during exercise is about 1 gram per minute—still not fast enough to replace what's being lost during hard exercise. As muscle glycogen stores become depleted, you're forced to slow down because the remaining fat stores require more oxygen to be burned. This reduced oxygen efficiency of fat compared with glucose is precisely why you must reduce your intensity once muscle glycogen reserves are severely depleted.

There is still a way out of this bottleneck. You can slow muscle glycogen loss by increasing how efficiently you burn fats and by increasing your IMT stores. Fats play a key role in how well you will perform in ultra-endurance events and bicycle road races. In long,

TABLE 5.3

Total Body Carbohydrate Stores in a Nontrained Person

SOURCE	AMOUNT (g)	CORRESPONDING CALORIES
Blood glucose	5	20
Liver glycogen	100	400
Muscle glycogen	400	1,600

moderate-intensity races such as these, not only do you deplete your carbohydrate reserves; you simply cannot metabolize ingested carbs (from drinks or energy bars) as fast as you are losing them. Accordingly, if you can maximize both your muscle IMT and glycogen before the race, you will be in a lot better shape during the race. Michael Vogt, PhD, and colleagues from the University of Bern in Switzerland showed that athletes consuming a 53 percent fat diet for 5 weeks were able to double their IMT stores without compromising muscle glycogen stockpiles. Further, the athletes' endurance performance at moderate to high intensities was maintained with a significantly larger contribution of fat to energy output. These results have been consistently confirmed in the ensuing 7 years since the publication of the first edition of *The Paleo Diet for Athletes*. Interested readers may consult these scientific references listed in the References.

Your individual dietary strategy will depend upon the length and intensity of your race. If ultra-endurance events are your thing, then you may want to give a higher-fat diet a try—but make sure it contains healthy fats, not trans fats that are found in most processed and fast foods. Shorter, high-intensity races require more carbs and less fat, but it is still important that you try to maximize both IMT and muscle glycogen stores.

Now let's tie up the loose ends. Our ancestral dietary patterns couldn't have allowed us to restore muscle glycogen day in and day out. High glycemic load carbs on a year-round basis simply did not exist. Additionally, Stone Age people typically did not eat three meals a day. Contemporary studies of the Aché hunter-gatherers in Paraguay show that men usually ate only a single large meal in the evening. About 10 days a month they took breakfast, but they almost never had a midday meal. Women and children, on the other hand, stayed closer to camp and ate frequently throughout the day. In modern scientific experiments, the conditions the Aché men experienced (long fasting periods) have been shown to increase IMT, as have high-fat diets. Consequently, our Paleolithic relatives were much more reliant upon IMT when it came to running down animals or doing long, drawn-out, heavy work. You, on the other hand, have the luxury of adding performance-enhancing high glycemic load carbs to your diet whenever you want. But remember the take-home message that we emphasize throughout this book: moderation and quality. Avoid refined grains and sugars and replace them with better choices at the right time, as outlined in Chapters 4 and 9.

Macronutrient Balance: Protein

One of the striking differences between ancestral and modern diets is the protein content. Protein makes up about 15 percent of the calories in the US diet, whereas in hunter-gatherers' diets it was between 19 and 35 percent of total energy. Compared with fat and carbohydrate, protein is a relatively negligible fuel source during rest. Even with moderate to strenuous exercise lasting up to 2 hours, protein accounts for less than 5 percent of the energy cost of the activity. However, during the end stages of prolonged endurance events, protein can contribute up to 15 percent of the total energy cost.

The building blocks of all proteins are smaller compounds called amino acids. Before proteins can be used to produce energy in muscles, they must first be broken down into their constituent amino acids. One of these amino acids, alanine, is then released into the bloodstream, where it travels to the liver and can be converted to glucose in a process known as gluconeogenesis. However, the conversion of alanine to glucose amounts to only about 4 grams per hour—just a trickle, compared with values as high as 3 grams of glucose per minute needed during very high-intensity exercise.

Does this mean that you should forget about protein and worry only about carbs and fat when it comes to improving performance? Absolutely not. As explained in Chapters 1, 2, and 9, upping your protein intake may positively influence fatigue, muscle protein synthesis during recovery, and immune function. Also, don't forget that meats, fish, and seafood are rich sources of zinc, iron, and vitamin B_6—trace nutrients that will almost certainly be low if you are following a starch and refined carb diet.

FATTY ACID BALANCE

When you adopt the Paleo Diet for Athletes, you will want to get rid of the bad fats and concentrate on the health-promoting ones. As you have seen, increasing fat in your diet may not be a bad thing when it comes to endurance performance. Getting the right kinds of fat into your diet may also improve your immune system and help lower the risk of many inflammatory diseases, heart disease, certain autoimmune diseases, and some cancers.

Chemical Structure of Fats

Like any other specialty area, you have to take some time to master the language before you can get a handle on how things work. Most athletes are concerned with their diet and know a little bit about the three major types of dietary fats: saturated, monounsaturated, and polyunsaturated. Let's get into just a bit more detail.

Technically, all fats are called acylglycerols; each is composed of a glycerol molecule bound to 1, 2, or 3 acyl molecules. A more familiar term for an acyl molecule is "fatty acid." So if a saturated fatty acid is attached to a glycerol molecule, it can legitimately be called a fat. If the saturated fatty acid is not connected to glycerol, then it formally is not a fat but, rather, a free fatty acid. The same holds for monounsaturated and polyunsaturated fatty acids: If they are bound to glycerol, they are fats. If not, they are free fatty acids. All free fatty acids aren't really free; they must be linked to a protein molecule to travel in the blood.

If a single fatty acid is connected to a glycerol molecule, it is called a monoacylglycerol or monoglyceride. Two fatty acids connected to glycerol make a diacylglycerol (or diglyceride), and three fatty acids attached to glycerol are called a triacylglycerol or, more commonly, a triglyceride. Virtually all the fats you eat and almost all the fats you store in adipose (fat) tissue are triglycerides. Storage triglycerides in your fat cells can be used to fuel your muscles, but the fatty acids have to be first cleaved from the glycerol molecule and then bound to a protein molecule (albumin) to be transported in the bloodstream as free fatty acids.

Next, let's discuss the three major types of dietary fats, how they are labeled, how their structures vary, and how they affect your health and performance.

Saturated Fatty Acids

Saturated fatty acids are the simplest of the three major families of fatty acids because they contain no double bonds between carbon atoms in the backbone of the molecule. Consequently, each carbon atom is fully "saturated" with hydrogen atoms. Figure 5.2 is a schematic diagram of a saturated fatty acid called lauric acid, which is given the technical designation of 12:0; it contains 12 carbon atoms and 0 double bonds between the carbon atoms. It also has an omega end and a carboxyl end. (You'll see why knowing which end is which is important when we talk about differences between omega-6 and omega-3 fatty acids.)

FIGURE 5.2

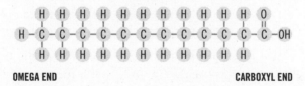

OMEGA END   CARBOXYL END

The other major dietary saturated fatty acids are 14:0 (myristic acid), 16:0 (palmitic acid), and 18:0 (stearic acid). Of all of these, 12:0, 14:0, and 16:0 raise blood cholesterol levels, whereas 18:0 is neutral. Both 12:0 and 14:0 are found in relatively small concentrations in fatty foods, so 16:0 is the primary fatty acid in butter, cheese, lard, bacon, salami, and other fatty meats responsible for elevating blood cholesterol. However, because it (16:0) also simultaneously elevates the "good" HDL cholesterol, the most recent meta-analyses (large population studies) show saturated fats in general to be minor risk factors for heart disease. I came up to a similar conclusion in a book chapter I wrote in 2006 that analyzed the amounts of dietary saturated fats in 229 hunter-gatherer societies.

Monounsaturated Fatty Acids

Compared with saturated fatty acids, monounsaturated fatty acids lower total blood cholesterol levels. They are labeled "mono" unsaturated because there is a single double bond in their carbon backbone. Figure 5.3 is a diagram of oleic acid, also known as 18:1v9. The "v" symbol stands for "omega." Again, "18" means that there are 18 carbons in its backbone; the "1" means there is one double bond, which is located 9 carbon molecules down from the omega end. Monounsaturated fatty acids are found in nuts, avocados, olive oil, and other oils listed in Chapter 11. These are some of the healthful fatty foods you want to include in your diet if you decide to up your fat intake.

FIGURE 5.3

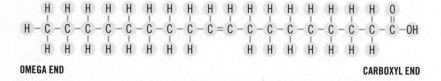

OMEGA END   CARBOXYL END

Polyunsaturated Fatty Acids (Omega-6s)

Polyunsaturated fatty acids are called "poly," meaning "many," because they contain two or more double bonds between the carbon atoms in their backbone. Figure 5.4 illustrates linoleic acid, or 18:2v6. By now, you probably are getting the drift of this naming scheme: Linoleic acid contains 18 carbon atoms and 2 double bonds, and the last double bond is located 6 carbon atoms down from the omega end of the fatty acid backbone.

FIGURE 5.4

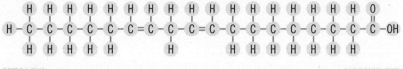

OMEGA END   CARBOXYL END

Linoleic acid is a member of the omega-6 family of polyunsaturated fatty acids and is found in high concentrations in corn oil, safflower oil, and other salad oils and processed foods made with vegetable oils. Excessive intake of omega-6 polyunsaturated fats may promote heart disease, inflammation, and certain cancers; and the typical American diet contains way too much of this fat. In Chapter 11, you'll learn how to achieve just the right balance of this fat on your menu.

Polyunsaturated Fatty Acids (Omega-3s)

Almost anyone who has an interest in diet and health has heard of omega-3 fatty acids, but most people really don't know what they are. This will change for you in about 2 seconds, now that you are becoming an accomplished lipid chemist with this tutorial. The simplest omega-3 polyunsaturated fatty acid is called alpha-linolenic acid (ALA), abbreviated 18:3v3. If you have been following along, you know that ALA contains 18 carbon atoms in its backbone and 3 double bonds, the last of which is 3 carbon atoms down from the omega end. Figure 5.5 on page 92 shows a diagram of this fatty acid. These diagrams are helpful in understanding the structure and names of the various fats, but they don't tell you everything. The carbon-to-carbon bonds in their backbones are not straight (180 degrees) but form a 109-degree angle. Hence, their actual physical structures look different from these diagrammatic representations.

FIGURE 5.5

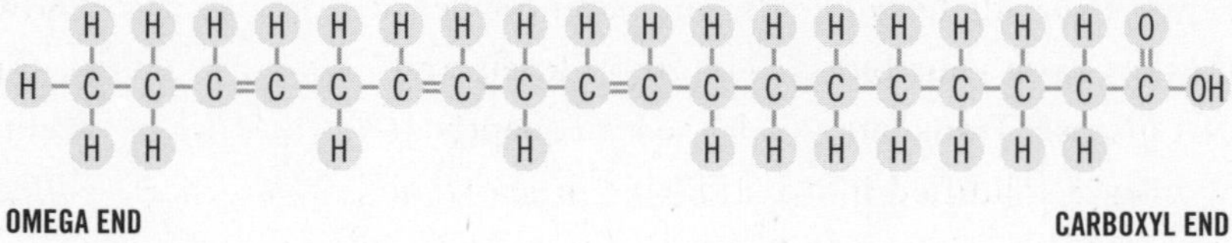

H-C-C-C=C-C-C=C-C-C=C-C-C-C-C-C-C-C-OH

OMEGA END   CARBOXYL END

ALA is the simplest omega-3 fatty acid and is found in high concentrations in flaxseed and canola oils. In the body, the liver can turn ALA from flaxseed or canola oil into longer chain omega-3s such as eicosapentaenoic acid (EPA), or 20:5v3, and docosahexaenoic acid (DHA), or 22:6v3. However, this process is quite inefficient, and only less than 1 percent of ALA is turned into DHA. Most of the beneficial biological effects of omega-3 fatty acids result from the long chain metabolites of ALA, which are EPA and DHA. You're better off getting your omega-3s from fish and seafood, which are rich sources of both EPA and DHA.

A few recent human experiments suggest that omega-3 fatty acids may have few performance enhancing effects; nevertheless, literally thousands of scientific experiments have shown that these fatty acids promote good health. Omega-3s are potent anti-inflammatory agents comparable or superior to aspirin. In one study of 10 elite endurance athletes, by Dr. Tim Mickleborough at Indiana University, dietary fish oil supplementation proved to be highly effective in reducing exercise-induced constriction of the airways leading to the lungs. This isn't of interest only to elite athletes: Exercise-induced asthma (EIA) is a real problem that may affect as much as 10 percent of the general population. If that includes you, then increasing your dietary intake of omega-3s not only makes sense but also may be essential medicine. Even if you don't suffer symptoms of EIA, your long-term health will benefit in many ways if you get more of these highly therapeutic fatty acids into your diet.

Trans Fatty Acids

Trans fatty acids have been in the news for decades, so you may know that they raise your blood cholesterol levels and increase your risk for heart disease. Trans fatty acids most frequently are formed when vegetable oils are solidified into margarine or shortening by a process called hydrogenation. Consequently, hydrogenated or partially hydrogenated vegetable oils contain trans fatty acids. European scientists participating in a large clinical trial called the TransLinE Study showed that trans fatty acids can also be formed when vegetable oils are deodorized. Careful deodorizing prevents the formation of trans fatty acids. So, when you buy vegetable oil, make sure the label guarantees that the product is trans fat–free.

Trans fatty acids are isomers of normally occurring fatty acids—meaning that they have the same molecular weight as a normal fatty acid but a slightly different structure. We've already talked about oleic acid, a mono-unsaturated fat labeled 18:1v9 or, more precisely, 18:1v9 cis. That means the hydrogen atoms adjacent to the single double bond are on the same side (cis). Figure 5.6 shows a trans fatty acid designated 18:1v9 trans. It is called a "trans" fatty acid because the hydrogen atoms about the double bond are on opposite sides. This specific trans fatty acid is also known as trans elaidic acid and is the bad guy responsible for the cholesterol-raising and other adverse health effects of trans fatty acids found in margarine and shortening. The deodorization of vegetable oils produces trans isomers of 18:3v3 (ALA), which also negatively affect your blood lipid profile. Do yourself a favor and keep these nasty fats out of your diet.

FIGURE 5.6

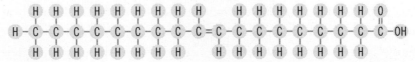

OMEGA END   CARBOXYL END

POTASSIUM/SODIUM BALANCE

In the typical US diet, we get almost 10 grams of salt per day. Because salt is made up of sodium and chloride, this translates into a daily intake of 3.5 grams of sodium and 6.5 grams of chloride. Most people know that the sodium part of salt is not good for health, particularly when we get too much of it. But few people have a clue that the chloride portion is also problematic (more on this later). Consider the ratio of potassium to sodium in the average American diet: Because our average daily potassium intake is a paltry 2.6 grams, the ratio (2.6:3.5) is 0.74. One of the reasons we have so little potassium in our diets is that in the United States we simply eat too few fruits and veggies, the richest sources of this element. Ninety-one percent of the US population does not meet the USDA recommendation of two to three daily servings of fruit and three to five daily servings of vegetables. In stark contrast, a modern-day Paleo diet, like that outlined in Chapter 1, contains 9 grams of potassium and 0.7 gram of sodium, for a ratio of 12.5. From hundreds of computer simulations of modern-day Paleo diets, we have found the ratio of potassium to sodium is always greater than 5, whereas in the typical US diet, it is always less than 1.

This complete inversion of the Paleo potassium/sodium ratio may produce a number of potential health problems that may hurt your race-day performance. Similar to the effects of having too few omega-3 fatty acids in your diet, excessive sodium also worsens exercise-induced asthma symptoms. Experiments from our laboratory and Dr. Mickleborough's at Indiana University in both humans and animals show beyond a shadow of a doubt that reducing dietary salt for those with EIA is therapeutic. This strategy won't eliminate EIA, but it will vastly improve symptoms. Similarly, if you suffer from hypertension or osteoporosis, lowering the salt and upping the fruit and veggies in your diet may prove helpful. For athletes training or racing long distances in heat, we don't suggest eliminating salt completely but, rather, using it moderately and following the guidelines established in Chapters 2, 3, and 4.

ACID/BASE BALANCE

Most athletes and many nutrition experts alike are unaware of the concept of dietary acid/base balance and how it may affect health, well-being, and athletic performance. All foods after digestion report to the kidney as either acid or base (see Table 4.4 on page 59). If the diet produces a net metabolic acidosis, then the kidney must buffer this acid load with stored alkaline base. Ultimately, alkaline base can come from calcium salts in the bones. Alternatively, more acid can be excreted in the urine by the muscles breaking down and releasing more of the amino acid glutamine. Over the long haul, both effects may hurt your performance. Accelerated bone mineral loss increases the likelihood of stress fractures—clearly a liability in your training schedule.

Accelerated glutamine loss from a net acid-producing diet may adversely affect exercise performance through a wide variety of mechanisms. Glutamine supplementation has been shown to increase growth

TABLE 5.4

Acid/Base Balance in Average US Diet

Net Acid-Yielding Foods
Cereal grains = 23.9% energy

Meats, fish = 15.7% energy

Dairy = 10.6% energy

Nuts, legumes = 3.1% energy

Eggs = 1.4% energy

Salt = 9.6 g/day

Net Alkaline-Yielding Foods
Vegetables = 4.8% energy

Fruits = 3.3% energy

Neutral (But Displace Alkaline Foods)
Refined sugars = 18.6% energy

Refined oils = 17.9% energy

Values represent percentage of the total daily energy consumed.

hormone and help spare muscle mass in critically ill patients and in some animal experiments. Also, like alanine, glutamine can be converted to glucose in the liver and may provide an additional carbohydrate source during prolonged exercise. Finally, depleted blood glutamine levels in endurance athletes are a symptom of overtraining and increase the likelihood of infection and upper respiratory illness. Because most endurance athletes eat a net acid-producing diet similar to the typical American diet outlined in Table 5.4 on page 95, chances are good that glutamine reserves will be compromised. By following the Paleo Diet for Athletes, you will be getting plenty of glutamine from fresh meats, fish, and seafood.

FIBER INTAKE

The average person in the United States does not get enough fiber. Current intakes (15 grams per day) fall way short of recommended levels (about 25 to 35 grams per day). When you adopt the Paleo Diet for Athletes, fiber will become a nonissue because you will get it almost entirely from fresh fruits and vegetables. A common perception is that whole grains are excellent sources of fiber. Think again. Figure 5.7 shows this not to be the case in its depiction of the average total fiber content in a 1,000-calorie serving of 3 refined cereals, 8 whole grain cereals, 20 fresh fruits, and 20 nonstarchy vegetables. When it comes to soluble fiber, whole grains are lightweights compared with fruits and veggies.

Fiber has little influence upon exercise performance, but it helps to normalize bowel function and prevent constipation, and it may help to avert "runner's trots," which can be more embarrassing than detrimental to performance. Increased fiber consumption may also slightly improve your blood chemistry and over the course of a lifetime may prevent varicose veins, hemorrhoids, hiatal hernia, and other illnesses associated with the gastrointestinal tract.

FIGURE 5.7

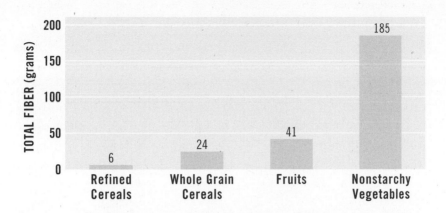

TRACE NUTRIENT DENSITY

In Chapter 1 we showed you what a nutritional lightweight the USDA
Food Pyramid/MyPlate diet is compared to the Paleo Diet for Athletes,
particularly when we get down to the issue of vitamins and minerals.
Most people in the United States would be lucky to eat as well as the
USDA Food Pyramid/MyPlate designers would like us to eat. In fact, we
don't do very well at all. Table 5.5 on page 98 shows that more than half
of the US population gets insufficient vitamin B_6, vitamin A, magnesium,
calcium, and zinc. The problem comes not only from our avoidance of
fruits and veggies but also our consumption of so many empty calories
in the form of refined sugars and grains in processed foods. Refined
sugars make up 18 percent of our daily calories yet have absolutely zero
vitamins and minerals. Grains compose 24 percent of our daily food
intake, but, unfortunately, 85 percent of the grains consumed in the
United States are taken as refined grains. Figures 5.8 and 5.9 (see pages
98 and 99) show how the refining process strips whole wheat of most of
its vitamins and minerals.

TABLE 5.5

US Individuals Age 2 and Older Meeting RDAs

NUTRIENT	PERCENTAGE
Vitamin B_{12}	82.8
Protein	79.5
Vitamin B_3	74.1
Vitamin B_2	70
Vitamin B_1	69.8
Folate	66.8
Vitamin C	62
Iron	60.9
Vitamin B_6	46.4
Vitamin A	43. 8
Magnesium	38.4
Calcium	34.9
Zinc	26.7

These are the 13 nutrients most lacking in the US diet (1994–96), according to 1989 RDAs.

FIGURE 5.8

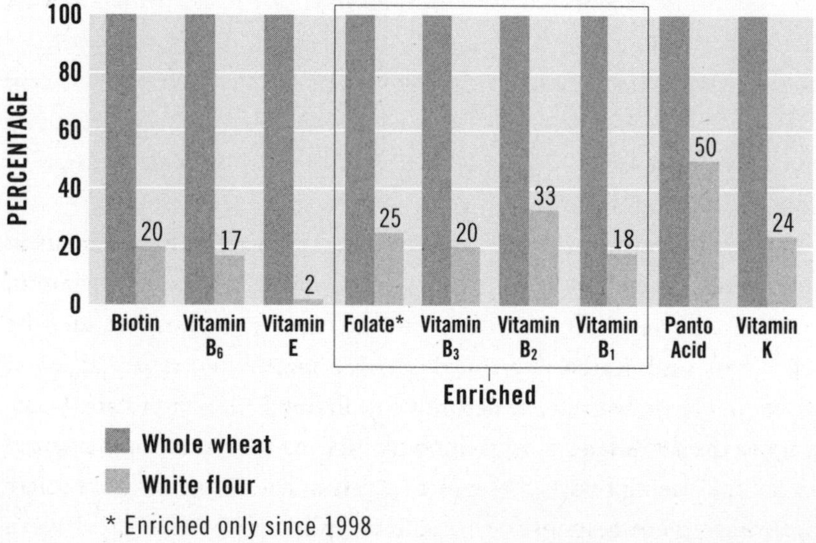

Whole wheat

White flour

* Enriched only since 1998

FIGURE 5.9

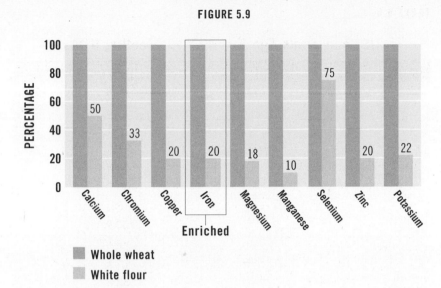

These figures give you a pretty good idea that white flour is a nutrient-depleted mess! Even governmental agencies understand that white flour isn't such a good thing. Starting shortly after World War II, all white flour was required by law to be enriched with vitamins B_1, B_2, B_3, and iron. It's almost inconceivable to call this stuff "enriched" when at least 18 vitamins and minerals are severely depleted during the refining process, yet only 4 are added back. Wait, make that 5. In 1998, legislation by the Food and Drug Administration (FDA) and the Centers for Disease Control and Prevention (CDC) mandated further supplementation of white flour with folic acid.

Folic acid is an artificial compound first synthesized by scientists at Lederle Labs in 1947. After ingestion, it is converted into the B vitamin folate by the liver. Note that folic acid and folate are not one and the same compound. Rather, folic acid is metabolized in a slightly different manner in the body than the naturally occurring B vitamin folate. Leading up to the 1998 federal legislation mandating folic acid supplementation, an increasing body of scientific literature had suggested that folate deficiencies were responsible for the crippling and often fatal birth defects known as neural tube defects. Accordingly, the governmental rationale for folic acid fortification in the US food supply was to reduce the incidence of neural tube defects, of which spina bifida is most well known.

In a 6-year period (1990–1996) before mandatory folic acid fortification, the average number of neural tube defects per year in the United States was 1,582. In the first year (1998–1999) following fortification, neural tube defects dropped to 1,337, so 245 cases of this disease were prevented. The problem with population-wide folic acid supplementation was that it had never been adequately tested in large randomized, controlled human trials to determine if this artificial compound had any adverse health effects. I would be the first person to congratulate governmental agencies for mandating a national policy that could reduce or eliminate neural tube defects. Unfortunately, this shotgun approach put the entire US population (300 million people) at risk for death and disability from other more serious diseases.

In the last decade, an accumulating body of scientific evidence now makes it clear that the FDA's mandatory folic acid fortification program represents a terrible blunder in US public health policy. An alarming number of human clinical trials, animal experiments, and epidemiological studies show that excess folate via folic acid fortification has resulted in population-wide increases in the risk for breast, prostate, and colorectal cancers. Although scientists aren't completely sure how excess folate and folic acid promote cancer, animal experiments indicate that these compounds induce a cancer-causing reaction called hypermethylation in the DNA of cancer cells.

Because the Paleo Diet for Athletes recommends that you should severely restrict or eliminate all grains, the nationwide folic acid fortification program becomes a nonissue for Paleo Dieters, providing you do not take folic acid–containing vitamins or supplements. As we have made it clear throughout this revision, supplementation (except for fish oil and vitamin D) is unnecessary, and antioxidant supplements may actually prevent the health promoting effects of exercise and hamper training adaptations in endurance performance.

It would appear that you are a whole lot better off eating whole grains to get calcium, iron, magnesium, and zinc. Wrong! Whole grains contain numerous substances called antinutrients that can impair nutrient absorption or adversely affect health in a wide variety of ways. Phytic acid, otherwise known as phytate, is an antinutrient found in all whole grains and legumes that binds calcium, iron, magnesium, and zinc and severely inhibits their absorption. Whether whole or refined, grains are an inferior food when it comes to vitamins and minerals. Do yourself a favor and get the bulk of your carbs from fresh fruits and veggies.

CHAPTER 6

FITNESS AND FOOD

There are three factors that contribute to fitness. The first, and most important, is a sound training program that focuses on the demands of high performance. Without physical stress as created by challenging workouts, your body will not have the stimulus to adapt and grow stronger. The second contributor to performance is rest, especially adequate sleep. It's during sleep that your body experiences the process of adaptation. Workouts provide the potential for fitness, but it's realized while you are resting and sleeping. During rest and sleep your body requires resources to rebuild. These are the macronutrients (protein, fat, and carbohydrate) and the micronutrients (vitamins and minerals). This is the third factor in fitness. These dietary contributors make growth and adaptation to the stress of training possible. If these nutrients are not adequate in your diet, then not only will your athletic performance suffer, but also your health. There are several other ways that your diet affects fitness. We will examine them here. Let's start with the most basic question.

WHAT IS FITNESS?

Athletes talk about fitness a lot. So what is it? Endurance athletes usually discuss fitness in terms of performance. Runners talk about their 10-km pace or a recent marathon time. Cyclists lay claim to high-power outputs. While these are actually quite good ways to define fitness, they don't tell us anything about the mechanisms responsible for it—which may provide clues regarding how to go about improving it. That, of course, is the ultimate goal of athletic training.

Exercise physiologists are a bit more precise when it comes to "fitness." For decades they have proposed that there are only three things you can do to become more fit for endurance sports. You can increase your aerobic capacity, elevate your anaerobic threshold, and become more economical. That's it. Nothing else. All of your training comes down to these three elements. And they are what ultimately produce your fast 10-km run and high-power output. So what are they, what can you do in training to improve them, and how are they affected by what you eat?

Aerobic Capacity

You probably know this as "max VO_2." It's a measure of how much oxygen your body uses when working at a maximal aerobic effort. Physiologists define it as the maximal volume of oxygen consumed in milliliters per kilogram of body weight per minute (the formula is ml O2/kg/minute). The higher your max VO_2, the more likely you are to perform at a high level in endurance events.

Your aerobic capacity is unique to each sport. If you have a high max VO_2 for swimming it won't necessarily be high for cycling or running.

To raise your max VO_2, do highly intense intervals. This workout would be something along the lines of 3-minute intervals at an intensity you could hold for only about 5 or 6 minutes. Do four to six of these intervals in a session with 3 minutes of recovery between them at least once each week. Doing one to three of these sessions weekly in the last 12 weeks before a priority A race has been shown in the research to produce significant gains in aerobic capacity.

Aerobic capacity is also raised by losing excess body weight. In the formula above, oxygen consumed is divided by body weight, so as body weight goes down, max VO_2 rises. This is undoubtedly obvious to you.

At those rare times when your body weight has increased, riding your bike up a hill or running became a bit harder. Your aerobic capacity had decreased. Later in the chapter we'll get into this issue of body weight and performance along with the related benefits of eating the Paleo Diet.

Anaerobic Threshold (AT)

You may know this as "lactate threshold" or even "ventilatory threshold." Sport scientists differentiate among these three thresholds, but for the average athlete the differences are not critical to training or performance. Basically, this is the highest intensity you can maintain for about an hour. Another way of thinking of AT is that it's the intensity at which you begin to "redline." When you cross this threshold as you speed up, you sense the effort becoming *hard*. On a perceived-effort scale of 1 to 10, with 10 being *very, very hard,* AT occurs at about 7.

A high AT is very important for endurance performance. Among athletes with similar aerobic capacities, AT plays a major role in determining the outcome of a race. Many studies have shown it to be the better predictor. In other words, you really can't predict who will win an endurance race based only on aerobic capacity (max VO_2). But we know that people with a high max VO_2 will cross the finish line first. That person is likely to have the highest AT among those with high aerobic capacities.

In the lab, AT is measured as a percentage of aerobic capacity. During a high-intensity workout or race, a highly fit athlete will experience AT at about 85 percent of max VO_2. Less fit athletes will have lower ATs at around 75 to 80 percent. The higher the AT as a percentage of max VO_2, the faster the athlete will be.

In workouts AT can be gauged using heart rate, pace, or power. This can be done using a heart rate monitor, a runner's GPS device for pace, or a bike power meter. Your average heart rate, pace, or power for an all-out 30-minute effort is a good predictor of your AT intensity.

To improve AT do long intervals at your AT pace, power, or heart rate with short recoveries between them. The high-intensity interval duration could be 5 to 20 minutes long with 20 to 60 minutes of accumulated AT time within a session. For example, a common AT workout may be 5-minute intervals at AT pace, power, or heart rate five times (5 x 5 min @ AT). This workout could be 300-meter swim intervals, 2-mile bike intervals, or 1,200-meter run intervals. The recovery time between intervals is about one-fourth the duration of the work interval. So for 5-minute intervals the easy recoveries would be 75 seconds.

As your AT rises with increasing fitness you will go faster at your AT heart rate or have a lower heart rate at your AT pace or power. You're becoming more fit. When this change occurs, it's time to retest your AT.

Training and racing at your AT or slightly below it, as in races lasting about an hour or longer, can be improved by becoming better at burning fat for fuel. We'll take a closer look at what that means in relation to your diet later in this chapter.

Economy

Sport scientists understand less about economy than about aerobic capacity and anaerobic threshold. Yet it may be the most important of the three when it comes to performance in long endurance events.

I'm certain you understand the concept. Your automobile has an economy rating—how many miles it gets per gallon of gas. Your body also has an economy rating—how far it can go on a given amount of energy (or oxygen, which is an indirect indicator of energy use). While your car runs on gasoline, for humans the primary fuels are fat and glycogen (stored carbohydrate). Highly economical endurance athletes use their stored energy sparingly.

Many variables affect economy. Some of these are the result of genetics—the physical characteristics your parents gave you. For example, good swimmers tend to have long arms and big hands. Most of the best cyclists have long femur (thigh) bones relative to the lengths of their legs. Economical runners tend to have long tibias (shin bones). In general, the best endurance athletes have more of the slow-twitch muscles than do power-sport athletes, who inherited lots of fast-twitch muscles. The list of such genetic traits common to the best endurance athletes by sport is quite long.

Economy isn't just the result of the athlete's physiological makeup, however. It is also improved by using lightweight, aerodynamic, and hydrodynamic equipment (shoes, bikes, skis, swimsuits), having well-honed skills, and improving sport-specific strength.

In terms of your diet, the most important component of economy is your body's fuel preference. A body that prefers to use fat for fuel, as opposed to carbohydrate, is economical. Even the skinniest athlete has enough fat stored away to exercise for hour after hour. But our bodies store relatively little carbohydrate. Training the body to burn fat while sparing carbohydrate improves economy.

FAT BURNERS AND CARB BURNERS

Are you a fat burner or a carbohydrate burner? Most athletes don't know, yet this is valuable information, especially if you compete in endurance events lasting longer than about 2 hours. The longer your event, the more critical this concept is to performance.

A limiting factor for such events is carbohydrate intake. If you don't take in enough sugar (the common form of carbohydrate found in sports drinks, bars, gels, and other sport nutrition products) during the event, you are likely to run low, which ultimately means your name in the results will be followed by the letters DNF (did not finish). On the other hand, take in too much sugar and your gut can't process it—possibly resulting in bloating and nausea.

To further complicate the matter, there is a considerable amount of individual variation when it comes to using carbohydrate during such events. Some people's bodies burn more carbohydrate as a percentage of total calories used. They are "sugar burners" and need to be very concerned with carbohydrate intake. The "fat burner" has a body that prefers to use fat for fuel and so spares stored carbs. This person is metabolically ready for long endurance. That may be the result of fortunate genetics, effective training, wise nutrition, or some combination of these variables.

How do you know if you're a sugar burner or a fat burner? And how do you determine if you are taking in the right amount of carbohydrate? The answers are found in your respiratory equivalency ratio (RER), sometimes also called the respiratory quotient (RQ). They aren't exactly measures of the same factor, but are close. Once you know your RER, you have a better idea of your fat- versus sugar-burning preference and what your carb-intake needs are during exercise. If you find you're a sugar burner, it is possible to change your body so that it relies more heavily upon fat. More on this later.

RER is determined by doing a metabolic assessment or max VO_2 test. Until recently you had to go to a medical clinic or university lab to have such a test done, but now there are boutique testing centers popping up around the country in health clubs, bike shops, and running and triathlon stores. A few coaches even offer this service. You can probably find a test facility somewhere near where you live. The test generally costs between $150 and $250.

RER testing is most common for cycling and running. There are a few facilities that can test rowers, Nordic skiers, and swimmers. If you're a triathlete and can afford only one test, I'd suggest doing it on the bike, as your nutrition here generally has a greater impact on your race performance than when you are swimming or running, since half of the race is on the bike.

The typical test protocol is simple. It starts you out at a very easy effort and increases the intensity every few minutes until you fatigue and can no longer continue. In order to get good data, you need to treat the test like a race by resting for a couple of days before. Doing this test with accumulated fatigue from several days of hard training will muddle the results and what you learn from them.

There will be several pieces of information resulting from such a test. One is the all-important RER. As the intensity of the test increases, you will gradually burn more carbohydrate (stored as glycogen) for fuel. The RER closely estimates how much of the energy came from carbs and

TABLE 6.1

Carbohydrate and Fat Utilization as a Percentage of Total Calories Relative to Respiratory Equivalency Ratio (RER)

RER	CARB %	FAT %
0.71	0.0	100.0
0.71	1.1	98.9
0.72	4.8	95.2
0.73	8.4	91.6
0.74	12.0	88.0
0.75	15.6	84.4
0.76	19.2	80.8
0.77	22.8	77.2
0.78	26.3	73.7
0.79	29.9	70.1
0.80	33.4	66.6
0.81	36.9	63.1
0.82	40.3	59.7
0.83	43.8	56.2
0.84	47.2	52.8
0.85	50.7	49.3
0.86	54.1	45.9
0.87	57.5	42.5
0.88	60.8	39.2
0.89	64.2	35.8
0.90	67.5	32.5
0.91	70.8	29.2
0.92	74.1	25.9
0.93	77.4	22.6
0.94	80.7	19.3
0.95	84.0	16.0
0.96	87.2	12.8
0.97	90.4	9.6
0.98	93.6	6.4
0.99	96.8	3.2
1.00	100.0	0.0

how much from fat. Table 6.1 may be used to determine your percent of energy burned from these two nutrients throughout the test.

The fat burner will start the test with an RER of around 0.80, meaning that he or she is already using about 33 percent carbohydrate and 67 percent fat for fuel (see Table 6.1). That's good. An otherwise similarly fit sugar burner, in terms of aerobic capacity, may start the test at the same low intensity but with an RER of perhaps 0.90 or higher. At this RER he or she is burning 67 percent carbs and 33 percent fat. That's not so good. When they reach their anaerobic thresholds, both the fat burner and sugar burner will be at about 1.00 RER, which means 100 percent carbohydrate and zero percent fat. (Fatigue will typically end the test at an RER of about 1.1 to 1.2 for both.)

Notice that the sugar burner has a much narrower RER range (0.90–1.00) than has the fat burner (0.80–1.00). So at moderate intensities, as are common in long-distance events, the sugar burner needs to be very aware of carbohydrate intake as he or she risks running low on this precious fuel. If that happens, the athlete bonks. Some athletes are such gigantic sugar burners that they find it difficult to take in enough carbohydrate during the competition. They must go slow to lower their use of stored glycogen. They're using sugar faster than their stomachs can process it from sports drinks. That often means a gut "shutdown" and nausea.

If you discover from a test that you are a sugar burner, you may be able to modify this condition somewhat. I say "may" because there is some research indicating that there is an element of genetics involved. This probably has to do at least in part with your muscle makeup, especially your percentage of slow-twitch or "endurance" muscles. This factor, for the most part, is an inherited trait over which you have no control. But there is also no way of knowing if your high RER is genetic or the result of something else, such as how you train.

Doing workouts that focus heavily on anaerobic effort trains the body to preferentially use sugar for fuel. Long-duration, low- to moderate-intensity aerobic workouts promote fat burning. As you become more aerobically fit, your RER will drop, and, related to that, research has shown that as training volume increases, RER is also reduced.

The other chief determinant of RER is your usual diet. Simply put, the more high glycemic load carbohydrate foods you eat (starches are the most prevalent in this category), the more your body will rely on sugar during exercise. Conversely, the more fat and protein in your diet, the lower your RER will be. Eating starch or taking in glucose in a sports drink before the start of the metabolic test, workout, or the race may also slightly shift your RER to the sugar-burning side. (This is why we recommended in Chapter 2 not consuming anything other than water in the last 2 hours prior to starting exercise, with the exception of the last 10 minutes prior to exercise.)

It is even possible to determine how much carb you need to take in during a race from an RER test. All you need to do is find your goal race intensity—heart rate, power, or pace—for your event in the test's raw data results and determine, also from the results, how many calories you were burning at that point. Then check RER at that same intensity (see Table 6.1 on page 108) to see what percentage of those calories came from sugar. You will need to replace much of this expended, carb-based energy during long events (see Chapter 3 for details). The test technician can help you figure this out.

Knowing your RER and, more important, keeping it on the low side through diet and training have the potential to improve your performance in long-distance endurance events.

Lowering your RER so that you are more economical is a good starting point for using food to improve your fitness. But there is much more to be gained from what you eat and when you eat it. As discussed in Chapters 2, 3, and 4, this is something that changes throughout the day. But there are also dietary shifts going on throughout the season that have a strong influence on fitness and race performance.

PERIODIZATION OF DIET

In working with athletes from novices to elites, we have found that varying the Stage V diet along with training volume and intensity produces the best performances. By varying the macronutrient intake, it is possible to enhance the benefits sought in different types of training at certain points in the season. For example, if a purpose of the base (general preparation) period is to train the athlete's body to preferentially use fat for fuel, thus sparing carbohydrate, and we know that eating a diet higher in fat and lower in carbohydrate also promotes such a metabolic shift, then it seems reasonable to have the athlete eat more fat and less carbohydrate at this time in the season. We have used this strategy with athletes and observed changes in RER as described above indicating that glycogen, the muscles' storage form of carbohydrate, was being spared, compared with pretests in which carbohydrate was relatively high and fat low in the diet. There is a growing body of research in this area that supports the notion that aerobic training, along with a greater intake of fat, produces increased benefits in the form of glycogen sparing.

In the same way, when the intensity of training increases to become more racelike while volume stabilizes or perhaps decreases slightly in the build (specific preparation) period, the athlete uses more carbohydrate for fuel. During this period, which occurs about 6 to 12 weeks before priority A races, it is wise to increase the carbohydrate content of the diet slightly, while decreasing fat intake. This means being particularly focused on carb intake in Stages III and IV following workouts and eating plenty of fruits and vegetables in Stage V. Protein stays stable relative to the total training workload throughout the season.

Before going into more detail on this subject, it is important that we explain some basic tenets of periodization. Periodization is a system in which the athlete's training program is modified over time so that a high level of fitness is typically achieved two or three times in a season. This system of training, largely developed by Eastern bloc countries in the 1960s, has been prevalent in Western countries since the 1970s and is widely employed by serious athletes around the world. In periodization, the season is divided into periods that may be 1 to 12 weeks in duration; each has a purpose and a unique method of training associated with it.

In the classic periodization model, the training year begins with general preparation made up of the "preparation" and "base" periods. The purpose of training for endurance athletes at this time is to produce gains in the areas of general aerobic endurance, muscular strength, and sport skills. The training at this time in the season is not specific to the intensity and duration demands of the targeted event, but rather general in nature.

Following this is specific preparation for competition during the "build" and "peak" periods when training becomes increasingly specific to the demands of the coming event. This is usually marked by a shift in emphasis from general endurance to higher-intensity training, although this is determined by the targeted race's characteristics. For example, for very long events, workout intensity is relatively low, and moderate-intensity endurance training continues much as in general preparation—although there may be race-specific training adjustments made relative to terrain, weather conditions, and equipment used. In the 1- to 2-week peak period just prior to the competition, it is common for the athlete to significantly reduce the training volume while completing a "dress rehearsal" workout every 2 or 3 days. During these periods, the gains made in the general preparation period are maintained, with reduced frequency of training for endurance, strength, and skills.

Next comes the competition or "race" period. This is what you've trained for. It's when the all-important priority A races are scheduled. For most athletes, the race period is best kept quite short—no more than 1 week. A few athletes—most likely elites, who have greater capacity when it comes to devoting themselves to extensive training and limited recovery—may be able to hold a peak of fitness for a few weeks. Attempting to maintain a peak level for too long will result in a gradual erosion of fitness due to the emphasis on rest.

The race period is followed by the "transition" period, when physical and mental rejuvenation is the goal. This may last from a few days at midseason to a few weeks at the end of the race season.

Just as the duration, frequency, and intensity of training are adjusted throughout the season, so must the types of foods and when they are eaten, as well the amount of calories consumed. Table 6.2 summarizes these objectives and unique nutritional requirements. When the workload is the greatest, in the base and build periods, the volume of food eaten and subsequent calories consumed are also at the highest levels for the year. With these as the standard, or 100 percent level, the other periods will require fewer calories since the recovery demands are not as great. As previously explained, there should be a shift between carbohydrate

TABLE 6.2

The Parallel Purposes of Training and Nutrition While Following a Classic Periodization Model

PERIOD	DURATION	WORKLOAD	EXERCISE EMPHASIS	NUTRITION EMPHASIS
Preparation (general preparation)	2 6 weeks	Moderate	General aerobic, cross-training, general strength training	Fat increased, carbohydrate decreased, protein stable, calories low
Base (general preparation)	8–12 weeks	Increasingly high	Increasing volume, moderate intensity, usually aerobic, skills emphasis, specific strength training	Fat increased, carbohydrate decreased, protein stable, calories increasing to match workload
Build (specific preparation)	6–8 weeks	High	Reduced volume, race-like intensity, base fitness maintained	Fat decreased, carbohydrate increased, protein stable, calories stable
Peak (specific preparation)	1–2 weeks	Moderate and decreasing	Tapering volume, race simulation every 2–3 days, base fitness maintained	Fat, carbohydrate, and protein stable, calories decreased
Race (competition)	1 week	Low	Increasingly reduced volume, maintenance of race-like intensity, rest, mental preparation	Fat, carbohydrate, and protein proportions maintained as calorie consumption is reduced in parallel with training reduction
Transition	3 days– 4 weeks	Very low	Mental and physical rejuvenation, general aerobic	Fat increased, carbohydrate decreased, protein stable

TABLE 6.3

An Example of Caloric Breakdown by Training Period

TRAINING PERIOD	CALORIES (% of Peak Intake)	CARBOHYDRATE CALORIES (%)*	PROTEIN CALORIES (%)	FAT CALORIES (%)
Preparation	90	40–50	20–25	30–40
Base	100	40–50	20–25	30–40
Build	100	50–60	20–25	20–30
Peak	90	50–60	20–25	20–30
Race	80	50–60	20–25	20–30
Transition	80	30–50	20–25	30–50

* Carbohydrate calories are consumed primarily in Stages I, II, III, and IV.

and fat according to the demands of the training sessions and races. Protein remains about the same throughout the year. Table 6.3 demonstrates these caloric and macronutrient adjustments.

Now that we've laid out the general outline for eating relative to exercise throughout the season, let's see what the menu might look like for a day in the life of a serious athlete. Table 6.4 provides a breakdown of calories by source and recovery stage. Table 6.5 provides further detail on the athlete's food choices on this same day.

TABLE 6.4

An Example of Daily Caloric Breakdown During the Build Period for a 150-Pound Athlete Doing a 2-Hour Workout While in a 15-Hour Training Week

RECOVERY STAGE	CARBOHYDRATE CALORIES	PROTEIN CALORIES	FAT CALORIES	TOTAL CALORIES
Stage I	200	0	0	200
Stage II	300	0	0	300
Stage III	432	108	0	540
Stage IV	200	180	13	393
Stage V	539	311	550	1,400
Totals for day	1,671	599	563	2,833
% of total calories	59	21	20	100

TABLE 6.5

Food Choices Relative to Exercise for a Day in the Build Period for a 150-Pound Athlete

TIME	ROUTINE	FOOD CHOICES	TOTAL CALORIES
Stage I			
4:45–5:15 a.m.	Arise, stretch, preworkout snack (10 minutes prior)	2 gel packets	200
		12 oz water	0
Stage II			
5:15–7:15 a.m.	2-hour workout	12 oz sports drink	300
Stage III			
7:15–7:45 a.m.	Stretch, recover	Recovery drink	540
Stage IV			
7:45–9:00 a.m.	Shower, dress, breakfast, commute	6 oz turkey breast	187
		1 apple	100
		6 oz grape juice	100
		1 cup coffee	6
Stage V			
9:00–11:30 a.m.	Work, snack	2 oz dried fruit with nuts	300
11:30–12:30 p.m.	Lunch	4 oz cod	111
		1 cup fruit salad	170
		2 carrots	62
12:30–5:30 p.m.	Work, snack	1 banana	100
5:30–9:00 p.m.	Family time, supper, bedtime snack	4 oz salmon	200
		1 cup broccoli	30
		Small spinach salad w/ dressing	200
		8 oz herbal tea	2
		2 oz dried fruit with nuts	300
		3½ oz wine	75
Total calories			**2,833**

As can be seen from the examples in these tables, our hypothetical athlete focuses on appropriate recovery foods throughout the day. Before, during, and in the 30 minutes immediately following exercise

(Stages I, II, and III), his food choices are intended to replace carbohydrate used in exercise and provide protein to prevent loss of muscle. In Stages IV and V he concentrates on eating foods that encourage a lower RER and shift blood pH levels toward greater alkalinity to preserve bone and muscle tissue. He also includes foods such as nuts and fish that are rich in omega-3 oils to reduce the risk of inflammation and protein for continuing muscle recovery.

BODY WEIGHT AND PERFORMANCE

Endurance athletes intuitively understand that their body weight has an impact on performance. Some find it necessary to shed excess weight, especially fat, in order to perform at a higher level. Here we will examine the known effects of weight and how the Paleo Diet can help in managing yours.

The Effects of Gravity and Heat

Nearly all endurance sports are affected by gravity. Any time there is vertical movement the combined weight of your body and equipment detracts from performance. Going up a hill while Nordic skiing or on a bike requires overcoming the force of gravity. The lighter you and your equipment are, the faster you will climb it. It's the same for running uphill. But running has the added burden of dealing with gravity even when the course is flat due to the small vertical oscillation associated with running technique.

The sports in which gravity has little effect are swimming and any activity involving strictly horizontal movement on flat terrain, such as riding a bike, ice skating, or Nordic skiing.

When riding a bike uphill, every extra pound "costs" about 1.5 watts of power whether due to a heavy bike or excess body weight. An extra pound slows a runner by about 2 seconds per mile. Even a few ounces can be significant in a closely contested race. That's why companies that make running shoes, bicycle equipment, skis, and other sports gear are always seeking to reduce product weight. It's also a good reason for endurance athletes to maintain their body weights at a low yet healthy level.

There's another downside to carrying excess body weight. The more weight you carry, the more likely you are to be affected by heat and humidity. The bigger the athlete, the more of a problem heat is. A few years ago Frank Marino and associates at Charles Sturt University in Australia had men of different sizes run 8-mile time trials on a treadmill on three separate occasions. The only thing that changed on the three runs was the room temperature, which was either cool (59°F), moderate (77°F), or hot (95°F). In the hottest condition the bigger athletes slowed down by about 12 percent compared with their pace in the coolest temperature. The smaller runners experienced very little change and far outperformed the bigger ones on the hottest run. Their times were about the same on the cooler runs. Why is this? More heat is produced by larger athletes and they have a harder time dissipating it, so more is stored. This factor has the potential to cause overheating and a slower performance.

Reducing excess body weight has the potential to pay off with better race performances. But there's risk associated with such weight reductions. If you lose muscle, especially the muscles that are used to propel you, you are likely to perform slower. And if too much fat is lost, your health may well be compromised. The trick here is to avoid becoming too lean while also maintaining an effective amount of muscle. The Paleo Diet, especially in Stage V of your training day (see Chapter 4), is an excellent way to accomplish these body composition changes.

Weight Management

In the final analysis, decreased body fat is the result of both exercise and a targeted eating program. But, of the two, the more effective way to lose body fat is by changing your diet. Training more hours every week without replacing all of the expended calories has a positive result when you step on the scales, but the changes will be quite small. On the other hand, changes in your diet are likely to produce much greater losses of excess weight. When a slight increase in exercise workload and dietary change occur simultaneously, the benefits are multiplied.

Realize, however, that you don't necessarily have to change anything about your training. You may be at a high workload now and so adding more is likely to be counterproductive due to increased fatigue and reduced workout quality. You may not even need to reduce your caloric intake. Many athletes experience a change in body weight by merely adopting a Paleo diet. Others find that they need to also reduce the amount of calories eaten daily, usually by a small amount, to see a positive change in weight.

When first adopting the Paleo Diet, wait a couple of weeks to see how your body responds. If you start with a complete reversal of your old diet to Paleo, you may well find you are frequently tired and don't recover as quickly following hard training sessions. This is a sign that your body is going through some changes. Be patient, as it takes a couple of weeks to adapt. If making the change during the last few days prior to your race, it's best to make rather small dietary adjustments to Paleo over several weeks instead of going "cold turkey." In this case your weight may not change at all until after your race season ends. That's all right, as weight loss and final race preparation are not generally a good combination. This is why we recommend making such a change early in the base (general preparation) period.

When immediately switching from a high-carb to a Paleo diet, there may be a rather rapid loss of weight, especially if you are in the base period of the season, when the emphasis is on dietary fat with a reduced carbohydrate intake. The rather rapid drop in weight at this time is primarily due to the loss of water, which is stored along with glycogen. Your body may give up some its glycogen stores along with its stored water in the first few days after the dietary change. As your body adjusts to the change, your glycogen stores will be replenished and water weight will return to normal. You can rest assured that subsequent reductions in weight will predominantly be the result of excess fat losses.

When you are trying to lose weight, energy intake must be adequate to meet the demands of training in order to continue producing positive changes in fitness. The greatest concern must especially be shown for the volume and timing of carbohydrate and protein. Glycogen stores must be maintained and adequate protein provided for the repair of exercise-damaged tissues. The body also needs a balance of omega-3 and omega-6 fatty acids, the "essential fatty acids," for long-term health, which is an important component of the Paleo Diet. Each of these demands is met by following the guidelines for eating relative to exercise as described in Chapters 2, 3, and 4.

Eating a higher-fat and higher-protein diet than you may normally eat probably raises two key questions: Will I gain weight? Will I train and race as well? Let's address these issues.

Will I gain weight? There have been several studies showing that eating a diet rich in both fat and protein produces about the same or increased weight loss over time as eating a conventional diet.

One such study conducted by Brown and associates at the University of Otago, in Dunedin, New Zealand, fed 30 cyclists either a diet of high fat (50 percent) or high carb (69 percent) for 12 weeks. They were training between 6 and 25 hours per week. The cyclists did not gain weight when eating mostly fat. (An interesting side note to this study is that the subjects increased their bone density on the high-fat diet.)

The bulk of such studies typically show the same thing: The key element in weight loss is calorie restriction and expenditure through exercise, not the type of food eaten. So, no, you won't gain weight eating a Paleo diet in Stage V every day unless you eat excessive calories or exercise less than you did before the dietary change.

In fact, many athletes report a decrease in weight when they switch over to Paleo even without changing their caloric intakes or training routines. This probably has to do, at least in part, with the insulin response common to high-carb diets. Eating high glycemic load foods such as starches in Stage V releases insulin into the bloodstream, which in turn causes the body to store calories as fat. This phenomenon is much less likely to happen during and immediately after exercise (Stages II and III), when the body's demand for carbohydrate in the form of glycogen is high to fuel exercise and restock expended glycogen stores. But by the time this exercise-related demand for glycogen is reduced in Stage V, sugar spikes in the blood will result in the release of insulin and the conversion of the carbohydrate to stored body fat. This factor is why the timing of your food intake relative to exercise is so important.

Another reason following a Paleo diet in Stage V may produce a loss of excess body weight without your focusing upon calories has to do with satiety. People are simply not as hungry when they eat "real" foods such as fruits, vegetables, and animal protein instead of highly processed foods made with starch, sugar, and salt. Putting away a dozen cookies is easy for most people. But how about a dozen carrots? A turkey breast is very filling, so you stop eating when satisfied. Can the same be said for pizza? Real foods are high in fiber and protein. These nutritional elements have been shown in numerous research studies to be hunger satisfying. The same can't be said of highly processed foods. You'll simply eat less without the psychological stress of "dieting" when you focus your Stage V diet on real food.

Will I train and race as well? You may experience a drop in performance, especially in your rate of recovery, in the first 2 or 3 weeks after making a sudden change in your diet. This change is normal. You need to hang in there beyond this initial period to experience a positive adaptation. If you do that, then your training will return to normal and may even exceed your prior levels. Here's an example of that.

A study conducted at the University of Copenhagen, as reported in *Medicine and Science in Sports and Exercise,* had 15 men eat either a high-fat or high-carbohydrate diet for 4 weeks. At the end of each 4-week period they were tested with a run to exhaustion on a treadmill at 80 percent of max VO_2. The research team found that there was no difference in total time until they had to stop. Additionally, the improvements in max VO_2 were the same. The only significant difference was that the subjects' RERs were lower on the high-fat diet, which is a good thing. That means their bodies were conserving glycogen and using greater amounts of fat for fuel. This study is like many others showing similar results.

The downside of most dietary changes intended to reduce body weight is the loss of muscle mass along with fat loss. Several studies have shown that reducing daily calories while eating a conventional, high-carb diet results in a significant loss of muscle. While there is no research using athletes who lost weight, most studies with nonathletic populations have shown that weight reduction on a high-protein diet, similar to Paleo, results in little or no loss of muscle compared with a conventional diet. This positive change probably has to do with the abundance of branched-chain amino acids in the Paleo Diet.

As discussed in Chapter 4, how much protein you eat on a daily basis depends on your training load. The more hours you work out weekly, the more protein is needed in your diet. If weight loss is an objective and you find it necessary to cut back on calories, be sure to keep your protein intake, especially from animal sources, at the recommended level.

CHAPTER 7

OVERTRAINING AND DIET

Recovery is one of the keys to high performance in sports but is little appreciated by most athletes. The commonly accepted road to success is hard workouts, and the more the better. That isn't entirely wrong, but without paying close attention to the recovery side of the training equation, hard workouts spaced closely together are not possible. If you recover quickly and more completely following hard training sessions, then your body is ready to go hard again sooner. That leads ultimately to peak performances.

As a highly motivated athlete who pays only lip service to recovery, you may experience a deep and compelling fatigue following a few weeks of high-workload training. You wake up in the morning tired. You are unable to complete even the easiest workouts. Fatigue haunts your every step throughout the day. And this goes on relentlessly for days or even weeks. You're overtrained.

How could this situation have been avoided? The answer is recovery. Recovery has several components, the two most critical being rest and nutrition. What you eat plays as great a role in your day-to-day performance as anything else in your training arsenal does, yet many athletes get it wrong. Let's take a closer look at overtraining and how food choices impact your capacity for quick recovery.

BEYOND FATIGUE

Effective training is more than workouts. It is a carefully balanced state of well-being between stress and rest. When this balance is achieved, your fitness improves at a steady rate. When rest exceeds stress (a rare occasion for serious athletes), the body quickly achieves a high level of readiness to race. This takes only a few days and is referred to as tapering or peaking. The result is what athletes call "form"—a readiness to race at a high level of performance due to the elimination of fatigue. Go beyond these few days of reduced training stress and fitness quickly erodes. You may have experienced the latter situation if you were injured or sick and couldn't work out.

When stress only just exceeds rest for a few days, the body adapts and becomes more fit. This is the purpose of training: Overload the body with the right amount of stress, then allow it to rest. During rest, the body's adaptive processes take place—muscles grow stronger, enzymes become more abundant, the heart increases its ability to pump blood, and other seminal physiological and psychological changes occur. This is the ultimate goal of the endurance athlete.

On a more sinister note, when stress greatly exceeds rest for more than a few days, the athlete begins to experience unrelenting fatigue and exhaustion. The body's capacity to adapt is compromised, and the defense mechanisms intended to prevent death are initiated. This is overtraining.

Overtraining may not result simply from too much exercise and too little rest. The stress component could also be related to work, school, relationships, finances, relocating, or a myriad of other stressors that make up your nonathletic life. Such stress when combined with what may otherwise be a perfectly appropriate level of exercise will produce overtraining if rest is inadequate, just as surely as too much exercise produces overtraining. In this case, you are "overliving" rather than overtraining. Regardless, the body experiences much the same negative consequences.

All of this is not to say that you shouldn't push yourself in training or that you should never experience fatigue. In order to grow as an athlete,

(continued on page 126)

WHAT IS FATIGUE?

Fatigue is a primary limiter standing between you and better performance. If you could delay or resist the sensations of fatigue, you would go faster and last longer at a given effort level—the ultimate purpose of training. Yet we never rid ourselves of fatigue, which is actually a good thing because this prevents us from damaging our bodies or perhaps needlessly expending physiological resources. But understanding what brings on fatigue during a race or workout may point to strategies that could raise your fatigue threshold, allowing you to go faster or farther.

Fatigue seems to vary according to the duration and intensity of exercise. An 800-meter runner and a marathon runner may both fatigue greatly during their races, slow down, and struggle to the finish lines, but their specific reasons for fatigue aren't the same. Or are they? What causes their fatigue? Currently there are three ways of explaining fatigue.

Catastrophe theory. This is the oldest model, having been around since the 1920s. It's the one accepted by most exercise physiologists. This model proposes that exercise stops when something catastrophic occurs in the body, especially in the working muscles.

Other than overheating and severe dehydration, which can obviously limit performance, the catastrophe model proposes that there are at least two common physiological reasons for fatigue during endurance events: the accumulation of metabolic by-products such as hydrogen ions, especially from lactic acid release (the 800-meter runner); and the depletion of energy stores such as glycogen and glucose (the marathoner). The catastrophe model proposes that when either of these situations occurs, the body is forced to slow down. It's much like a car running out of gas or the fuel lines becoming clogged. A catastrophe has just happened and the body stops functioning normally.

Central Governor theory. The second way of explaining fatigue originated in the physiology lab at the University of Cape Town in South Africa in the 1990s. Here, noted exercise physiologist Tim Noakes, PhD, proposed that fatigue occurs in the brain, not in the muscles.

In this model the body is constantly sending signals to the subconscious brain regarding the current status of the working muscles. For example, fuel levels and metabolic by-product buildup are being monitored by the brain. This is a bit like the operation of the thermostat in your home, which gauges the temperature and turns the heating or air-conditioning system on or off as needed. At some point the brain may make a decision, again subconsciously and the result of perceived exertion, to slow down due to the current status of the body. It's proposed that this central governor for fatigue evolved to protect the body from damage caused by excessively hard work.

Psychobiological theory. This theory is a bit like the central governor model, but with a twist. Samuele Marcora, PhD, at the University of Wisconsin proposed in the early 2000s that it is indeed perceived exertion, a subconscious calculation made by the brain during exercise, that limits performance. He proposed that exercise stops well before fuel levels and metabolic by-product accumulation suggest it is absolutely necessary.

In a part of the forebrain known as the anterior cingulate cortex (ACC), subconscious decisions are made regarding conflict resolution and response inhibition. Essentially, this means that during exercise the ACC is weighing the cost of continuing at a given intensity versus the reward for doing so. Dr. Marcora has shown that "fatigued" athletes are able to overcome the sensation at what appears to be the end of exercise to failure and produce a greater output if the reward is big enough.

You have probably experienced this at the end of a race. You may have been slowing down, but when you saw the finish line, you had the capacity to somehow speed up or even sprint. You were willing to overcome the suffering because the reward, an awe-inspiring finish or perhaps a slightly faster time or higher finishing place, was great enough to overcome the suffering you were feeling. He further suggests that this system evolved to keep us from needlessly wasting energy in the pursuit of food when the prospect of success in finding it was low. But should food appear (perhaps a deer on the horizon), increasing the likelihood of getting it, then the suffering becomes tolerable.

you must regularly flirt with overtraining. You will have days when you are tired and even some when you can't (or at least know you shouldn't) complete the workout. This state of fatigue is called "overreaching" and is an early point on the path to both greater fitness and, if allowed to continue for too long, overtraining. Some amount of overreaching is necessary for the serious athlete. The difference between overreaching and overtraining is that when you are overreached, you quickly recover with a day or two of rest. By paying close attention to the elements of recovery, especially sleep and nutrition, you can avoid overtraining and steadily improve your fitness.

How long does it take to progress from being overreached to overtrained? The answer, as with most such questions, starts with "It depends." Many variables may influence the answer. Studies that have dramatically increased the training volume for 5, 7, and 10 days were unable to produce a significant decline in performance, although the athletes showed signs of overreaching. In other research, it took 15 days to produce verifiable overtraining in a group of cyclists who increased their volume by 50 percent. And in one study with young, highly fit rowers, it took 3 weeks to fully achieve overtraining. It may well be that youth and a high level of fitness provide some immunity from overtraining and may delay its onset for up to 3 weeks. On the flip side, older or less fit athletes, including novices, may well achieve an overtrained state in 2 weeks or even less if the stress of overreaching is great enough.

IF IT ISN'T OVERTRAINING, WHAT IS IT?

Some common signs of overtraining in endurance athletes are listed in Table 7.1. Note that not all of these signs will be present if you allow yourself to become overtrained, and some symptoms that you experience may not even be listed. Overtraining is a condition that is unique to individual circumstances, although certain characteristics are common, such as decreased performance and chronic fatigue.

It's also quite possible that some of these symptoms, including decreased performance and chronic fatigue, signal an illness such as chronic fatigue syndrome, Lyme disease, mononucleosis, or another viral infection. Even if you're certain your symptoms are caused by overtraining, it's wise to consult your physician just to be sure you don't have some other health condition.

OVERTRAINING AND DIET

Overreaching that spirals downward to overtraining often starts, in part, with diet. You train hard to achieve very high performance goals. Knowing that several hard workouts are needed weekly for success, you repeatedly push yourself to the limit. The vigorous exercise may result in a decreased appetite for hours afterward. Or you restrict calories in an

TABLE 7.1

Common Symptoms of Overtraining

Physiological

Decreased performance

Decreased strength

Decreased maximum work capacity

Changes in heart rate at rest, exercise, and recovery (high or low)

Increased frequency of breathing

Insomnia

Loss of appetite

Increased aches and pains

Chronic fatigue

Psychological

Depression

Apathy

Decreased self-esteem

Emotional instability

Difficulty concentrating

Irritability

Immunological

Susceptibility to illness

Slow healing of minor scratches

Swollen lymph nodes

Biochemical

Negative nitrogen balance

Flat glucose tolerance curves

Reduced muscle glycogen concentration

Delayed menarche

Decreased hemoglobin

Decreased serum iron

Lowered total iron-binding capacity

Mineral depletion

Elevated cortisol levels

Low free testosterone

attempt to achieve a predetermined racing weight. Combined with incomplete recovery, the reduced caloric intake leads to greater fatigue and lackluster training. Being highly motivated, you continue this pattern of hard workouts, limited food, and inadequate recovery for 2 to 3 weeks—and you're overtrained. One consequence of the early stages of overtraining is even less appetite, which further exacerbates the all-too-common state of the overtraining syndrome you've managed to create.

This lesson is driven home quite effectively in a study conducted by David Costill, PhD, and his colleagues at Ball State University. The researchers doubled the training workload of a group of competitive collegiate swimmers for 10 days. After a few days, about 30 percent of the swimmers experienced much greater difficulty in maintaining the quality of the training sessions than did the others. The scientists found that the swimmers who were merely muddling through with the high workload were eating almost 1,000 calories per day less than those who were successfully coping. The low-calorie swimmers were well along the path to excessive overreaching in a matter of days. Had the study continued longer, there is little doubt that those taking in the fewest calories would eventually have wound up overtrained.

Besides intense exercise, other training factors that may contribute to a reduced appetite are high temperatures and humidity. Emotions related to stress and mood may also produce this effect, as may acute exposure to training at high altitude. Don't ignore a poor appetite when, following exercise, you experience fatigue that is not reduced after a day or more of complete rest or much lighter workouts. Be cautious with your training at this time, and carefully monitor your food intake to ensure that you are getting adequate calories and nutrients.

MACRONUTRIENTS AND OVERTRAINING

While many studies implicate nutrition in the process of becoming overtrained, none specifically addresses the dietary requirements of avoiding this condition. However, some research does suggest likely dietary scenarios associated with overtraining.

Carbohydrate

Depending on body size, a well-trained and properly fed endurance athlete may have up to about 2,000 calories stored away as carbohydrate. Most of this resides in the muscles as glycogen, with smaller amounts in the liver (glycogen) and blood (glucose). Compared with the potential energy available from fat and protein, glycogen and glucose are quite limited, representing only 1 to 2 percent of the body's total energy stores. Nevertheless, this fuel source is critical to success in endurance activities. As previously mentioned, there is an old saying in exercise physiology that illustrates this phenomenon: "Fat burns in a carbohydrate flame." As stored carbohydrate is depleted, the body can no longer efficiently use fat, the body's most abundant fuel, for energy; it must turn to protein to keep the fat-burning flame flickering. This is a time-consuming metabolic process associated with heavy fatigue and rapidly decreasing pace despite a high effort. Failure to maintain glycogen and glucose stores can easily lead to poor performance and perhaps to overtraining.

During intensive endurance exercise, the body shifts from primarily using glycogen to keep the flame burning to relying on blood glucose and, finally, on liver stores of glycogen as fuel slowly depletes. This process of shifting the energy source may take 60 to 90 minutes, depending on your fitness level and exercise intensity. The most common form of exhaustion in extensive endurance sports is closely related to this depletion of carbohydrate fuel. Carbohydrate intake both during and immediately following exercise is critical to success in endurance sports.

There is considerable research showing that consistently low carbohydrate intake during and following exercise may contribute to overreaching and eventually to overtraining. As the training intensity increases, this becomes even more critical. High glycemic load foods are a necessity in Stages II, III, and IV of recovery, as described in Chapters 3 and 4, in order to maintain glycogen and glucose stores and help prevent overtraining. Just a few days of inadequate eating at these critical times, when training intensity increases, can easily set you up for a disastrous season.

While most athletes have no difficulty eating carbohydrate, especially from starchy sources, a few overly zealous recent adherents to the Paleo Diet do. It is not unusual for those new to the Paleo concept to overdo it and omit all starches and sugars from their diets including during Stages II, III, and IV. For the athlete exercising less than about an hour a day this is unlikely to result in overtraining. In fact, at this level of training volume there is little need for sugar and starch. A 24-hour adherence to the Paleo Diet as suggested for Stage V will work just fine. As the volume of training increases, however, the need for carbohydrate to replenish fuel stores also increases. For the athlete training 3 or more hours per day including intensities approaching and exceeding the anaerobic threshold, consuming adequate carbohydrate, especially from starchy sources, is critical to avoiding overtraining.

Fat

If carbohydrate is so important for avoiding overtraining, you might wonder why the Paleo Diet for Athletes suggests eating more fat and less carbohydrate during the base (general preparation) period of training— might not this set you up for overtraining? No, it won't. Plenty of research indicates that well-trained endurance athletes actually continue to have good results on a diet that is somewhat higher in fat and lower in carbohydrate than is typically recommended by nutritionists, especially when intensity is low, as in the base period.

A classic study reported in the prestigious journal *Medicine and Science in Sports and Exercise* used well-trained runners as subjects. The runners spent 7 days eating each of three diets, then tested at the end of each 7-day period for running time to exhaustion at a fixed intensity just below anaerobic threshold. On their "normal" diet, they ate 61 percent of their daily calories as carbohydrate and 24 percent as fat. Their "fat" diet was made up of 50 percent carbohydrate and 38 percent fat—similar to the diet recommended here for your base period. The runners' "carbohydrate" diet included 73 percent carbohydrate and 15 percent fat. Protein stayed about the same (12 to 14 percent) in all three trials. The testing revealed that the fat diet produced the best average times to exhaustion (91.2 minutes), compared with the carbohydrate (75.8 minutes) and normal (63.7 minutes) diets.

In another, more recent study, 11 duathletes ate high-fat (53 percent fat) or high-carbohydrate (17 percent fat) diets for 5 weeks each. At the end of these periods, they completed a 20-minute time trial on a bicycle ergometer and ran a half marathon. There were no significant differences in performance between the two sets of test data, regardless of the diet. On the bikes there was a 1-watt difference, and for the run there was a 12-second difference in finishing times.

The take-home lesson from these studies and others is that substituting fat for carbohydrate in the base (general preparation) period will not harm your training or promote overtraining, so long as you use the post-workout recovery methods in Chapter 4 to replenish carbohydrate stores. In fact, a higher-fat diet proves to be beneficial because the body becomes more efficient at burning fat for fuel while sparing glycogen, one of the same benefits we seek in doing long, low-intensity endurance training in the base period. But as the intensity of training rises in the build (specific preparation) period, more carbohydrate is necessary to restock the significantly depleted glycogen stores in the muscles. Shifting your diet between carbohydrate and fat in the base and build periods of the season, with protein remaining relatively constant, will not contribute to overtraining and will boost your fitness.

Of course, as described in Chapter 4, the fat you add to the diet in Stage V of your daily recovery during the base period should be largely monounsaturated and polyunsaturated, especially omega-3. These fats are found in foods such as fish, avocados, nuts, eggs enriched with omega-3, leafy green vegetables, meat from free-ranging animals, and in olive and flaxseed oils.

Protein

Recovery following challenging workouts is essential for avoiding over-training. If nutritional action is not taken after a hard training session, the body may not be ready to go by the next workout, leading to a grad-ual decline in performance over the course of a few days, followed by overreaching and, ultimately, overtraining. More and more research sug-gests that, as with consuming carbohydrate immediately after such ses-sions, taking in protein improves the recovery process. This enhancement is a result of greater glycogen stores that restock faster, along with quicker rebuilding of damaged muscle tissue. Including protein in your Stage III and IV nutrition, as described in Chapter 4, will go a long way in promoting recovery while helping to avoid overtraining.

In much the same way, taking in adequate protein throughout the day is quite beneficial to your physical well-being and capacity for training. It has been our experience that most endurance athletes eat far too little protein; instead they concentrate their diets around carbohydrate, espe-cially from starches and sugars. Such an amino acid–poor diet will even-tually catch up with these athletes. Protein is necessary to repair muscle damage, maintain the immune system, manufacture hormones and enzymes, replace the red blood cells that carry oxygen to the muscles, and provide energy for exercise when carbohydrate stores are tapped. The following indicators of inadequate dietary protein overlap consider-ably with the markers of overtraining listed in Table 7.1 on page 127.

Frequent colds and sore throats

Slow recovery from workouts

Irritability

Poor response to training (slow to get in shape)

Chronic fatigue

Poor mental focus

Sugar cravings

Cessation of menstrual periods

The highest-quality protein is that which is most available to the body for absorption and includes large amounts of all of the essential amino acids. Animal products fit that definition and should be included in meals throughout the day. And the more you train, the more critical this is for avoiding overtraining.

Of the essential amino acids, four stand out as being critical to recovery: leucine, isoleucine, valine, and glutamine. The first three are the branched-chain amino acids (BCAA). During exercise, blood levels of BCAA and glutamine decline, contributing to a unique type of weariness called central fatigue—common in events lasting several hours. A training program that is challenging will likely leave you feeling chronically fatigued for days and may well be the result of inadequate protein intake.

Water

Inadequate fluid intake during and after exercise may be a nutritional contributor to overtraining. But it's unusual for athletes, or nearly anyone for that matter, to fail to replace body water losses throughout the day when it's readily available.

The key to avoiding the overtraining consequences of dehydration is quite simple: Drink according to your thirst. If thirsty, drink. When no longer thirsty, don't drink. It's pretty simple. There is no reason for elaborate drinking schedules or daily water volume goals. Thirst does indeed work. For example, a study of 14 elite Kenyan runners whose water losses and rehydration were tracked for 5 days supports this notion. No instruction was given on how much to drink. During training they drank nothing and typically lost 2.7 percent of body weight daily. On average they took in 4 quarts (3.8 liters) of fluids daily based entirely on thirst. No changes were reported in daily hydration status, body weights, or responses to training over the course of 5 days.

It's not unusual for athletes to take in excessive amounts of water the day before a race to prevent hydration on race day. There is no reason for this. Your body does not store water like a camel's does. If you drink an excessive amount, meaning more than necessary to quench thirst, you will soon urinate to remove the excess. And by drinking excessively you temporarily dilute electrolyte stores. So there is nothing to be gained by drinking copious amounts of fluids the day before or the morning of a race. Here again, thirst is the key. Pay attention to your body.

How about the oft-repeated stipulation that none of the water you take in can come from caffeinated beverages, as they cause a net loss of body fluid? Research contradicts this oft-repeated belief. Athletes do not appear to lose any more body stores of water following caffeine ingestion in the hours preceding exercise than those who did not use a caffeinated drink. And also be aware that fluid comes not just from drinking but also from the food you eat.

Much of the research seems to support the notion that a yellow urine color is a good indicator of significant dehydration, but not all of the research is in agreement. More research is needed in this area. While having yellow urine may indicate some level of dehydration, such a color by itself is not proof of dehydration. Metabolites, the end products of metabolism such as urea, are often expelled in the urine and provide color even though you are well hydrated. The same goes for B vitamin supplements. They will provide a bright yellow color to your urine. The best indicator of dehydration is thirst. It works. Just pay attention.

MICRONUTRIENTS AND OVERTRAINING

Many studies have reported that athletes make poor dietary choices, contributing to low vitamin and mineral status that is compounded by normal losses during periods of increased training. For example, a study of Dutch elite athletes showed that the female swimmers had an inadequate iron intake, while cyclists were not getting enough vitamins B_1 and B_6. Similar research on women runners has shown repeatedly that due to restriction of calories, extremely high carbohydrate intake, or vegetarian eating patterns, these athletes are often low in iron, zinc, magnesium, and calcium. Among both male and female runners, dietary zinc and iron have been shown to be low. Inadequate iron intake has also been confirmed for a group of cross-country skiers; 50 percent of Nordic women skiers in a Winter Olympics had prelatent iron deficiency, and 7 percent were anemic. In a study of 1,300 German athletes in various sports, 21 percent had low levels of serum magnesium, and 14 percent lacked iron. There is little doubt that many athletes do not meet their nutritional needs when it comes to micronutrients. Such deficiencies may well contribute to the onset of overtraining.

An athlete who is deficient in vitamins A, B_6, C, or E is at high risk for a weakened immune system and illness related to overreaching. In the same manner, deficiencies of the minerals zinc, magnesium, copper, and iron may also result in impaired immunity. All of this once again underscores the importance of eating a diet that is rich in micronutrients once you are into Stage V of recovery. Macronutrients are no longer the issue.

The most micronutrient-dense foods are vegetables and meats, including fish and poultry. However, eating a lot of cereal grains negates the benefits because these foods contain high amounts of phytates, which decrease the body's absorption of minerals such as iron and zinc.

Just as eating an inadequate diet can set you up for overtraining, relying on supplements instead of nutrient-dense foods to provide vitamins and minerals can also be detrimental. For example, excessive amounts of vitamin A, vitamin E, and zinc have been shown to weaken the immune system, thus contributing to overtraining symptoms. An excessive intake of iron promotes bacterial growth and can induce a zinc deficiency. The best way to ensure a balanced diet is to eat plenty of vegetables, fruits, and meats—not to take pills or eat lab-designed food products marketed to athletes. Science has yet to catch up with Mother Nature when it comes to producing nutritious food.

OVERTRAINING PREVENTION AND TREATMENT

There are no preliminary symptoms to warn you when you have gone too far with an imbalance between stress and rest. The progression from a normal and recurring state of overreaching to full-blown overtraining is so gradual that you won't recognize the impending doom. By the time you realize that you've pushed too hard, it's too late, and your only recourse is loss of fitness by greatly reducing or even eliminating the training stress.

If you are overreached, as indicated by an unusually high level of fatigue and suspect overtraining, take 3 to 5 days of complete rest, and then do a short, low-intensity workout. If you feel normal, you were only in an advanced stage of overreaching and are free to gradually return to regular training (but do so cautiously). But if after several exercise-free days the test workout feels like a wearisome burden, you are probably overtrained or are sick and should see your doctor. Take another 3 to 5 days of complete rest before retesting your status as before. Continue this pattern until exercise becomes fun again, which may take weeks or even months. Throughout the process, be sure to eat a nutritious diet made up primarily of fruits, vegetables, and meats, including fish and poultry.

It is far better to prevent overtraining in the first place than to deal with it after the fact, especially when you consider that it can take weeks if not months to recover. So what must you do to avoid it?

At its essence, overtraining results from training mistakes, and two are particularly common. The first is an imbalance between stress and rest, which usually occurs when the athlete suddenly increases the training workload in either volume or intensity—or both. The second scenario involves cutting back on recovery by substituting more challenging workouts for easy ones. Athletes have even been known to do both: suddenly increase the workload and eliminate rest and recovery days. In either situation the increased stress at first will result in improving fitness but also in a lot of fatigue. A few days of such increased stress may actually be beneficial. It's when the pattern continues for several days or weeks, depending on the work capacity of the individual, that it becomes problematic. Given the work ethic, the motivation, and, in some serious endurance athletes, the obsession, such an extended period of high stress probably seems like a sure route to success. It is not; it is a sure route to failure.

The best way to avoid this pitfall is to follow a long-term, periodized training plan that schedules weekly rest and recovery days, monthly rest and recovery weeks, and annual rest and recovery months. This plan should also provide for a gradual progression in the training workload and fit your unique characteristics, including sport experience, age, susceptibility to illness and injury, and goals.

Nutrition often plays a role in the onset of overtraining. Even a suitably aggressive training regimen that leads to an acceptable level of overreaching may be undermined by a diet that does not encourage quick recovery. In our experience, such a diet is usually lacking in total calories, protein, or micronutrients. This is all too common for the serious endurance athlete who concentrates on sugar and starch, eats a vegetarian diet, or is concerned about body weight and so reduces calories despite a high workload. Any one of these scenarios will diminish recovery in what might be an otherwise appropriate training program.

PART III

OUR
STONE AGE
LEGACY

CHAPTER 8

WHY EAT LIKE A CAVEMAN?

MAKING SENSE OUT OF NUTRITIONAL CHAOS

As an athlete, you probably are aware that even small variations in your performance can significantly alter how well you place in any given race. However, you may never have considered how huge this effect can be.

Consider a 1 to 2 percent difference in your time for a 10,000-meter race. At first it sounds fairly insignificant. Whether you run 1 to 2 percent faster or slower in a 10-K race is immaterial, right? Wrong! At the US Outdoor Track and Field Championships in 2011, just 14.96 seconds (a mere 0.87 percent difference) separated the top 10 finishers in the men's 10-K final. Even more telling were the top three finishers' times. The winner, Galen Rupp, beat the second-place finisher, Matt Tegenkamp, by 1.8 seconds—in relative terms, a minuscule 0.10 percent difference in performance. The third-place finisher, Scott Bauhs, was 2.34 seconds behind the winner—only 0.14 percent slower than the winning time. These numbers graphically illustrate how very small differences in performance can have an enormous impact on how well you place. But more important, they emphasize how crucial it is for you to optimize every factor that can possibly influence your race-day performance.

Your basic training foundation (intensity, frequency, and duration of exercise) clearly is of utmost importance in shaping how well you will perform. Over the long haul, how well and how fast you can recover from each and every workout will determine how hard you can train over the course of an entire season. Also, there is little doubt that staying healthy and free from injury and illness are essential in permitting you to train at higher intensities for longer periods, which in turn will benefit your race performance.

Now, let's go back to that crucial 1 to 2 percent difference in performance and have a look at Rupp's top three race times for the 10-K during the 2010–2011 seasons. The slowest of those (27:26.84) is 2.42 percent slower than his top time (26:48.00), whereas his second-best finish (27:10.74) is 1.41 percent slower than the top time, which set the American record for the 10-K. You can see that not only do small performance differences emerge among athletes, but they also appear within individuals. Given similar wind, weather, and altitude conditions, why might your performance vary by 1 to 2 percent? What factors might be responsible for these tiny but important performance differences? How about your muscle glycogen stores—might they be involved? Does the ability of your muscles to overcome fatigue from a previous race or workout play a role? What's the effect of a slight upper respiratory illness or lingering tendinitis? How about your ability to maintain quality workouts between races? Without a doubt, any or all of these issues have the potential to influence your race-day performance by 1 to 2 percent— or even more.

Nutritionists, exercise physiologists, and physicians alike agree that athletic performance can go to hell in a handbasket very rapidly from a faulty diet. However, they have dogmatically argued for decades that a "balanced" diet is all that's needed to maximize athletic performance, provided an optimal training schedule is followed. But what exactly is a "balanced diet"? More precisely, what is the starting point for any athletic diet? Is it the same diet that optimizes your health and well-being? And what is the best diet to optimize immune function and prevent colds and upper respiratory illnesses or to speed recovery from—or even prevent—muscle strains or injuries? All of those questions raise a much larger and all-encompassing question, one that, when answered correctly, provides us with an elegant, grand organizing template that allows us to make sense out of all this nutritional and dietary confusion and chaos.

Nutrition is every bit as contentious as politics and religion. It seems like everybody's got an opinion about proper diet, including health agencies, the government, leading scientists, diet doctors, and popular nutritionists. From the consumer perspective, the study of nutrition appears jumbled and chaotic. One day you hear one thing; the next, the exact opposite. Margarine is good for your health; margarine contains trans fatty acids. Eggs increase your blood cholesterol; eggs don't increase your cholesterol levels. Fiber prevents colon cancer; fiber doesn't prevent colon cancer. Pizza is a healthful food; pizza is junk food.

The USDA MyPlate poster, espousing healthful eating, is found in almost every elementary school and hospital lunchroom in the country. Yet an article in the prestigious *Scientific American* magazine, written by scientists from the Harvard School of Public Health, loudly condemned the MyPlate dietary recommendations. A decade ago, almost 30 million Americans were following Dr. Atkins's advice to eat more fat, butter, and cheese to lose weight. In utter contrast, Dean Ornish, MD, and T. Colin Campbell tell us fat and meat cause cancer, heart disease, and obesity and that we would all be a lot healthier if we were strict vegetarians. Who's right and who's wrong? How in the world can anyone make any sense out of this apparent disarray of conflicting facts, opinions, and ideas?

In mature and well-developed scientific disciplines, universal paradigms guide researchers to fruitful end points as they design their experiments and hypotheses. For instance, in cosmology (the study of the universe), the guiding paradigm is the big bang theory that the universe began with an enormous explosion and has been expanding ever since. In geology, the continental drift model established that all of the current continents at one time formed a continuous landmass that eventually drifted apart to form the present-day continents. These central concepts serve as orientation points for all other inquiry within each discipline. Scientists do not know everything about the nature of the universe, but it is unquestionable that it has been and is expanding. This central knowledge then serves as a template that allows scientists to make much more accurate and informed hypotheses about factors yet to be discovered.

The study of human nutrition has no such guiding template or organizing paradigm. Except for a growing body of scientists and individuals who are privy to a new way of thinking about diet and nutrition, nutrition remains an immature discipline. Most of this field's leading scientists and major players are mainly unaware of a very powerful idea that could bring order to the fog of disarray and chaos. So, you may ask, what is the larger and all-encompassing question that, when asked and answered correctly, can provide us with the template, the holy grail, the magical looking glass desperately needed to fill this void in nutritional theory?

The question is a very simple question—a child's question: "Why?" That's right; the "why" question. Why do we have nutritional requirements in the first place? Humans, most other primates, the guinea pig, and a few species of bats must obtain vitamin C from their diet, whereas all other mammals can synthesize vitamin C from glucose, a simple sugar found in the bloodstream of all mammals. Why in the world do humans have a dietary requirement for vitamin C when most other mammals do not?

For that matter, why do we have dietary requirements for any nutrient? What we are looking for here is not the proximate (nearby) answer but, rather, the ultimate answer. Every registered dietitian worth his or her degree knows that without vitamin C, we get scurvy. A dietitian who can remember the metabolic pathways well enough may even be able to tell you why scurvy causes all of its symptoms. But that is merely the proximate answer to "Why?" Do you know the ultimate answer to why we have a dietary vitamin C requirement? By answering correctly, you will be staring directly at the holy grail of nutritional science. The correct answer to this question represents the guiding template and the organizational paradigm that nutrition is so dearly missing.

THE GIFT FROM THE PAST

The selection of appropriate food for wild animals in zoos is no hit-or-miss business. Zookeepers at state-of-the-art facilities like the San Diego Zoo's Wild Animal Park realized long ago that if they wanted animals to stay healthy and happy and even breed in captivity, they needed to replicate each animal's natural environment as closely as possible. That meant duplicating diet as well. When lions or any other purely carnivorous cats were fed only raw muscle meat, their health rapidly deteriorated, and they developed vitamin A deficiency and bone loss (osteoporosis) and eventually died. Careful observations of wild lions in their natural habitat revealed that they ate their prey's entire carcass, including the organs, liver (an excellent source of vitamin A), and calcium-rich ribs. Accordingly, both vitamin A deficiency and osteoporosis were averted when these wild animals ate the diet that they were genetically adapted to eat. Lions are not only endowed with sharp fangs and claws to take down their prey, but their digestive tracts are also much shorter than those of herbivores (plant eaters), which accommodates their calorically dense food. Additionally, lions' livers and other metabolic machinery have become specifically modified to cope with an all-flesh diet. Pure carnivores like cats are literally genetically programmed to eat the flesh of other animals—it would make about as much sense to feed these animals cereal grains and berries as it would to feed them antelope meat.

All species of animals—whether cats, antelope, or tropical fish—occupy and exploit specific ecological niches and are well suited to their place in the environment. Their genetic makeup reflects their adaptation to their ecological niche, including not only their outward appearance but also the foods they are genetically programmed to eat. When new and different foods are fed to these animals, it almost invariably results in ill health or disease. Zookeepers know that exotic species of South American monkeys can be kept alive on cereal-based chow, but these animals don't do well, are prone to disease, and will not reproduce under these conditions. Only when they are fed their normal diet of insects, leaves, and tropical fruit do they thrive and produce offspring in captivity. Similarly, successful tropical fish hobbyists understand the superiority of live food over dry flaked fish food for getting certain exotic fish to breed in their aquariums.

Human nutritional requirements were determined in the exact same manner as those for lions, exotic monkeys, and tropical fish. As a species, we are genetically well adapted to the foods and food types that we typically encountered in our original and natural ecological niche. What, then, is the native human niche, and what foods and food types are typically encountered?

HOW WE KNOW WHAT PALEOLITHIC PEOPLE ATE

You likely realize by now that the original and natural human ecological niche was that of a hunter-gatherer, and you probably deduce that hunter-gatherers ate wild plant and animal foods. Well, right you are! However, the essence of the question—what did hunter-gatherers eat?— lies in the precise details. The Introduction discussed the foods and food types that couldn't have been eaten by our Stone Age ancestors, but now let's talk about what they ate—and how we know this.

Except for certain rare bits and pieces of tangible evidence, such as fossilized human feces (coprolites) and a few isolated cases of mummified bodies found with stomach contents intact, almost all estimates of Stone Age diets must be inferred from circumstantial evidence. The four main sources of circumstantial evidence are (1) studies of other primate diets; (2) studies of fossils and their isotopic element signatures; (3) anthropological accounts of modern-day hunter-gatherers, called ethnographic studies; and (4) examination of our own, present-day biochemical and metabolic pathways.

Before we look at these four lines of circumstantial evidence, it is important to make it clear from the outset that there was no single, standardized Stone Age diet. The Paleolithic Age (Old Stone Age) began with the manufacture of the first crude stone tools, some 2.6 million years ago in Africa, and ended 10,000 years ago with the development of agriculture in the Middle East. The Stone Age ended a little later (5,000 to 8,000 years ago) for most Europeans and Asians, as agriculture spread from its origins in the Middle East. For some isolated hunter-gatherers, the Stone Age ended only within the last century. During the Paleolithic Age, perhaps as many as 20 distinctive species of the human tribe existed (see Figure 8.1 on page 148). The best available information tells us that their diets were as varied as the environments they inhabited. However, of utmost importance to us are the universal dietary characteristics that transcend time, geographic locale, and even species. These worldwide dietary similarities established the range and limits of foods that shaped our modern genome and represent the range and limits of foods to which we are now genetically adapted.

1. Other Primate Diets

By analyzing a special kind of DNA called mitochondrial DNA, found in all living primates, scientists have determined that our closest living relative is the chimpanzee. Even though our outward appearance is quite different from that of chimps, there actually is only about a 1.6 percent difference between our genome and theirs. A careful look at Figure 8.1 reveals that the earliest member of our tribe (*Sahelanthropus tchadensis*) lived between 6 million and 7 million years ago in Africa. Scientists aren't completely sure if this primate was an ape or a hominin (a primate that walks upright on two legs). Nevertheless, it was during this time or slightly later that the "last common ancestor" existed before the evolutionary split between chimps and hominins.

From field observations of chimpanzee eating habits and analysis of their feces, anthropologists have a pretty good handle on what they eat. In the wild, a chimp's diet contains about 93 percent plant food, primarily ripe fruit. However, the wild fruit they eat would gag us. These fruits are tough, fibrous, and, by modern standards, definitely not sweet. Many contain substances that taste like turpentine. For wild chimps, a

FIGURE 8.1

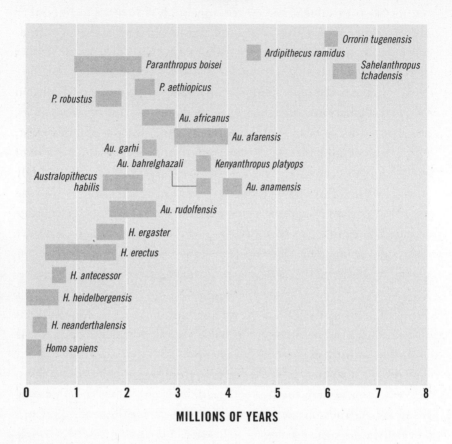

succulent apple or orange would be a candylike treat and voraciously gobbled up. You may be surprised to learn that wild chimps hunt, kill, and eat small monkeys and antelope. During the dry season in Africa, meat can account for almost 25 percent of a male chimp's diet.

If you have seen pictures of wild chimps, you may have noticed their large, protruding guts. A chimp has a big gut not because it is fat (like the average American couch potato) but because it needs a large, metabolically active gut to handle all of that tough, fibrous fruit. Chimps are relative geniuses in the animal world; however, their average brain size (400 cubic centimeters) is about a third the size of ours.

The difference between their brains and guts and ours—and the reason for it—forms one of the most eloquent ideas in all of evolutionary anthropology. It also gives us a good clue to the kind of diets we modern humans are genetically programmed to eat. Let's see how this works.

The brain is the most metabolically active organ in our bodies. In fact, at rest it uses nine times more energy than any other organ does. So, in order for us to have evolved a large brain, two possibilities exist: Either our overall metabolism increased, or the metabolism and size of another organ decreased. Think about it this way: If your entire body were made up of brains, it would have an overall metabolic rate nine times higher than it actually has. Of course, that's not the case, but we do have a body that contains three times more brain relative to our body size than a chimp does. It seems reasonable to conclude that the evolution of our large brains caused our overall metabolic rate to increase. Right? Wrong! Our net metabolic rate at rest is exactly as predicted for our body size. So the first possibility is out, leaving the second—that another organ got smaller. And, indeed, a human's gut is about half the size it should be, compared with a chimp's.

Anthropologists call this concept the expensive tissue hypothesis. This evolutionary brain/gut energy trade-off could have occurred only when the demands placed upon the gut to digest a bulky, fibrous, plant-based diet were reduced by the consumption of more energetically dense foods. Slightly before the fossil record shows brain size increasing, hominins began to manufacture the first stone tools that were used to butcher and dismember animal carcasses. Taken together, these facts verify that starting about 2.6 million years ago, hominins began to eat more and more animal food. It was this energetically dense food (meat, marrow, and organs) that allowed natural selection to relax the former selective pressure that had required a large, metabolically active gut. Literally, without meat, marrow, and organs in the diets of our ancient ancestors, we would not be here now. And the take-home message for you, the athlete, is that animal food (meat and organs) has been part of our ancestral diet from the get-go.

2. The Fossil Record

One of the most important clues we have in trying to piece together what our Stone Age ancestors ate is the fossil record. These are the items our prehistoric relatives left behind: their garbage, possessions, tools, weapons, and, less frequently, bones and teeth. Unfortunately, the fossil record is biased and will never allow us to peer into archaic diets with exacting precision. You don't have to be an archaeologist to figure this out. Animal remains such as hard teeth and bones resist decomposition in the soil and, thus, have a much greater chance of becoming fossilized than do soft plant remains. So when archaeologists dig up the remains of an ancient campsite, they rarely, if ever, find any evidence that plant foods were consumed. What they do find, typically, are bones of prey animals embellished with stone cut marks and sometimes the stone tools themselves. Does this mean that our Paleolithic relatives were total carnivores? Hardly. Our hunter-gatherer ancestors were opportunists: If it could be eaten, it probably was. But a few emerging themes play out in the fossil record, even with this preservation bias favoring animal remains.

The very earliest hominins who made stone tools were small (full-grown adults weighed 60 to 80 pounds and stood about 4½ feet tall) and probably not much more intelligent than chimps. Consequently, they probably weren't very good hunters of large animals. Many anthropologists believe that stone tool marks found on bones of large animals such as the zebra, wildebeest, and hippo came about from scavenging rather than hunting.

By about 1.7 million to 2 million years ago, hominins had achieved modern-day body proportions from the neck down. A remarkable, nearly complete male skeleton found in Kenya and dated to 1.6 million years ago would have stood 6 feet tall as an adult, with a slender body and narrow hips similar to the bodies of modern-day champion runners from Kenya. Slightly later, toolmaking became a bit more sophisticated, and medium to large prey animals became the preferred target. At one particularly amazing archaeological site in Kenya, called Olorgesailie,

400 stone hand axes were found along with the butchered remains of 65 extinct gorilla-size baboons. At another site in Germany, dated to 400,000 years ago, seven wooden spears were discovered with the butchered bones of more than 10 horses.

Just as in politics, there are smoking guns in the fossil record; these show beyond a shadow of a doubt what was going on. A few examples: In 1950, German anthropologists found an 8-foot thrusting spear, dated to 125,000 years ago, lodged between the ribs of an extinct straight-tusked elephant. How do you think that spear got there? A similar find was made in August 1951, when summer rains brought heavy flooding to the Greenbush Creek a mile northwest of Naco, Arizona. Erosion in the arroyo exposed part of a skull with teeth and the tusk of a large mammoth. Further excavation revealed eight razor-sharp stone spear points embedded between the animal's ribs. Because there were no stone cut marks on any of the mammoth's bones, anthropologists deduced that "this one got away."

How incredible would it be if we could have just a single photograph of our Paleolithic relatives going about their hunting and food collecting activities? We do have the next best thing—a highly detailed drawing, "The Shaft of the Dead Man," which you can see at the Web site www.culture.gouv.fr/culture/arcnat/lascaux/en/. This drawing, made 17,000 years ago in the famous Lascaux Cave in France, depicts a wounded European bison with its entrails spilling out and a spear stuck between its ribs. The enraged animal is in the process of goring a human armed with a spear-throwing device called an atlatl.

Now, why would our ancestors have risked life and limb to kill large, ferocious beasts to get meat? Couldn't they have gone after much less dangerous small prey like rabbits, partridges, clams, and fish? Why would anyone in their right mind lunge a flimsy wooden spear between the ribs of a 6- to 8-ton elephant? They did it because they had to. At the time, they were aware of no other alternative solution to survive. Why is that?

Believe it or not, you can get too much of a good thing, and protein is good for you only up to a certain point. You can include as much carbohydrate and fat in your diet as you like with no immediate ill effects, but the same can't be said for protein. In the typical US diet, protein makes up about 15 percent of our daily calories, whereas in hunter-gatherer diets, it would have been considerably higher, ranging from 25 to 40 percent of the daily energy intake. Laboratory studies in humans show that the maximum amount of protein we can ingest on a regular basis is about 40 percent of our daily calories. Anything above this and we get sick—a lesson our hunter-gatherers knew quite well. Early frontiersmen and explorers also knew exactly what happened when they were forced to eat only the lean meat of fat-depleted animals. They called this sickness "rabbit starvation." After eating enormous quantities of very lean meat, they would become nauseated and irritable, lose weight, develop diarrhea, and eventually die. They were better off starving than continuing to eat only lean meat. The only way around this situation: Get either fat or carbohydrate into the diet to dilute the protein level to below 40 percent.

In the modern world, it is easy to change the fat content of any food. Lobster is extremely lean (84 percent of its energy is protein) and would quickly cause protein poisoning if that's all you ate. Most of us prefer to dip our lobster in melted butter, which allows us to eat all we want and never develop symptoms of protein excess. Hunter-gatherers weren't so lucky. Fat and protein came in a single packet—the animal's carcass. Either the animal had fat or it didn't. There was no such thing as adding fat to a food. Similarly, if you were to eat a carbohydrate source such as brown rice or potatoes along with the lobster, you'd dilute the protein below the crucial 40 percent protein ceiling and have no problems whatsoever. However, until the development of agriculture and domestication of cereal grains, hunter-gatherers, particularly those living at higher latitudes, had no reliable year-round source of carbohydrate.

Now let's answer the question of why Stone Age hunters risked life and limb on a regular basis to kill large, unruly beasts. Large animals are fat animals. The larger a species, the more body fat it has. The average body fat content of a small animal like a squirrel (1 pound) is 5.2 percent by weight, whereas a large animal such as a musk ox (900 pounds) has 20.5 percent body fat by weight. If we look at the squirrel's body fat by total calories rather than weight, it's clear why the sole consumption of squirrels would cause protein poisoning. A squirrel's entire body is 35 percent fat by energy (calories) and 65 percent protein—way over the 40 percent ceiling. In contrast, the musk ox's body is 73 percent fat and 27 percent protein. A carcass containing only 27 percent protein can easily be consumed in its entirety without even coming close to the protein ceiling.

The fossil record unmistakably tells us that ancestral humans have always included meat and animal foods in their diets, but there is tantalizingly little evidence showing how much meat was eaten. And there is even less evidence to reveal how much plant food was typically consumed. Fortunately, anthropologists have developed a clever procedure that can give us a rough approximation of the dietary ratio of animal to plant by measuring stable isotopes in the fossilized bones and teeth of long-dead hominins. Stable isotopes are elements like carbon 13 and nitrogen 15 that vary slightly from the normal versions. Julia Lee-Thorp, PhD, and her colleagues from the University of Cape Town in South Africa have measured stable isotopes in many of the very first hominins who were living in Africa 1 million to 3 million years ago, and she concluded that all ate significant quantities of both animal and plant foods. Using stable isotopes to examine the diets of Neanderthals living in Europe 30,000 years ago, Mike Richards, PhD, of the University of British Columbia in Canada, concluded, "The isotope evidence overwhelmingly points to the Neanderthals behaving as top-level carnivores." In a similar study of Stone Age people living in England 12,000 years ago, he summarized, "We were testing the hypothesis that these humans had a mainly hunting economy, and therefore a diet high in animal protein. We found this to be the case."

Dr. Richards's isotopic data are interesting but come from very specialized groups of our ancestors, whose diets may have significantly varied from the mainstream. The Neanderthals generally lived in Europe during the Ice Age, when very little plant food would have been available on a year-round basis. Consequently, they may have had no choice but to eat animal food. Similarly, many anthropologists believe that modern humans living in Europe 12,000 to 40,000 years ago may have developed animal-based diet strategies because of the relative abundance of large game animals. There is another avenue available to us that can help to solve the riddle of how much plant and animal food was typically found in our ancestors' diets.

3. Ethnographic Studies

Hundreds, if not thousands, of descriptions of hunter-gatherers and what they ate have been written throughout historical times. These accounts were penned by explorers, sailors, trappers, frontiersmen, physicians, anthropologists, and others who encountered native peoples during their travels. Fortunately, an industrious anthropologist, George Murdock, PhD, took it upon himself to compile and organize historical accounts not only of hunter-gatherers but also of all the world's cultures and how they lived. His enormous database included more than 100 specific data points for each society. In 1967, Dr. Murdock completed his life's work with the publication of a massive volume called the *Ethnographic Atlas,* a work that allows anybody to easily compare and contrast any society or culture on earth.

One year after the publication of Dr. Murdock's massive volume, a young anthropologist at Harvard, Richard Lee, PhD, utilized some of the hunter-gatherer data from the *Ethnographic Atlas* to establish the plant-to-animal composition in the average hunter-gatherer diet. Dr. Lee concluded that hunted animal foods composed 35 percent of the energy in the average hunter-gatherer diet and that plant foods made up the balance (65 percent). For the next 3 decades, Dr. Lee's conclusion became the unquestioned dogma in anthropological circles. Unfortunately, his analysis was flawed, and it wasn't corrected until 32 years later with our publication of a reanalysis of the *Ethnographic Atlas*'s hunter-gatherer data. Let me show you how I came to this conclusion.

It's pretty hard to overeat raw carrots and celery—in fact, most of us have had enough after one or two carrots or celery stalks. Can you imagine eating 65 percent of your daily calories from celery? An active man who takes in 3,000 calories a day would have to eat 27 pounds of celery to obtain 65 percent of his daily calories from this plant food. Okay, perhaps celery is an extreme example. How about tomatoes? Try 20 pounds! Cantaloupe, maybe? Twelve pounds! Perhaps potatoes would work: To get 65 percent of 3,000 calories (1,950 calories), you would have to eat 4 pounds. This is a doable situation. But the problem is that most wild tubers and roots bear little resemblance to today's thoroughly domesticated potatoes. Compared with their modern counterparts, wild tubers are smaller, usually more fibrous, less starchy, and, therefore, not nearly as calorically dense.

It became increasingly clear to me that only a very few wild plant foods could be consumed at quantities approaching 65 percent of the daily caloric intake. These were oily nuts and seeds, tubers, and cereal grains. Grains were out of the equation because they were rarely, if ever, consumed by hunter-gatherers, as explained in the Introduction. Also, when hunter-gatherers forage for food, they need to make some critical decisions. First, they must get more energy from the food they are hunting or gathering than the energy they expend to obtain it. It would be a losing proposition to run around all day using up 800 calories, only to bring back 500 calories. Second, hunter-gatherers prioritize food choices relative to their energy return rate. These are the foods that give them the most "bang for their foraging buck"—large animals are preferred over small, and animal foods are almost always preferred over plant foods. Anthropologists have dubbed these hunter-gatherer decisions "optimal foraging theory."

At any rate, all of this information made me suspicious. It seemed unlikely that plant foods could have made up the majority of daily calories in the typical hunter-gatherer diet. So I went back to the original *Ethnographic Atlas,* plugged all the data points for the 229 hunter-gatherer societies into a spreadsheet, and reanalyzed the whole kit and caboodle. I completed my analysis on Christmas Day 1997 and could not believe my eyes. Not only were the results different from Richard Lee's analysis; they were exactly reversed. Plant foods represented about 35 percent of the total calories, while animal foods stood out at 65 percent! How could this be? I carefully checked all of the more than nearly 23,000 data points—no errors there. Hmm! What was going on?

At last I saw it. Dr. Lee had failed to include fished animal foods along with hunted animal foods in determining the overall animal-to-plant subsistence ratio.

One of the huge problems with ethnographic studies is that they are almost entirely subjective. We went back to some of the original studies that Dr. Murdock had used to estimate the subsistence ratios and were dumbfounded at how he did it. There were absolutely no concrete data in many of these accounts of hunter-gatherers to show how much meat or plant food was consumed. Using some of the accounts as a starting point, my research team and I rooted out each and every quantitative study in which the foods were weighed and the caloric content known. It turned out that 13 reports could be used. Two of them involved Eskimos, who have no choice but to eat animal food, so we were down to 11 reports. These more robust, quantitative studies were in agreement with our earlier analysis and once again demonstrated that animal foods made up two-thirds of the average energy intake in hunter-gatherer diets.

So, three separate lines of evidence (other primate diets, the fossil record, and ethnographic studies) now independently point to the notion that meat, organs, and animal foods have always been a significant part of the diet to which we are genetically adapted. But, as you'll see in Chapter 9, wild animals and domesticated, feedlot-produced animals are worlds apart nutritionally. A modern diet with 65 percent of its energy coming from processed fatty meats (bologna, salami, hot dogs, sausages, bacon, etc.) produced from grain-fed animals bears little resemblance to our ancestral diet.

Let's take a brief look at another piece of the puzzle that shows the types of foods Mother Nature intended for us.

4. Biochemical and Metabolic Pathways

Within our own body's biochemical machinery lie clues to the way in which diet has changed in the 5 million to 7 million years since our evolutionary split from the apes. It may come as a surprise to you, but we humans have evolved a number of biochemical adaptations that are parallel to those found in pure carnivores. Obviously, we are not pure carnivores. We are omnivores who are genetically adapted to eating a mixed diet of both plant and animal foods. However, substantial biochemical evidence suggests that, during the past 2.6 million years, we have made a significant evolutionary shift that has brought us closer to a meat-based diet than to a plant-based diet.

Pure carnivores, such as cats, must obtain all of their nutrients from the flesh of other animals. Because of this requirement they have evolved certain biochemical adaptations that demonstrate their total dietary dependence upon animal-based foods. Most of these adaptations involve either the loss or reduced activity of certain enzymes required to build essential nutrients. These losses occurred because the evolutionary selection pressure to maintain these enzymes and metabolic pathways was no longer needed. Let me give you a few examples and show you how humans have moved down a similar evolutionary pathway.

Taurine is an amino acid that is not found in any plant food and is an essential nutrient in all cells of the body. Herbivores, such as cows, are able to synthesize taurine from precursor amino acids found in plants, whereas cats have completely lost that ability. Since all animal foods (except cow's milk) are rich sources of taurine, cats have been able to relax the evolutionary selective pressure required for taurine synthesis because they obtain all they need from their exclusive meat-based diet.

Humans, unlike cats, still maintain the ability to synthesize taurine in the liver from precursor substances. However, this ability is limited and inefficient—so much so that infant formula must be supplemented with taurine. Without taurine supplementation in infant formula, bottle-fed babies are more susceptible to visual and hearing problems as they grow. Even adults don't fare much better if they stop eating meat. Studies show that vegan vegetarians have low levels of blood and urinary taurine—levels that indicate our poor ability to synthesize taurine from vegetable amino acids. Similar to that of cats, our inefficiency to build taurine from plant amino acids occurred because of our long reliance upon taurine-rich animal food.

A second example, similar to the taurine story, is the situation with long-chain fatty acids. Cats have almost completely lost the ability of the liver to convert 18-carbon to 20-carbon fatty acids. All cells in the bodies of mammals require 20-carbon fatty acids to make localized hormones called eicosanoids and prostaglandins. Herbivores have no choice but to synthesize 20-carbon fatty acids in their livers from plant-based 18-carbon fatty acids, since 20-carbon fatty acids occur only in animal food and are not found in any plant foods. Again, cats have nearly lost the ability to build 20-carbon fatty acids from their 18-carbon precursors because there was no need for it; they got all the preformed 20-carbon fatty acids they required from the flesh of their prey. Similarly, humans maintain very inefficient pathways to convert 18- to 20-carbon fatty acids because of our more than 2-million-year history of meat consumption.

In the Introduction, we discussed the foods that couldn't have been consumed by our Stone Age ancestors; in this chapter, we illustrated those that were eaten. By putting both of these pieces of the puzzle together, we get a much clearer picture of the foods that we are genetically programmed to eat. These are the foods that provide us with optimal health and well-being. By mimicking the nutritional characteristics of the ancestral human diet with commonly available modern foods, it is entirely possible to eat a Stone Age diet in the 21st century. In the next chapter, we will explain how easily this can be accomplished.

CHAPTER 9

THE 21ST-CENTURY PALEO DIET

SPECIAL DIETARY NEEDS OF MODERN ATHLETES

As a serious athlete, you have a lifestyle and an activity level that are far different from that of the average American. Chances are your training patterns also vary significantly from the daily activity patterns of our Paleolithic ancestors. They were unlikely to ever run 26.2 miles as fast as they could, nonstop. Nor would they work and run at high-intensity levels day after day, week after week. The only reason they would have done so would have been under extreme conditions in which their lives were continually at risk, and the only way to survive was to run far and fast every day. Such situations were rare. As you will see in the next chapter, the more typical manner of "exercise" for the Paleolithic athlete would have involved long, steady hunts and foraging expeditions conducted at a moderate pace until the kill was imminent or the gathered foods were hauled back to camp. At these times their effort would increase, but they would no doubt rest at every opportunity. Ceremonial dance would also provide nearly continuous "exercise," but the intensity would be relatively low.

What all of this means for you is that your diet must be modified slightly to accommodate your "unusual" high-level training patterns that are a requisite for peak performance during competition. These modifications, as you are now well aware, involve exactly when and what you eat before, during, and immediately following exercise. These critical dietary nuances were discussed extensively in Chapters 2, 3, and 4.

Now let's get down to the crux of this chapter: What should you eat for the remainder of your day, from the time short-term recovery ends until just before the next workout begins? During this period, you should be eating in a manner similar to that of your Paleolithic ancestors. You'll quickly discover that your day-to-day recovery is greatly enhanced and, as a result, your performance will improve.

21ST-CENTURY DIETARY TWEAKS

Let's make it clear from the start: It would be nearly impossible for any athlete or fitness enthusiast living in a typical modern setting to exactly replicate a Paleolithic hunter-gatherer diet. Many of those foods are unavailable commercially, no longer exist, or are totally disgusting to modern tastes and cultural traditions. Do brains, marrow, tongue, and liver sound appealing to you? Probably not, but to hunter-gatherers, these organs were mouthwatering treats that were gobbled up every time an animal was killed. For hunter-gatherers, the least appetizing part of the carcass was the muscle tissue, which is about the only meat most of us ever eat.

Produce for the Paleo Athlete

Most of the familiar fruits and veggies that we find in the produce section of our supermarkets bear little resemblance to their wild counterparts. Large, succulent, orange carrots of today were nothing more than tiny purple or black fibrous roots 1,000 years ago. The numerous varieties of juicy, sweet apples that we enjoy would have resembled tiny, bitter crab apples a few thousand years ago. Thanks to thousands of years of selective breeding, irrigation, and, later, fertilizers and pesticides, we now eat domesticated fruits and veggies that are larger and sweeter and

FIGURE 9.1

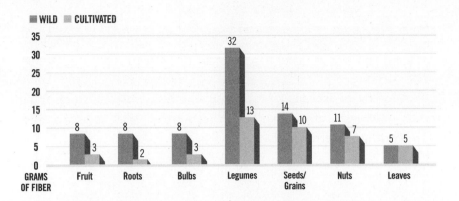

have less fiber and more carbohydrate than their wild versions. Figure 9.1 contrasts the fiber content of wild and cultivated plants in a 100-gram sample, and Table 9.1 compares the vitamin and mineral content of wild plant foods and their domesticated counterparts. You can see that the B vitamins, iron, and zinc concentrations are comparable between the two, whereas wild plants have more calcium and magnesium, and domesticated plants are better sources of vitamin C. Unless you are fortunate enough to live where you can harvest Mother Nature's nuts, berries, or other uncultivated plant foods, most of us will rarely eat wild plant foods on a regular basis. Nevertheless, it matters little because the overall nutritional differences between wild and domesticated plants are small and generally insignificant.

TABLE 9.1

Comparison of the Vitamin and Mineral Content of Wild and Domesticated Plants

	Vitamin B₁	Vitamin B₂	Vitamin C	Magnesium	Calcium	Iron	Zinc
Wild	0.19 mg	0.11 mg	8.1 mg	98 mg	117 mg	7.6 mg	3.5 mg
Domesticated	0.15 mg	0.10 mg	22.5 mg	67 mg	49 mg	7.4 mg	1.5 mg

TABLE 9.2

Sugar Content in Dried and Fresh Fruits

DRIED FRUITS	
Extremely high in total sugars	**Total sugars per 100 grams**
Dried mango	73.0
Raisins, golden	70.6
Zante currants	70.6
Raisins	65.0
Dates	64.2
Dried figs	62.3
Dried papaya	53.5
Dried pears	49.0
Dried peaches	44.6
Dried prunes	44.0
Dried apricots	38.9
FRESH FRUITS	
Very high in total sugars	**Total sugars per 100 grams**
Grapes	18.1
Banana	15.6
Mango	14.8
Cherries, sweet	14.6
High in total sugars	**Total sugars per 100 grams**
Apples	13.3
Pineapple	11.9
Purple passion fruit	11.2
Moderate in total sugars	**Total sugars per 100 grams**
Kiwifruit	10.5
Pear	10.5
Pear, Bosc	10.5
Pear, D'Anjou	10.5
Pomegranate	10.1
Raspberries	9.5
Apricots	9.3
Orange	9.2

FRESH FRUITS—continued	
Moderate in total sugars	**Total sugars per 100 grams**
Watermelon	9.0
Cantaloupe	8.7
Peach	8.7
Nectarine	8.5
Jackfruit	8.4
Honeydew melon	8.2
Blackberries	8.1
Cherries, sour	8.1
Tangerine	7.7
Plum	7.5
Low in total sugars	**Total sugars per 100 grams**
Blueberries	7.3
Star fruit	7.1
Elderberries	7.0
Figs	6.9
Mamey apple	6.5
Grapefruit, pink	6.2
Grapefruit, white	6.2
Guava	6.0
Guava, strawberry	6.0
Papaya	5.9
Strawberries	5.8
Casaba melon	4.7
Very low in total sugars	**Total sugars per 100 grams**
Tomato	2.8
Lemon	2.5
Avocado, California	0.9
Avocado, Florida	0.9
Lime	0.4

Fresh produce is an essential element of contemporary Paleo diets, and I encourage you to eat as much of these healthy foods as you possibly can. The only excluded vegetables are potatoes, cassava root, sweet corn, and legumes (peas, green beans, kidney beans, pinto beans, peanuts, etc.). Fruits are Mother Nature's natural sweets, and the only fruits you should totally steer clear of are canned fruits packed in syrups. Dried fruits should be consumed sparingly by most nonathletes, as they can contain as much concentrated sugar as candy does. Nevertheless, most trained endurance athletes can eat dried fruit with few adverse health consequences because athletes in general maintain sensitive insulin metabolisms. If you are obese or have one or more diseases of the metabolic syndrome (hypertension, type 2 diabetes, heart disease, or abnormal blood lipids), you should sidestep dried fruit altogether and eat sparing amounts of the "very high" and "high" sugar fruits listed in Table 9.2 on page 162. Once your weight returns to normal and disease symptoms fade away, eat as much fresh fruit as you please.

So you can see there is no need to go out and forage for wild plants and animals to stock your pantry for this lifetime nutritional plan. Nearly all of the performance rewards and health benefits of the Paleo Diet for Athletes can easily be achieved from modern-day foods and food groups that had a counterpart in Stone Age diets.

The fundamental dietary principle of the Paleo Diet for Athletes is simplicity itself: unrestricted consumption of fresh meats, poultry, seafood, fruits, and vegetables. Foods that are not part of modern-day Paleolithic fare include cereal grains, dairy products, high-glycemic fruits and vegetables, legumes, alcohol, salty foods, processed meats, refined sugars, and nearly all processed foods.

The exceptions to these basic rules are fully outlined in Chapters 2, 3, and 4. For instance, immediately before, during, and after a workout or competition, certain nonoptimal foods may be eaten to encourage a quick recovery. During all other times, meals that closely follow the 21st-century Paleolithic diet described here will promote comprehensive long-term recovery and allow you to come within reach of your maximum performance potential.

ANIMAL AND PLANT FOOD BALANCE

A crucial aspect of the 21st-century Paleolithic diet is the proper balance of plant and animal foods. How much plant food and how much animal food were normally consumed in the diets of Stone Age hunter-gatherers? There is little doubt that whenever and wherever it was ecologically possible, hunter-gatherers preferred animal food over plant food. In our study of 229 hunter-gatherer societies, published in the *American Journal of Clinical Nutrition,* my research team showed that 73 percent of these cultures obtained between 56 and 65 percent of their daily subsistence from animal foods. In a follow-up study published in the *European Journal of Clinical Nutrition,* involving 13 additional hunter-gatherer groups whose diets were more closely analyzed, we found almost identical results. Our colleague, Mike Richards, PhD, of the University of British Columbia in Canada, has taken a slightly different approach in determining the plant-to-animal balance in Stone Age diets. He has measured chemicals called stable isotopes in skeletons of hunter-gatherers that lived during the Paleolithic era. His results dovetailed nicely with ours and confirmed that hunter-gatherers living 12,000 to 28,000 years ago consumed the majority of their daily calories from animal sources.

Based upon the best available evidence, you should try to eat a little more than half (50 to 55 percent) of your daily calories from fresh meats, fish, and seafood. Avoid fatty processed meats (bologna, hot dogs, salami, sausages, bacon, etc.), but fatty fish such as salmon, mackerel, and herring are perfectly acceptable because of their high concentrations of healthful omega-3 fatty acids.

Meats and Animal Foods for the Paleo Athlete

One of the crucial ideas woven throughout *The Paleo Diet for Athletes* is that you should eat animal foods at virtually every meal. But the important point here is one of quality and freshness. At all times try to eat your meat, seafood, and poultry as fresh as you can get them. Fresh is always best, followed by frozen—avoid processed, canned, tinned, or salted animal foods. When it comes to beef, chicken, and pork, grass-fed, free-ranging, or pasture-produced meats are superior, although a bit expensive. Check out your local farmers' market or visit my friend Jo Robinson's Web site (http://eatwild.com/) to locate a farmer or rancher in your locale who can provide you with untainted, grass-fed meats.

Feedlot- and Grain-Fed Meats

Ninety-nine percent of the beef, pork, and chicken consumed in the United States is produced in colossal feedlots, frequently containing up to 100,000 animals. The motivating force behind feedlot-produced meat is purely financial. The singular goal of these enormous corporate agri-businesses is to produce the largest, heaviest animals possible with the smallest amount of feed. To accomplish this objective, the animals are restricted to tiny spaces where they get little or no exercise and are fed unlimited quantities of grain.

The final outcome is not pretty. Feedlot-produced cattle have a thick fat layer covering their entire body. These artificial creations of modern agriculture are obese and unhealthy and produce second-rate meat laced with hormones, antibiotics, and other toxic compounds. Their muscles are frequently interspersed with fat, which we call marbling, a trait that enhances flavor but makes cattle insulin-resistant and in poor health, just like us. Since feedlot-raised animals are fed solely grains (corn and sorghum), their meat is concentrated with omega-6 fatty acids at the sacrifice of healthful omega-3 fatty acids.

The take-home point is that the nutritional qualities of feedlot-produced meat are second-rate compared with those of meat from grass-fed or free-ranging animals. Nevertheless, I still believe that some, but not all, of these meats can be incorporated into the Paleo Diet for Athletes, especially if you try to eat leaner cuts and concurrently eat fatty fish like salmon, mackerel, herring, or sardines a few times a week. Fattier cuts of feedlot-produced meats are not ideal, because they contain not only more omega-6 fats, but also much less protein than leaner cuts contain. This characteristic in turn lowers your total intake of vitamins

TABLE 9.3

Protein and Fat Content
(Percentage of Total Calories in Lean and Fatty Meats)

LEAN MEATS	% Protein	% Fat	FATTY MEATS	% Protein	% Fat
Skinless turkey breasts	94	5	T-bone steak	36	64
Buffalo roast	84	16	Chicken thigh/leg	36	63
Roast venison	81	19	Ground beef (15% fat)	35	63
Pork tenderloin lean	72	28	Lamb shoulder roast	32	68
Beef heart	69	30	Pork ribs	27	73
Veal steak	68	32	Beef ribs	26	74
Sirloin beef steak	65	35	Fatty lamb chops	25	75
Chicken livers	65	32	Dry salami	23	75
Skinless chicken breasts	63	37	Link pork sausage	22	77
Beef liver	63	28	Bacon	21	78
Lean beef flank steak	62	38	Bologna	15	81
Lean pork chops	62	38	Hot dog	14	83

and minerals because the lean (muscle) protein component of meats is a richer source of vitamins and minerals than is the fat component. In Table 9.3, you can see for yourself the differences in the total protein and fat content between lean and fatty cuts of meat.

PROCESSED MEATS

In the first edition of *The Paleo Diet for Athletes,* I was adamant in my recommendation that you should avoid fatty processed meats like bologna, bacon, hot dogs, lunch meats, salami, and sausages. That suggestion remains, and from Table 9.3 on page 167 you can see that processed meats are really more like fat disguised as meat. Processed meats are man-made concoctions of meat and fat synthetically blended at the meatpacker or butcher's whim with no concern for the authentic fatty acid profile or protein content of the wild animals our Stone Age ancestors ate. In addition to their unnatural fatty acid compositions (high in omega-6 fatty acids, low in omega-3 fatty acids) and low protein content, processed fatty meats contain preservatives called nitrites and nitrates, which are converted into potent cancer-causing nitrosamines in our intestinal tracts. Further, these unnatural meats are characteristically laced with salt, sugar, high-fructose corn syrup, grains, and other additives that have many objectionable health effects.

With the Paleo Diet for Athletes I encourage you to consume as much high-quality "real" meat as you can afford. Clearly, the nearer you can get to "wild," the better off you'll be when it comes to the fat, protein, and nutrient profile of your meats. Game meat is not required for the Paleo Diet for Athletes, but if you are looking for a culinary adventure, try some. It's highly nutritious and adds a unique flavor to any Paleo meal. Game meat is pricey (unless you hunt or know hunters) and usually is found only at specialty markets or butcher stores.

WHAT ABOUT EGGS?

Despite being a comparatively high-fat food (62 percent fat, 34 percent protein) and one of the most concentrated sources of cholesterol (212 mg per egg), virtually all recent scientific studies conclude that ordinary egg consumption (seven per week) does not increase the risk for heart disease. You can now find eggs at your local supermarket that are enriched with the healthful long-chain omega-3 fatty acids EPA and DHA. Alternatively, seek out local growers whose chickens are cage-free, free-ranging and eat insects, worms, bugs, and wild plants. So please, enjoy this extremely nutritious food.

HOW ABOUT FATTY MEATS?

In the original version of *The Paleo Diet for Athletes,* we suggested that you should avoid fatty cuts of meat such as T-bone steaks, spareribs, lamb chops, and pork ribs because these cuts of meat contain more saturated fat than leaner cuts do. Further, it is known beyond a shadow of a doubt that increases in dietary saturated fat raise total blood cholesterol levels. This information has been known for more than 50 years from human metabolic ward studies, in which diet is strictly controlled and subjects are allowed to eat only the foods provided in the experiment. However, the next supposition, that increases in total blood cholesterol levels elevate the risk for heart and blood vessel disease, has been hotly debated by scientists since the original edition of our book was published. The consensus that is emerging from meta-analyses in which the results of multiple studies are combined indicates that dietary saturated fats have little or no effect upon the risk for cardiovascular disease. I quote Dariush Mozaffarian, MD, MPH, DrPH, and Renata Micha of the Harvard School of Public Health, who published the results of their meta-analysis in 2010, "*These meta-analyses suggest no overall effect of saturated fatty acid consumption on coronary heart disease events.*"

There is absolutely no doubt that hunter-gatherers favored the fattiest parts of animals. There is incredible fossil evidence from Africa, dating back to 2.5 million years ago, showing this scenario to be true. Stone-tool cut marks on the inner jawbone of antelope reveal that our ancient ancestors removed the tongue and almost certainly ate it. Other fossils show that Stone Age hunter-gatherers smashed open long bones and skulls of their prey and ate the contents. Not surprisingly, these organs are all relatively high in fat. Analyses from our laboratories showed the types of fat in the tongue, brain, and marrow are healthful. Brain is extremely high in polyunsaturated fats, including the health-promoting omega-3 fatty acids, whereas the dominant fats in tongue and marrow are the cholesterol-lowering monounsaturated fats.

Most of us would not savor the thought of eating brains, marrow, tongue, liver, or any other organ meat on a regular basis; therefore, a few 21st-century modifications of the original Paleolithic diet are necessary to get the fatty acid balance right. First, we suggest you limit your choice of meats to fresh, nonprocessed types, preferably grass-fed, and try to eat fatty fish a few times a week—it's good for you, just like the organ meats our ancestors preferred. Second, we recommend that you add healthful vegetable oils to your diet. If you follow these simple steps, together with the other nuts and bolts of this plan, the fatty acid balance in your diet will approximate what our Stone Age ancestors got.

From our analyses of 229 hunter-gatherer diets and the nutrient content of wild plants and animals, our research team has demonstrated that the most representative fat intake would have varied from 28 to 57 percent of total calories. To reduce risk of heart disease, the American Heart Association and the USDA MyPlate recommend limiting total fat to 30 percent or less of daily calories. On the surface, it would appear that, except for the extreme lower range, there would be too much fat in the typical hunter-gatherer diet—at least according to what we (the American public) have heard for decades: Get the fat out of your diet! The USDA's MyPlate cautions us to cut out as much saturated fat as possible and replace it with grains and carbohydrate. Not only is this message misguided; it is flat-out wrong. Recent meta-analyses have shown that when used to replace saturated fats, carbs increased the risk for heart disease by elevating blood triglycerides and lowering HDL cholesterol levels. More important, these meta-analyses demonstrated that, compared with carbs, saturated fats were neutral and neither increased nor decreased the risk for heart disease.

Now let's get back to the fat content of our ancestral hunter-gatherers' diet. They frequently ate more fat than we do, but they also ate lots of healthy fats. Using computerized dietary analyses of the wild plant and animal foods, our research team has shown that the usual fat breakdown in hunter-gatherer diets was 55 to 65 percent monounsaturated fat, 20 to 25 percent polyunsaturated fat (with an omega-6-to-omega-3 ratio of 2:1), and 10 to 15 percent saturated fat (about half being the neutral stearic acid). This balance of fats is exactly what you will get when you follow our dietary recommendations.

FOODS NOT ON THE PALEOLITHIC MENU

Let's get down to the specifics of the diet. Table 9.4 on page 172 includes an inventory of modern foods that should be avoided. These recommendations might at first seem like a huge laundry list, with seemingly needless elimination of entire food groups. Most dyed-in-the-wool nutritionists wouldn't object to our advice to cut down or eliminate sugars and highly refined, processed foods. They would have no problem with our suggestions to reduce trans fats and salt, and they would be ecstatic about our recommendations to boost fresh fruit and vegetable consumption. But they would, guaranteed, react violently to the mere thought of eliminating "sacred" whole grains from your diet. If they heard we also advocate reducing or eliminating dairy products, they almost certainly would brand this diet unhealthful, if not outright dangerous. You may wonder why, just because hunter-gatherers did not regularly eat grains or dairy products, you should follow suit. After all, aren't whole grains healthful, and isn't milk good for everybody? How can you get calcium without dairy? And won't eating a lot of meat increase blood cholesterol levels?

In science, decisions should be made based upon what the data tell us and not upon human bias and prejudice. With these ground rules in mind, let's take a look at the reasons for and potential benefits of eliminating or severely restricting entire food groups with the Paleo Diet for Athletes. One of the major goals of any diet, for both athletes and non-athletes alike, is to supply you, the consumer, with a diet rich in nutrients

Modern Foods to Avoid

DAIRY FOODS

Milk

Cheese

Butter

Cream

Yogurt

Ice cream

Ice milk

Frozen yogurt

Powdered milk

Nonfat creamer

Dairy spreads

All processed foods made with dairy products

CEREAL GRAINS

Wheat (bread, rolls, muffins, noodles, crackers, cookies, cake, doughnuts, pancakes, waffles, pasta, tortillas, pizza, pita bread, flat bread, and all processed foods made with wheat or wheat flour)

Rye (bread, crackers, and all processed foods made with rye)

Barley (soup, bread, and all processed foods made with barley)

Oats (instant oatmeal, rolled oats, and all processed foods made with oats)

Corn (corn on the cob, corn tortillas, cornstarch, corn syrup)

Rice (including brown, white, wild, and basmati; ramen and rice noodles; rice cakes; rice flour; and all processed foods made with rice)

Millet

Sorghum

CEREAL GRAIN–LIKE SEEDS

Amaranth

Chia seeds

Quinoa

Buckwheat

LEGUMES

All beans (kidney, pinto, navy, white, lima, black, and broad beans) including string beans

Lentils

Peas, snow peas

Peanuts (peanuts are legumes, not nuts)

Soybeans and all soybean products

Chickpeas and garbanzo beans

STARCHY TUBERS

Potatoes

Cassava roots

YEAST-CONTAINING FOODS

Breads, doughnuts, rolls, muffins

All fermented foods (beer, wine, pickled foods, foods containing vinegar, and tofu)

PROCESSED AND CANNED MEATS AND FISH

Sausages, bacon

Processed meats (lunch meats, deli meats, preserved or smoked meats such as ham and turkey, and smoked or dried and salted fish)

Canned or pickled meats and fish (tuna, sardines, herrings, smoked oysters and clams, canned salmon and mackerel, chicken, and beef)

ALCOHOLIC BEVERAGES

All alcoholic beverages (permitted in moderation; see Chapter 11)

SWEETS

All candy

Honey

Dried fruit (permitted in moderation; see Chapter 11)

Note that these foods are not forever banned from your diet, but are to be regularly avoided; see Chapter 11.

(vitamins, minerals, and phytochemicals) that promote good health, which in turn promotes good performance. Table 9.5 on page 174 shows the nutrient density of seven food groups.

From top to bottom, here's the ranking of the most nutritious food groups: fresh vegetables, seafood, lean meats, fresh fruits, whole grains and milk (tied for second to last), and nuts and seeds. Why in the world would the USDA include grains in MyPlate if the goal is an adequate intake of vitamins and minerals? This strategy makes no sense for the average American, much less for athletes like you. Had we included refined grains in the list, they would have ended up dead last because the refining process strips this nutrient-poor food group even further of vitamins and minerals. Unfortunately, in the United States, 85 percent of the grains we eat are highly refined, and grains typically make up 24 percent of our daily calories.

Grains and dairy foods are not only poor sources of vitamins and minerals; they also retain nutritional characteristics that clearly are not in your best interest, whether you're an athlete or not. From Chapter 5, you now know all about the glycemic index and acid-base balance in foods, along with how they impact your performance. Virtually all refined grains and grain products yield high glycemic loads. Further, all grains, whether whole or refined, are net acid-producing. Dairy products are one of the greatest risk factors for heart disease in the American diet, and cheeses produce the highest acidic loads of any foods. If that's not bad enough, recent studies have found that dairy products, despite having low glycemic indices, spike blood insulin levels similar to the way white bread does and cause insulin resistance in children. Do yourself a favor—get the grains and dairy out of your diet and replace them with more healthful fruits, veggies, lean meats, and seafood.

If you, like most Americans, have been swayed by those milk mustache ads, you probably are part of the mass hysteria, largely generated by the dairy industry, suggesting there is a nationwide calcium shortage that underlies osteoporosis. Not true! Calcium intake from dairy, or any other food, is only part of the story behind bone mineral health. More important is calcium balance, the difference between how much calcium

TABLE 9.5

Nutrient Density for Various Food Groups
(100 kilocalorie samples)

	WHOLE GRAINS	WHOLE MILK	FRUITS	VEGETABLES	SEAFOOD	LEAN MEATS	NUTS/ SEEDS
Vitamin B12 (mcg)	0.00[4]	0.58[5]	0.00[4]	0.00[4]	7.42[7]	0.63[6]	0.00[4]
Vitamin B3 (mg)	1.12[4]	0.14[1]	0.89[3]	2.73[5]	3.19[6]	4.73[7]	0.35[2]
Phosphorus (mg)	90[3]	152[5]	33[1]	157[6]	219[7]	151[4]	80[2]
Vitamin B2 (mg)	0.05[3]	0.26[6]	0.09[4]	0.33[7]	0.09[4]	0.14[5]	0.04[2]
Vitamin B1 (mg)	0.12[5]	0.06[2]	0.11[4]	0.26[7]	0.08[3]	0.18[6]	0.12[5]
Folate (mcg)	10.3[3]	8.1[2]	25.0[6]	208.3[7]	10.8[4]	3.8[1]	11.0[5]
Vitamin C (mg)	1.53[3]	74.2[5]	221.3[7]	93.6[6]	1.9[4]	0.1[1]	0.4[2]
Iron (mg)	0.90[4]	0.08[1]	0.69[2]	2.59[7]	2.07[6]	1.10[5]	0.86[3]
Vitamin B6 (mg)	0.09[3]	0.07[1]	0.20[5]	0.42[7]	0.19[4]	0.32[6]	0.08[2]
Vitamin A (RE)	2[3]	50[5]	94[6]	687[7]	32[4]	1[2]	2[3]
Magnesium (mg)	32.6[4]	21.9[2]	24.6[3]	54.5[7]	36.1[6]	18.0[1]	35.8[5]
Calcium (mg)	7.6[2]	194.3[7]	43.0[4]	116.8[6]	43.1[5]	6.1[1]	17.5[3]
Zinc (mg)	0.67[4]	0.62[3]	0.25[1]	1.04[5]	7.6[7]	1.9[6]	0.6[2]
Sum Rank Score	44	44	48	81	65	50	38

Superscripts represent relative ranking per nutrient (7 = highest; 1 = lowest).

Nutrient values represent average of food types within each food group: 8 whole grains, 20 fruits, 18 vegetables, 20 types of seafood, 4 lean meats, 10 seeds and nuts. Food types within food groups were based upon the most commonly consumed foods in the US diet for the 13 vitamins and minerals most frequently lacking or deficient in the US diet.

goes into your body from diet and how much leaves in urine. You will be out of balance if more calcium leaves than what comes in, no matter how much milk you drink. What we really need to pay attention to is the other side of the equation—the calcium leaving our bodies. Dietary acid-base balance is the single most important factor influencing calcium loss in the urine. Net acid-producing diets overloaded with grains, cheeses, and salty processed foods increase urinary calcium losses, whereas the Paleo Diet for Athletes is rich in alkaline-yielding fruit and vegetables that bring us back into calcium balance and promote bone mineral health.

DIETARY STAPLES: MEATS

With the Paleo Diet for Athletes, you'll be eating fresh meat and seafood, and lots of it, at almost every meal. Consequently, your protein intake will rise significantly. This is a good thing.

Experiments by Bernard Wolfe, MD, at the University of Western Ontario, have decisively shown that when animal protein replaces dietary saturated fat, it is more effective in lowering blood cholesterol and improving blood chemistry than are carbohydrates. In nutritional interventions such as Dr. Wolfe's, the key to scientific credibility is replication—replication, replication, replication! It is absolutely essential that other scientists get similar results from comparable experiments. To the surprise of some party-line nutritionists, a series of papers from independent researchers around the world confirmed Dr. Wolfe's earlier work.

Is there a limit to a good thing? You now know that lean animal protein lowers your blood LDL (bad) cholesterol levels, increases HDL (good), and provides muscle-building branched-chain amino acids. How much protein should—or can—you eat?

There is a limit to the amount of protein you can physiologically tolerate. Nineteenth- and 20th-century explorers, frontiersmen, and trappers who were forced to eat nothing but the fat-drained flesh of wild game in late winter or early spring developed nausea, diarrhea, and lethargy and eventually died. Studies conducted in the laboratory of Daniel Rudman, MD, at Emory University, have examined the causal mechanisms underlying the protein ceiling and found that toxicity occurs when the liver can't eliminate nitrogen from the ingested protein fast enough. Nitrogen is normally excreted as urea in the urine and feces, but with protein toxicity, ammonia and excessive amino acids from protein degradation build up in the bloodstream and produce adverse symptoms.

For most people, the maximum dietary protein limit is between 200 and 300 grams per day, or about 30 to 40 percent of the normal daily caloric intake. On the Paleo Diet for Athletes, you will never have to worry about protein toxicity, as you will eat unlimited amounts of carbohydrates in the form of fruits and vegetables. Further, in the postexercise window, as fully explained in Chapters 2, 3, and 4, you will be encouraged to consume high glycemic, alkaline-yielding carbohydrates to fully replenish your glycogen stores.

From our analyses of hunter-gatherer diets and the nutrient content of wild plants and animals, our research team has shown that the protein intake in the average hunter-gatherer diet would have ranged from 19 to 35 percent of daily calories. Since the protein intake in the normal US diet is about 15 percent of daily energy, we recommend that for peak performance during Stage V of recovery (the period following short-term recovery, lasting until your next preexercise feeding), you boost your protein intake to between 25 and 30 percent of daily calories. At values higher than 30 percent of energy, some people may begin to experience symptoms indicative of the physiologic protein ceiling.

MACRONUTRIENT BALANCE

We've already mentioned that the fat content in Paleolithic diets (28 to 57 percent total calories) was quite a bit higher than values (30 percent or less) recommended by the American Heart Association and the

USDA's MyPlate. We suggest consuming between 30 and 40 percent of your Stage V energy as fat. How about carbohydrate? In hunter-gatherer diets, carbohydrate normally ranged from 22 to 40 percent of total daily energy. Because of your special need as an athlete to restore muscle glycogen on a daily basis, you should boost these values a bit higher. We suggest that Stage V carbohydrate intake should typically range from 35 to 45 percent of calories. As you personalize the Paleo Diet for Athletes to your specific training schedule and body needs, you will be able to fine-tune your daily intake of carbohydrate, fat, and protein.

NUTRITIONAL ADEQUACY

Regardless of your final ratio of protein to fat to carbohydrate, you will be eating an enormously enriched and nutrient-dense diet, compared with what you were probably eating before. We've partially addressed this concept in Chapter 1, where we compared the Paleo Diet for Athletes with the recommended USDA Food Pyramid/MyPlate diet, and also in Table 9.5 on page 174. An even better way to appreciate how much more nutritious your diet will become when you adopt the Paleo Diet for Athletes is by looking at what the average American eats. Figure 9.2 on page 178 shows the breakdown by food group in the typical US diet. Notice that grains are the highest contributor to total calories (23.9 percent), followed by refined sugars (18.6 percent) and refined vegetable oils (17.8 percent). When you add in dairy products (10.6 percent of total energy) to grains, refined sugars, and refined oils, the total is 70.9 percent of daily calories. None of these foods would have been on the menu for our Paleolithic ancestors, as fully discussed in Chapter 8.

Refined sugars are devoid of any vitamins or minerals, and except for vitamins E and K, refined vegetable oils are in the same boat. Think of it: More than a third of your daily calories come from foods that lack virtually any vitamins and minerals. When you add in the nutrient lightweights we call cereals and dairy products (check out Table 9.5 on page

174), you can see just how bad the modern diet really is. The staple foods (grains, dairy, refined sugars, and oils) introduced during the agricultural and industrial revolutions have displaced more healthful and nutrient-dense lean meats, seafood, and fresh fruits and vegetables. Once you begin to get these delicious foods back into your diet, not only will your vitamin, mineral, and phytochemical intake improve, but so will your performance.

FIGURE 9.2

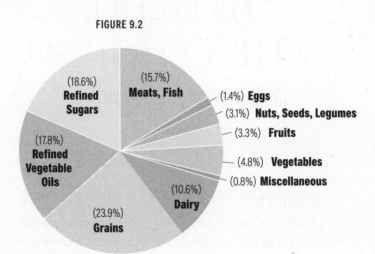

CHAPTER 10

THE PALEOLITHIC ATHLETE: THE ORIGINAL CROSS-TRAINER

Ten thousand years sounds like a long, long time ago. But if you think about it in terms of how long the human genus (*Homo*) has existed (2.3 million years), 10,000 years is a mere blink of the eye on an evolutionary time scale. Somewhere in the Middle East about 10,000 years ago, a tiny band of people threw in the towel and abandoned their hunter-gatherer lifestyle. These early renegades became the very first farmers. They forsook a mode of life that had sustained each and every individual within the human genus for the previous 77,000 generations. In contrast, only a paltry 333 human generations have come and gone since the first seeds of agriculture were sown. What started off as a renegade way of making a living became a revolution that would guarantee the complete and absolute eradication of every remaining hunter-gatherer on the planet. At the dawn of the 21st century, we are at the bitter end. Except for perhaps a half dozen uncontacted tribes in South America and a few others on the Andaman Islands in the Bay of Bengal, pure hunter-gatherers have vanished from the face of the earth.

So what difference does that make? Why should 21st-century endurance athletes care one iota about whether or not there are any hunter-
gatherers left? Because once these people are gone, we will no longer be
able to examine their lifestyle for invaluable clues to the exercise and
dietary patterns that are built into our genes. When I was a track athlete
in the late 1960s and early '70s, runners rarely or never lifted weights,
and no runners worth their Adidas or Puma flats would even think
about swimming. Fast-forward 40 years. What progressive coach now
doesn't know the value of cross-training? Those benefits might have been
figured out much earlier had we only taken notice of clues from our
hunter-gatherer ancestors.

Very few modern people have ever experienced what it is like to "run
with the hunt." One of the notable exceptions is Kim Hill, PhD, an
anthropologist at Arizona State University who has spent the last 30
years living with and studying the Aché hunter-gatherers of Paraguay
and the Hiwi foragers of southwestern Venezuela. His description of
these amazing hunts represents a rare glimpse into the activity patterns
that would have been required of us all, were it not for the agricultural
revolution.

> I have only spent a long time hunting with two groups, the Aché
> and the Hiwi. They were very different. The Aché hunted every
> day of the year if it didn't rain. Recent GPS data I collected with
> them suggests that about 10 km per day is probably closer to their
> average distance covered during search. They might cover another
> 1–2 km per day in very rapid pursuit. Sometimes pursuits can be
> extremely strenuous and last more than an hour. Aché hunters
> often take an easy day after any particularly difficult day, and
> rainfall forces them to take a day or two a week with only an
> hour or two of exercise. Basically they do moderate days most of
> the time, and sometimes really hard days usually followed by a
> very easy day. The difficulty of the terrain is really what killed me
> (ducking under low branches and vines about once every 20 sec-
> onds all day long, and climbing over fallen trees, moving through

tangled thorns, etc.). I was often drenched in sweat within an hour of leaving camp, and usually didn't return for 7–9 hours with not more than 30 minutes rest during the day. The Aché seemed to have an easier time because they "walk better" in the forest than me (meaning the vines and branches don't bother them as much). The really hard days when they literally ran me into the ground were long distance pursuits of peccary herds when the Aché hunters move at a fast trot through thick forest for about 2 hours before they catch up with the herd. None of our other grad students could ever keep up with these hunts, and I only kept up because I was in very good shape back in the 1980s when I did this.

The Hiwi on the other hand only hunted about 2–3 days a week and often told me they wouldn't go out on a particular day because they were "tired." They would stay home and work on tools, etc. Their travel was not as strenuous as among the Aché (they often canoed to the hunt site), and their pursuits were usually shorter. But the Hiwi sometimes did amazing long distance walks that would have really hurt the Aché. They would walk to visit another village maybe 80–100 km away and then stay for only an hour or two before returning. This often included walking all night long as well as during the day. When I hunted with Machiguenga, Yora, Yanomamo Indians in the 1980s, my focal man days were much much easier than with the Aché. And virtually all these groups take an easy day after a particularly difficult one.

By the way, the Aché do converse and even sing during some of their search, but long distance peccary pursuits are too difficult for any talking. Basically men talk to each other until the speed gets up around 3 km/hour which is a very tough pace in thick jungle. Normal search is more like about 1.5 km/hour, a pretty leisurely pace. Monkey hunts can also be very strenuous because they consist of bursts of sprints every 20–30 seconds (as the monkeys are flushed and flee to new cover), over a period of an hour or two without a rest. This feels a lot like doing a very long session of wind sprints.

Both my graduate student Rob Walker and Richard Bribiescas of Harvard were very impressed by Aché performance on the step test. Many of the guys in their mid 30s to mid 50s showed great aerobic conditioning compared to Americans of that age. (V02 max/kg body weight is very good.) While hunter-gatherers are generally in good physical condition if they haven't yet been exposed to modern diseases and diets that come soon after permanent outside contact, I would not want to exaggerate their abilities. They are what you would expect if you took a genetic cross section of humans and put them in lifetime physical training at moderate to hard levels. Most hunting is search time not pursuit, thus a good deal of aerobic long distance travel is often involved (over rough terrain and carrying loads if the hunt is successful). I used to train for marathons as a grad student and could run at a 6:00 per mile pace for 10 miles, but the Aché would run me into the ground following peccary tracks through dense bush for a couple of hours. I did the 100 yd in 10.2 in high school (I was a fast pass catcher on my football team), and some Aché men can sprint as fast as me.

But hunter-gatherers do not generally compare to world class athletes, who are probably genetically very gifted and then undergo even more rigorous and specialized training than any forager. So the bottom line is foragers are often in good shape and they look it. They sprint, jog, climb, carry, jump, etc., all day long but are not specialists and do not compare to Olympic athletes in modern societies.

Dr. Hill's wonderful imagery and insight tell us part of the story, but not everything. In this day and age of gender equality, women are just as likely as men, if not more so, to be found at the gym, lifting weights, or out on the trails, running or riding a bike.

In stark contrast, hunter-gatherer women almost never participated in hunting large game animals. Nearly without exception, ethnographic accounts of hunter-gatherers agree on this point. Does this mean that women did no hard aerobic work? Absolutely not! Women routinely gathered food every 2 or 3 days. The fruits of their labors included not only plant foods but also small animals such as tortoises, small reptiles, shellfish, insects, bird eggs, and small mammals. They spent many hours walking to sources of food, water, and wood. Sometimes they would help carry butchered game back to camp. Their foraging often involved strenuous digging, climbing, and then hauling heavy loads back to camp, often while carrying infants and young children. Other common activities, some physically taxing, included tool making, shelter construction, childcare, butchering, food preparation, and visiting. Dances were a major recreation for hunter-gatherers and could take place several nights a week and often last for hours. Table 10.1 on page 184 shows the caloric costs of typical hunter-gatherer activities and their modern counterparts.

The overall activity pattern of women, like men's, was cyclic, with days of intense physical exertion (both aerobic and resistive) alternating with days of rest and light activity. What hunter-gatherers did in their day-to-day lives appears to be good medicine for modern-day athletes. When Bill Bowerman, a well-known track coach at the University of Oregon, advocated the easy/hard concept back in the '60s, it was thought to be both brilliant and revolutionary. Using his system of easy/hard, athletes recovered more easily from hard workouts and reduced their risk of injury. Ironically, Coach Bowerman's "revolutionary" training strategy was as old as humanity itself. Similarly, during the same decade, weight training combined with swimming was a stunning innovation at Doc Counsilman's world-famous swim program at Indiana University. Now it is the rare world-class endurance coach who doesn't advocate cross-training to improve performance, increase strength, and help prevent injury. Once again the rationale behind the success of cross-training can be found in the hunter-gatherer genes in all of us.

TABLE 10.1

Calories Burned per Hour in Hunter-Gatherer and Modern Activities

HUNTER-GATHERER		MODERN HUMAN	
Activity	Calories Burned	Activity	Calories Burned
Carrying logs	893	Carrying logs	670
Running (cross-country)	782	Running (cross-country)	587
Carrying meat (20 kg) back to camp	706	Climbing hills (20 kg load)	529
Carrying a young child	672	Climbing hills (10 kg load)	504
Hunting, stalking prey (carrying bows and spears)	619	Climbing hills (5 kg load)	464
Digging (in a field)	605	Digging (in the garden)	454
Dancing (ceremonial)	494	Dancing (aerobic)	371
Stacking firewood	422	Stacking firewood	317
Butchering large animal	408	Chopping slowly with ax	306
Walking (normal pace in fields and hills)	394	Walking (normal pace in fields and hills)	295
Gathering plant foods	346	Weeding garden	259
Archery	312	Archery	234
Scraping a hide	302	Scraping paint	227
Shelter construction	250	Carpentry	187
Flint knapping	216	Shoe repair	162

Calorie burn (kilocalories per hour) is based on a 176-pound man or 132-pound woman.

WHY WE ARE DESIGNED TO EXERCISE

It may seem obvious, but sometimes the obvious is rarely considered. Do you know why the Aché and, for that matter, all hunter-gatherers exercise? Before we go down this road, let's clarify the word "exercise." No adult hunter-gatherers in their right minds would have ever set off on a run or repeatedly lifted a heavy stone simply to expend energy and "get exercise." Virtually all of their movement resulted from the day's mandatory activities: food and water procurement, shelter building, journeys, tool making, wood gathering, escape from dangers, child rearing, and social activities. Hunter-gatherers had no choice but to do physical labor of all kinds, big and small, day in and day out, for their entire lives. There were no retirements, vacations, layoffs, career changes, or labor-saving devices. Except for the very young or the very old, everyone did labor of one form or another on a regular basis.

Let's get back to the obvious that you may never have considered. Hunter-gatherers "exercised" because they had to. They had no other choice—period! For all humans living before the agricultural revolution, energy input (food) and energy expenditure (exercise) were directly linked. If Stone Age people wanted to eat, they had to hunt, gather, forage, or fish. Now you can see what may have motivated the Aché hunters as they furiously chased that herd of peccaries hour after hour through the tropical forest in Paraguay. Whether you do a long, hard workout or none at all, food is always there for you at the end of the day. Wouldn't it be disappointing to do your long, hard workout and come home to an empty fridge? Would an empty belly motivate you even more on the next workout (hunt) if the intensity of the exercise were directly related to the amount of food in the refrigerator?

In the modern world, we have totally obliterated the ancient evolutionary link between energy expenditure and food intake. As you lazily stroll down the grocery aisle and throw one item after another into the cart, you don't give a single thought to "search time" or "pursuit" of your prey, as Dr. Hill graphically portrayed for us with his description of the Aché hunters. In a supermarket, the search and pursuit times are identical whether you toss a smoked ham or a head of lettuce into your cart.

The consequences of severing this primeval evolutionary connection between energy expenditure and intake are not pretty. When we eat more energy than we expend, we gain weight. And when we gain weight, our health suffers. Unless you pay no attention to printed or online news, you know that we are in the midst of an obesity epidemic in the United States. Two-thirds of all Americans are either overweight or obese, 40 million have type 2 diabetes, and cardiovascular disease is the leading cause of death in this country. There is little doubt in my mind that none of this would be possible without the uncoupling of energy intake and expenditure that was handed to us when we deserted our ancestral hunter-gatherer way of life.

COMPARING THE LIFESTYLES OF HUNTER-GATHERERS AND MODERN ATHLETES

After reading Dr. Hill's description of the Aché hunters (see page 180), you probably have a pretty good feel for how their daily workout compares with yours, whether you're a recreational athlete, an accomplished local and regional endurance athlete, or an elite athlete of national or international caliber. How would the average hunter-gatherer stack up when it comes to high-level endurance performance on race day?

First, let's take a look at the advantages on the hunter-gatherer's side. From the time of weaning until very old age, hunter-gatherer athletes would have done moderate to hard aerobic activity, month in and month out, for their entire lives. They would have regularly rotated hard days with easy ones, and strength activities would have commonly accompanied aerobic work. This pattern of movement would have diminished their chance of injury, so they could get up morning after morning to hunt and gather again and again.

In exercise physiology there is a well-known law stating that aerobic capacity (max VO_2) within an individual may increase based upon exercise frequency, intensity, and duration. Of these three factors, intensity is the most important feature in squeezing out the last bit of aerobic capacity from already trained subjects. The problem is that as intensity increases, the chances of injury and illness also increase. Hunter-gatherers were in it for the long haul. Their objectives were to obtain food day in and day out, year in and year out. Regular high-intensity exercise would have been a liability because injury and illness meant less food. On the other hand, today's endurance athletes don't have to worry about injuries or illness getting in the way of eating; food is always available, no matter what your condition. Accordingly, endurance athletes can take their chances with high-intensity training. As a matter of fact, high-intensity workouts (>85 percent max VO_2) are not an anomaly but rather a requisite to perform at the highest levels upon the world's stage.

As we previously outlined, it is virtually impossible to exercise at >85 percent max VO_2 for extended periods unless muscle glycogen stores are fully topped off. Without daily consumption of high glycemic load carbs, regular high-intensity workouts simply are not feasible. Since high glycemic load carbs were not on the hunter-gatherers' menus, they could not have eked out the last 2 to 5 percent of their genetic aerobic potential by doing high-intensity workouts, as can modern athletes. On the other hand, because they ate more fat and fewer daily meals than we do, their intramuscular triglyceride stores would have been much higher, thereby allowing them to do aerobic work at moderate intensity for extended periods—just what the doctor ordered if you need to go hunting daily and high glycemic carbs don't exist. For the modern-day endurance athlete who is solely interested in maximum performance, an alternative exists: Both can be done. You can maximize muscle glycogen and triglyceride stores by following the diet we have summarized in Chapters 2, 3, 4, and 9.

Because the protein content of their diet was higher than ours, the concentration of the anabolic branched-chain amino acids (leucine, isoleucine, and valine) would have been much higher. As pointed out previously, these dietary amino acids promote muscle resynthesis following exercise and may also delay the onset of fatigue. Unless you are eating lots of lean meats and fish, hunter-gatherers would have had the advantage here. The high protein content of our ancestral diet meant that another amino acid, glutamine, would also have been higher than what you get in a vegetarian diet of beans and brown rice, or simply the standard American junk-food diet. A classic symptom of overtraining in endurance athletes is low blood levels of glutamine.

The trick with glutamine is not just how much you are getting but also how much you are losing. Losing excess glutamine is just like not getting enough. If you are eating a high-carb, low-fat diet—pretty much the standard endurance-athlete fare—it is almost certain that your body will be in a slight state of net metabolic acidosis. As we have previously shown, a net acid-producing diet causes your body to excrete more and more of the muscles' glutamine in an attempt to restore acid-base balance. The loss of muscle glutamine from an acid-yielding diet and from insufficient intake of glutamine-rich foods (lean meats, fish, and seafood) may adversely affect performance. Chalk up another advantage to hunter-gatherers.

One of the most important variables leading to athletic success is staying healthy and free of illness and colds. There is little doubt that proper nutrition is absolutely essential for optimizing your immune system. Because hunter-gatherers ate no processed foods, cereal grains, or refined sugars or oils, their intake of trace nutrients (vitamins, minerals, and phytochemicals) was way higher than what the average US citizen gets. Also, they consumed more healthful omega-3 fatty acids than most of us now do. These dietary advantages would have again allowed our hunter-gatherer ancestors to go out day after day to hunt and forage without interruption from illness. For our species, natural selection had no interest in winning a 10-K or marathon; the name of the evolutionary game was adequate calories, not maximum exercise performance.

So let's get down to the nitty-gritty. Was there ever a hunter-gatherer who could have taken home the Olympic gold in any endurance event in the last 30 years? The answer is no. The average hunter-gatherer was clearly more fit than the average American couch potato, as we pointed out in the Introduction. Most foragers, both men and women, could have run any recreational runner into the ground. At the local and regional levels, their best athletes would have been competitive. But there is no comparison between them and elite national and international athletes for two basic reasons.

First are the numbers. The primary determinant of aerobic capacity is maximum oxygen consumption, or max VO_2. If you want to be a world-class endurance athlete, you better choose your parents well, because max VO_2 is almost entirely determined by genetics. One of the highest max VO_2 values ever reliably recorded for an elite male athlete in the United States is about 84 milliliters per kilogram per minute (ml/kg/min). Contrast this value to about 40 ml/kg/min for the average American male. So what happens if the 40 ml/kg/min guy wants to become world class and sets off upon an incredibly intense training program for years and years? Does he have a chance of getting to 84 ml/kg/min? Not even close! Max VO_2 can increase by about 10 to 15 percent in the best of all worlds, but no more. In the United States, we now have more than 300 million residents. Compare this with the fewer than 1,000 Aché hunter-gatherers that Dr. Hill accompanied. If only one person out of 1,000 has a genetically determined max VO_2 of greater than 70 ml/kg/min, then in the US population, there will be 30,000 people who have the genetic potential to perform at extremely high aerobic capacities. Among the Aché hunter-gatherers, only one person in their entire population will have this genetic capacity.

Hunter-gatherers wouldn't stand a chance against Olympian endurance athletes, not only because of the numbers game but also because they were limited to low-octane fuel. Intramuscular triglyceride is a great energy source for moderate to hard exercise lasting for hours, but it can't hold a candle to glycogen when it comes to high-level exertion at 85 percent or greater of the VO_2 required to make Olympic champions. Because hunter-gatherers ate less carbohydrate and more fat, along with fewer daily meals, their intramuscular triglyceride stores would have been higher than ours. But they also ate no high glycemic load carbs (except for occasional honey), so their muscle glycogen reserves would have always been lower than ours. They simply lacked the fuel injection of high glycemic load carbs to restore muscle glycogen concentrations following hard exercise. You now have this option. Not only can you increase muscle glycogen concentrations via careful dietary manipulation but, by following our nutritional plan, you can also increase intramuscular triglycerides.

You, as a 21st-century endurance athlete, are no longer reliant upon the current scientific status quo relating diet to performance—you have the added advantage of knowing how the wisdom of your ancestral dietary background can improve performance. When you combine the best of their world with the best of ours, your performance will soar.

PART IV

Putting It into Practice

CHAPTER 11

THE TRAINING TABLE

You won't need to buy any exotic foods to properly follow the Paleo Diet for Athletes. No matter if you live in a big city or in the country, the diet's mainstays (fresh meats, fish, and fruits and vegetables) are almost always on hand at your local grocery store or supermarket. In Chapter 9 we laid out a comprehensive list of the foods you should limit or exclude from your diet. In this chapter, we'll show you all the delicious, health-giving choices you have the luxury to eat. We'll also give you some practical pointers on how to pull off a Stone Age diet in the 21st century.

YOUR PRIORITY: FRESH FOODS

When you're hungry in the United States, getting something to eat is as easy as the nearest vending machine, fast-food restaurant, or convenience store. But you know what? You have to look long and hard to find "real" food—food that is not adulterated with sugar, salt, refined grains, and trans fats—at any of these places. The incredible overabundance and easy access to processed foods in this country make it easy to derail your plans to improve your diet—particularly when you're famished and need food now.

One of the keys to the Paleo Diet for Athletes is fresh foods. I repeat—fresh foods! They really are so much better for you than their canned, processed, frozen, and prepackaged counterparts that there is no comparison. Canned, sugar-laced peaches don't hold a candle to fresh peaches, either in taste or nutrition. A fatty hot dog with its added salt, sugar, and preservatives, whether it's ground from leftover pork or beef, bears little nutritional resemblance to fresh pork loin or beef flank steak.

As an athlete, you know that small but perceptible extra efforts during training, day in and day out, season in and season out, will pay off over the long haul. Pushing that last interval to the max hurts, but by doing so regularly, you will become fitter and stronger and your performance will improve—maybe by only 1 to 2 percent, but, as we pointed out in Chapter 8, that seemingly minuscule difference can be huge when it comes to racing. This same principle holds true with the foods you eat. By methodically eating fresh, wholesome foods whenever and wherever you can, the overall trace nutrient (vitamins, minerals, and phytochemicals) density of your diet will ultimately improve. And, as we have previously pointed out, there is a mountain of scientific evidence to show that your immune system functions better when properly nourished. A healthy immune system can more effectively ward off illness and help you to recover more rapidly from injuries, thereby allowing you to train at higher levels. Do yourself a favor—get fresh fruits, veggies, lean meats, and seafood into your diet whenever you can.

If you're like most Americans, fresh fruits and veggies occupy a small drawer in your fridge, where they get wilted, soft, and brown, and they end up thrown out more often than eaten. This will change with your new diet, and here are some practical pointers to help you get more fresh produce into your meal plans.

1. Thoroughly wash your fresh veggies and put them in storage bags or containers before you put them in your refrigerator. These simple steps will prevent wilting, increase storage life, and reduce contaminants.

2. Buy enough produce to last for no more than 5 to 7 days. It's better to get fresh supplies at least once a week.

3. If food preparation time is an issue, you can purchase a lot of produce that's packaged and ready to go with little or no prep. Examples include shredded lettuce and salad mixes; precut broccoli florets; baby spinach leaves; washed and peeled baby carrots; precut chunks of melon, pineapple, and other fruit; and shelled nuts. But remember, you'll pay a bit more for the convenience.

4. Make a very large mixed salad at the beginning of the week and put it in a large, sealed container; dish out portions as needed throughout the week.

Organic Produce

How about organic produce—any advantages to it? Should you pay the higher price? Table 11.1 is adapted from the results of a study that compiled numerous publications comparing the nutrient content of organic versus conventionally produced plant foods. Data from this study as well as other comprehensive reviews of the literature generally conclude that,

TABLE 11.1

Comparison of Organic versus Conventionally Grown Plant Foods. Percentage of Studies in Which Organic Crops Have Increased, Remained the Same, or Decreased Compared with Conventionally Grown Crops.

NUTRIENT	% INCREASED	% REMAINED SAME	% DECREASED	NO. OF STUDIES
Vitamin C	58.3	33.3	8.3	36
Beta-carotene	38.5	38.5	23.0	13
Zinc	25.0	56.3	18.7	16
B vitamins	12.5	75.0	12.5	16
Calcium	44.7	42.5	12.8	47
Protein	100	0	0	3
Magnesium	37.7	53.3	8.0	45
Nitrate	12.5	25.0	62.5	40
Iron	42.9	40.0	17.1	35

except for a slightly higher vitamin C content and possibly protein in organically produced vegetables (but not fruits), no differences exist for any other vitamins or minerals. So, if you're contemplating buying organic produce for its greater nutritional value, it's simply not worth it.

However, do note that the levels of nitrate in organically produced fruits and veggies are consistently lower than in conventional produce. Both the World Health Organization and the Environmental Protection Agency (EPA) in the United States have set limits for daily nitrate intake (1.6 milligrams/nitrate/kilogram body weight). Generally, both conventional and organic fruits and vegetables fall below acceptable limits. Similarly, some studies have demonstrated reduced amounts of pesticides in organic produce. Elevated environmental and dietary exposure to both nitrates and pesticides is associated with an elevated risk for developing certain cancers. If either of these issues is of concern to you, then go with organic produce.

Acceptable Fresh Vegetables

Potatoes maintain high glycemic loads and should be eaten only during the postexercise window, as explained in Chapter 4. If you have an autoimmune disease, you should proceed cautiously with potatoes, as they contain antinutrients that increase intestinal permeability, a significant step toward autoimmunity. Corn on the cob is a cereal grain and should therefore be excluded. Most of us have never tasted cassava roots, but they also should be avoided because of their high glycemic loads. Otherwise, virtually all fresh vegetables are perfectly acceptable: asparagus, parsnip, radish, broccoli, lettuce, mushrooms, dandelion greens, mustard greens, watercress, purslane, onions, green onions, carrots, parsley, squash of all varieties, all peppers, artichokes, tomatoes, cauliflower, cabbage, Brussels sprouts, celery, cucumbers, tomatillos, collards, Swiss chard, endive, beets, beet greens, rutabaga, kohlrabi, kale, eggplant, pumpkin, sweet potatoes, turnips, turnip greens, spinach, seaweed, yams.

Acceptable Fresh Fruits

As with vegetables, any fresh fruits you can get your hands on are fair game, except for people who are overweight or have one or more symptoms of metabolic syndrome (type 2 diabetes, high blood pressure, high cholesterol, or heart disease). In this case, you should follow the recommendations we have made for fruit in Chapter 9. For athletes, the only exceptions are dried fruits (such as raisins, dates, and figs), which, like potatoes, have high glycemic loads and should be limited to the postexercise window. Reach for these and other fruits anytime: apples, oranges, pears, peaches, plums, kiwifruit, pomegranates, grapes, watermelon, cantaloupe, honeydew melon, cassava melon, pineapple, guava, nectarines, apricots, strawberries, blackberries, blueberries, raspberries, avocado, carambola, cherimoya, cherries, grapefruit, lemon, lime, lychee, mango, papaya, passion fruit, persimmon, tangerine, star fruit, gooseberries, boysenberries, cranberries, rhubarb.

GETTING THE FATTY ACID BALANCE RIGHT

As you know by now, getting the fatty acid balance right is essential in replicating hunter-gatherer diets with modern foods. For our Stone Age ancestors, this problem was a no-brainer. Because their only food choices were wild plants and animals, the fatty acid balance always fell within healthful limits. By following our simple advice of eating fresh meats, seafood, and fatty fish along with healthful oils, you won't have to give a second thought to the correct balance, either.

Acceptable Domestic Animal Products

Always choose fresh meat, preferably free range or grass-fed. Almost all cuts of beef, pork, and poultry are good choices, and as we have outlined in Chapter 9, fattier cuts of meat can be included in your diet without increasing your risk for heart disease. Nevertheless, know that fatty meat contains less protein than leaner cuts do and hence is not as nutritionally dense as lean meat. A good financial strategy is to look for sales and buy your meat in bulk and then freeze it.

Eggs are high in protein, vitamins, and minerals and should be regularly included in your diet. Look for eggs produced by free-ranging chickens or for omega-3-enriched eggs. Virtually all recent human studies confirm that egg consumption will not increase your risk for cardiovascular disease.

Organ meats, except for marrow and brains, of commercially produced animals are quite lean. However, the liver and kidneys, which cleanse and detoxify the animal's body, frequently contain high concentrations of environmental contaminants. We recommend eating only calves' liver because virtually all calves slaughtered in the United States haven't found their way to the toxic feedlot environment; all are pasture fed. Brains contain high concentrations of omega-3 fatty acids and were relished by our hunter-gatherer ancestors. However, because of the small risk of developing prion disease (mad cow disease), we do not advise eating the brains of any animal, domestic or wild. Cholesterol-lowering monounsaturated fatty acids are the dominant (about 65 percent) fatty acids in marrow and tongue, both of which are quite healthful and tasty. Beef, lamb, and pork sweetbreads are infrequently eaten, but contain healthful fatty acids.

Grass-Fed or Free-Ranging Meats

If you can find it, grass-fed (or free-ranging) meat will always be a better choice than domestic beef, pork, or poultry because it is richer in healthful omega-3 fatty acids, higher in protein (like wild game), and less likely to be tainted with hormones and pesticides. Figure 11.1 contrasts the total fat percentage among wild game, grass-fed beef, and feedlot-produced beef, while Table 11.2 compares the differences in fatty acid content.

FIGURE 11.1

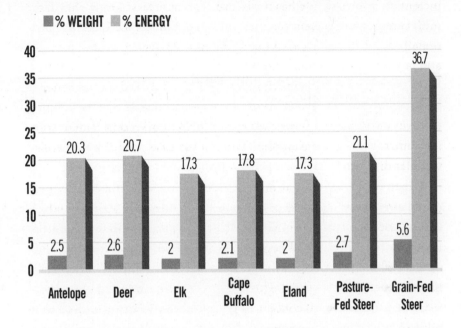

Jo Robinson's Web site, http://eatwild.com/, is the best and most comprehensive resource for locating farmers and ranchers in your locale that produce grass-fed meats.

You can often find organically produced beef and other meat items in health food stores or at farmers' markets. However, organic meat and

TABLE 11.2

Comparison of Animals' Muscle Fatty Acid Concentrations (mg fatty acids/100 g sample)

FATTY ACID	ELK	MULE DEER	ANTELOPE	PASTURE-FED STEER	GRAIN-FED STEER
SAT	610	989	895	910	1,909
MUFA	507	612	610	793	1,856
PUFA	625	746	754	262	341
Omega-3 PUFA	178	225	216	61	46
Omega-6 PUFA	448	524	536	138	243

SAT = total saturated fatty acids; MUFA = total monounsaturated fatty acids; PUFA = total polyunsaturated fatty acids grass-fed meat are not always one and the same. Frequently, organic beef or buffalo is fattened with "organically produced" grains, yielding the same poor ratio of omega-6 to omega-3 found in feedlot animals.

Commercially Available Game Meat and Other Exotic Meats

In the United States, the commercial sale of hunted wild game is prohibited. So, unless you are a hunter, the only way to obtain game meat is to purchase meat that has been produced on game farms or ranches—but even that, except for buffalo, is difficult to find. (One of the largest mail-order suppliers of game meat that can be found in the United States is Game Sales International.) Generally, this meat is superior to feedlot products, but it may not be as lean or as healthful as wild game. It is not an uncommon practice to feed grain to elk and buffalo to fatten them before slaughter.

Exotic meats you may want to try include kangaroo, venison, elk, alligator, reindeer, pheasant, quail, Muscovy duck, goose, wild boar, ostrich, rattlesnake, emu, turtle, African springbok antelope, New Zealand Cervena deer, squab, wild turkey, caribou, bear, buffalo, rabbit, and goat.

Fish, Seafood, and Shellfish

We no longer live in a healthy, pristine, unpolluted environment; pesticides, heavy metals, chemicals, and other toxic compounds frequently make their way into our food chain. No one knows precisely how low-level exposure to these toxins affects health over the course of a lifetime. It is prudent to try to reduce our exposure to toxic compounds whenever possible, but it is virtually impossible to eliminate exposure to environmental toxins because they now permeate even such places as the Antarctic. Fish frequently contain high concentrations of mercury and pesticides. To minimize your risk of eating contaminated fish, avoid eating freshwater fish from lakes and rivers, particularly the Great Lakes and other industrialized areas. Also avoid large, long-lived fish such as swordfish, tuna, and shark because they tend to concentrate mercury in their flesh.

Fish, seafood, and shellfish are a few of the most healthful animal foods you can consume and represent a foundation of the Paleo Diet for Athletes because they are enriched sources of the therapeutic, long-chain omega-3 fatty acids known as EPA and DHA. Fatty fish such as salmon, mackerel, sardines, and herring are particularly concentrated in both of these long-chain omega-3 fatty acids. Try to take in fish at least three times per week.

About 20 years ago, people with heart disease were advised to steer clear of shellfish, which was believed to have too much cholesterol. It's true that shellfish is high in cholesterol—but the good news is that we don't have to avoid it. It turns out that dietary cholesterol has a very small effect upon blood cholesterol when the food's total saturated fat content is low. Table 11.3 shows that all shellfish are quite low in both saturated and total fat, despite having relatively high cholesterol concentrations. We encourage you to eat as much shellfish as you enjoy.

TABLE 11.3

Cholesterol and Fat Content in Shellfish (100 g portions)

FOOD	CHOLESTEROL (mg)	SATURATED FAT (g)	TOTAL FAT (% total energy)
Shrimp	200	0.4	15
Crayfish	114	0.2	11
Lobster	95	0.2	9
Abalone	85	0.2	7
Whelk	65	0.03	3
Crab	59	1	10
Oysters	50	0.5	26
Clams	34	1	12
Scallops	33	0.1	8
Mussels	28	0.4	23

Here's a list of fish and shellfish that are important components in any modern-day variety of the Stone Age diet:

FISH

Bass

Bluefish

Cod

Drum

Eel

Flatfish

Grouper

Haddock

Halibut

Herring

Mackerel

Monkfish

Mullet

Northern pike

Orange roughy

Perch

Red snapper

Rockfish

Salmon

Scrod

Shark

Striped bass

Sunfish

Tilapia

Trout

Tuna

Turbot

Walleye

Any commercially available fish

SHELLFISH

Abalone

Calamari (squid)

Crab

Crayfish

Lobster

Mussels

Octopus

Oysters

Scallops

Shrimp

Besides being rich sources of EPA and DHA, fish and seafood represent some of our best high-protein foods. The high protein content of the Paleo Diet for Athletes is central to many of its performance benefits. Protein helps you lose weight more rapidly by raising your metabolism while concurrently curbing your appetite. Additionally, protein lowers your total blood cholesterol as it simultaneously increases the good HDL molecules that rid your body of excessive cholesterol. Protein also stabilizes blood sugar and reduces the risk of high blood pressure, stroke, heart disease, and certain cancers.

Healthful Oils, Nuts, and Seeds

Table 11.4 on page 204 provides you with all the information you need to pick out the most healthful oils. Oils you use for cooking need to be stable and more resistant to the oxidizing effects of heat, whereas those you use in your salads don't. Saturated fatty acids (SAT) are the most stable and heat resistant, followed by monounsaturated fatty acids (MUFA), then polyunsaturated fatty acids (PUFA). Your choice of cooking oils should be high in MUFA and relatively low in PUFA. For the price, olive oil is the best oil for cooking. All oils, regardless of their fatty-acid makeup, oxidize during cooking. Consequently, you should not fry at high or searing heats; instead, sauté at low to medium temperatures and cook for shorter periods.

The stability of oil is determined not only by its relative ratio of SAT to MUFA to PUFA but also by the type of PUFA. Omega-3 PUFA are more fragile than omega-6 PUFA because of the location and number of the double bonds in the fatty acid molecule. Consequently, flaxseed and walnut oils should not be used for cooking because of their high concentrations of total PUFA and omega-3 PUFA. However, both oils are good choices for dressing salads. Flaxseed oil is the richest vegetable source of omega-3 fatty acids. Pour it over steamed veggies or incorporate it into a marinade added to meat and seafood after cooking. Both strategies are great ways to get more omega-3 fatty acids into your diet.

Because of their high MUFA and low PUFA contents, olive, macadamia and avocado oils are good choices for cooking and add a wonderful flavor to any dish. However, macadamia and avocado oils are pricey and difficult to find. Notice that coconut oil also can be used for cooking because of its high SAT and low PUFA content. It is also a highly

TABLE 11.4

Fatty Acid Composition of Salad and Cooking Oils

TYPE OF OIL	OMEGA-6: OMEGA-3 RATIO	% MUFA	% PUFA	% SAT
Flaxseed	0.24	20.2	66.0	9.4
Canola	2.00	58.9	29.6	7.1
Walnut	5.08	22.8	63.3	9.1
Macadamia	6.29	77.7	2.0	15.9
Soybean	7.5	23.3	57.9	14.4
Wheat germ	7.9	15.1	61.7	18.8
Avocado	13.0	67.9	13.5	11.6
Olive	13.1	72.5	8.4	13.5
Rice bran	20.9	39.3	35.0	19.7
Oat	21.9	35.1	40.9	19.6
Tomato seed	22.1	22.8	53.1	19.7
Corn	83.0	24.2	58.7	12.7
Sesame	137.2	39.7	41.7	14.2
Cottonseed	258	17.8	51.9	25.9
Sunflower	472.9	19.5	65.7	10.3
Grape seed	696	16.1	69.9	9.6
Poppy seed	extremely high (no omega-3s)	19.7	62.4	13.5
Hazelnut	extremely high (no omega-3s)	78.0	10.2	7.4
Peanut	extremely high (no omega-3s)	46.2	32.0	16.9
Coconut	extremely high (no omega-3s)	5.8	1.8	86.5
Palm	extremely high (no omega-3s)	11.4	1.6	81.5
Almond	extremely high (no omega-3s)	70.0	17.4	8.2
Apricot kernel	extremely high (no omega-3s)	60.0	29.3	6.3
Safflower	extremely high (no omega-3s)	14.4	74.6	6.2

MUFA=monounsaturated fatty acids; PUFA = polyunsaturated fatty acids; SAT = saturated fatty acids concentrated source of a fatty acid called lauric acid, which has therapeutic effects upon gut bacterial flora. Numerous studies of indigenous traditional Pacific Island societies prior to westernization verify that coconut consumption has no adverse effects upon cardiovascular disease.

The oils we recommend are flaxseed, walnut, avocado, macadamia, coconut, and olive. Although soybean and wheat germ oils appear on paper to have acceptable fatty acid balances, both are concentrated sources of antinutrients known as lectins. Wheat germ oil is the highest dietary source of the lectin wheat germ agglutinin (WGA), and soybean oil contains soybean agglutinin (SBA). In animal models, both of those lectins have been shown to adversely influence gastrointestinal and immune function. Similarly, peanuts are not nuts but legumes. Peanut oil, just like soybean oil, is a concentrated source of the lectin peanut agglutinin (PNA).

What's Wrong with Peanut Oil and Peanuts?

If you look at peanut oil fatty acid composition in Table 11.4, you'll see that almost 80 percent is made up of cholesterol-lowering monounsaturated and polyunsaturated fats. Hence, on the surface, you might think that peanut oil would be helpful in preventing the artery-clogging process (atherosclerosis) that underlies coronary heart disease. Well, your idea is not a whole lot different from what nutritional scientists believed—that is, until they got around to actually testing peanut oil in laboratory animals. Starting in the 1960s and continuing into the 1980s, scientists found peanut oil to be unexpectedly atherogenic, causing arterial plaques to form in rabbits, rats, and primates—only a single study showed otherwise. In fact, peanut oil is so atherogenic that it continues to be routinely fed to rabbits to stimulate atherosclerosis to study the disease itself.

At first, it was not clear how a seemingly healthful oil could be so toxic in such a wide variety of animals. Then, in a series of experiments, David Kritchevsky, PhD, and colleagues at the Wistar Institute in Philadelphia showed that peanut oil lectin (PNA) was most likely responsible for the artery-clogging properties. A lectin is a fairly large protein molecule, and most nutritional scientists had assumed that digestive enzymes in the gut would degrade it into its component amino acids, so the intact lectin molecule would not be able to get into the bloodstream to do its dirty work. But they were wrong. It turned out that lectins were highly resistant to the gut's protein-shearing enzymes. An experiment conducted by Dr. Wang and colleagues and published in the prestigious medical journal *Lancet* revealed that PNA gets into the bloodstream intact in as little as 1 to 4 hours after participants ate a handful of roasted, salted peanuts. Even though the concentrations of PNA in the blood were quite low, they were still at amounts known to cause atherosclerosis in animal experiments. Lectins are a lot like superglue—it doesn't take much. Because these proteins contain carbohydrates, they can bind to a wide variety of cells in the body, including the cells lining the arteries. And indeed, it was found that PNA did its damage to the arteries by binding to a specific sugar receptor. So, the practical point here is to stay away from both peanuts and peanut oil. There are better choices.

How about Canola Oil?

Since the publication of *The Paleo Diet for Athletes* in 2005, I have now reversed my position on canola oil and can no longer support its consumption or use. Let me explain why. Canola oil is extracted from the seeds of the rape plant (*Brassica rapa* or *Brassica campestris*), which is a member of the broccoli, cabbage, Brussels sprouts, and kale family. Unquestionably, humans have eaten cabbage and its botanical relatives before historical times, and I still solidly support consumption of these healthy veggies. However, the concentrated oil from *Brassica* seeds is an entirely different proposition.

Before genetic modification by agronomists, rape plants produced a seed oil that maintained high levels (20–50 percent) of erucic acid (a monounsaturated fatty acid; lipid name: 22:1v9), which is toxic and causes tissue injury in many organs of experimental animals. In the 1970s, Canadian plant scientists developed a strain of rape plant that produced a seed with less than 2 percent erucic acid (hence the name canola oil). The erucic acid concentration of store-bought canola oil averages 0.6 percent. Nevertheless, several experiments in the 1970s demonstrated that even at low concentrations (2.0 percent and 0.88 percent), canola oil fed to rats could still cause small heart scarring that was deemed "pathological." A succession of current rat studies of low erucic canola oil performed by Dr. Naoki Ohara and colleagues at the Hatano Research Institute in Japan reported kidney injuries, elevations in blood sodium concentrations, and irregular alterations to a hormone (aldosterone) that controls blood pressure. Other adverse effects of canola oil consumption in animals at 10 percent of calories include decreased litter sizes, behavioral changes, and liver damage. A number of current human studies of canola/rapeseed oil by Sanna Poikonen, MD, and coworkers at the University of Tampere in Finland indicated it to be a potent allergen in adults and children that causes allergic cross-reactions from other environmental allergens. Based upon these brand-new findings in both humans and animals, I favor to err on the safe side, and can no longer recommend canola oil as a part of contemporary Paleo diets.

Nuts and Seeds

Except for peanuts, we recommend all nuts and seeds as healthful components of the Paleo Diet for Athletes. Many people have food allergies, and nuts are one of the more common ones. Always listen to your body; if you know or suspect that nuts do not agree with you, then don't eat them. This advice holds for all foods, including shellfish, which also frequently causes allergies. In Table 11.5 on page 208, you can see the fatty acid balance for commonly available nuts. Notice that except for walnuts and macadamia nuts, all other nuts maintain high ratios of omega-6 to omega-3. The ideal ratio in your diet should be about 2:1 or slightly lower. Because nuts are so calorically dense, they can very easily derail the best-laid dietary plans. If you use nuts as staples—rather than

TABLE 11.5

Fatty Acid Composition of Nuts and Seeds

NUT	OMEGA-6: OMEGA-3 RATIO	% MUFA	% PUFA	% SAT
Walnuts	4.2	23.6	69.7	6.7
Macadamia nuts	6.3	81.6	1.9	16.5
Pecans	20.9	59.5	31.5	9.0
Pine nuts	31.6	39.7	44.3	16.0
Cashews	47.6	61.6	17.6	20.8
Pistachios	51.9	55.5	31.8	12.7
Sesame seeds	58.2	39.5	45.9	14.6
Hazelnuts (filberts)	90.0	78.7	13.6	7.7
Pumpkin seeds	114.4	32.5	47.6	19.9
Brazil nuts	377.9	36.2	38.3	25.5
Sunflower seeds	472.0	9.2	69.0	11.0
Almonds	Extremely high (no omega-3s)	66.6	25.3	8.1
Coconut	Extremely high (no omega-3s)	4.4	1.3	94.3
Peanuts	Extremely high (no omega-3s)	52.1	33.3	14.6

MUFA = monounsaturated fatty acids; PUFA = polyunsaturated fatty acids; SAT = saturated fatty acids

lean meats, seafood, and fresh fruits and veggies—chances are that you will not get sufficient omega-3 fatty acids in your diet. Enjoy nuts, but use them carefully.

CHEATING

The Paleo Diet for Athletes is actually not a diet at all but, rather, a life-long pattern of eating that, besides improving athletic performance, will normalize body weight and reduce the risk for heart disease, cancer, and osteoporosis. It also plays a significant role in treating diabetes, hypertension, high blood cholesterol, inflammatory gut conditions, and certain autoimmune diseases. The positive health effects are thoroughly explained in *The Revised Paleo Diet* (2010, John Wiley & Sons) and in *The Paleo Answer* (2012, John Wiley & Sons).

In order for most people to make lifelong dietary changes, a number of behavioral techniques seem to be helpful. When giving up certain foods, most people do better psychologically when they know that they do not have to completely and forever ditch some of their favorites. The Paleo Diet for Athletes allows for what we call the 85:5 rule, which means that what you do infrequently will have little negative impact on the favorable effects of what you do most of the time.

Most people consume about 21 meals per week, plus snacks. It's perfectly acceptable and pleasurable if two or three of those meals include any food you want, as long as fresh meats, seafood, fruits, vegetables, healthful oils, and nuts and seeds make up roughly 85 percent of the balance of your weekly calories. The Paleo Diet for Athletes allows moderate alcohol and coffee consumption or occasional chocolates, bagels, or whatever your favorite food may be. Cheating and digressions now and then are of great emotional benefit, and—so long as they make up 15 percent or less of the overall diet—will have little impact on athletic performance and health effects. This recommendation, of course, does not include the non-Paleo foods that may be eaten immediately before, during, and after some workouts, as described in Chapters 2, 3, and 4.

EATING OUT AND ON THE ROAD

Many restaurants cater to vegetarians and increasingly more are offering menus for low-carb dieters. But, to date, very few offer Paleo meals. However, by ordering carefully, you can usually approximate the Paleo Diet for Athletes. The best strategy for breakfast is to order either an egg dish or some kind of fresh meat along with a bowl of fresh fruit. Poached eggs are a good bet because they will not be prepared with the wrong kinds of fat, which invariably accompany omelets and fried eggs. Also, poached or hard-boiled eggs are less likely to contain oxidized cholesterol, a by-product of fried eggs that especially promotes atherosclerosis in laboratory animals.

Lunch and dinner are usually no problem; most restaurants offer some kind of fish, seafood, or lean-meat entrée for these meals. Remember, the key is to get a big piece of animal protein as your main dish. Strive for simplicity: Forsake fancy entrées made with complicated sauces for simpler versions. To even out the acid load, order a salad (hold the croutons) and request steamed veggies instead of the compulsory bread or potatoes. For the salad dressing, vinegar and oil—particularly olive oil—are fine in a pinch. See if you can get fresh fruit for dessert.

For road trips, pack a cooler with fruits, veggies, salads, and leftover meats and seafood. A good strategy at dinnertime is to cook about two or three times as much meat or seafood as you will eat, and keep the rest for breakfast and lunch the next few days. For example, barbecue a big chunk of London broil for dinner one evening, refrigerate the leftovers, and the next day slice the beef into a mixed salad and toss with flaxseed oil and lemon juice. Voilà—an instant Paleo picnic lunch! If you don't have a cooler, check out the deli or seafood section of a supermarket to get cooked meat or shrimp. Proceed to the produce section and grab some fresh fruit, avocados, and crisp veggies. Always keep a sharp knife and some utensils in your car so that you don't have to deal with cutting up meat with a plastic knife.

CHAPTER 12

Paleo Recipes

The bottom line in creating Paleo Diet for Athletes recipes with modern foods is to keep it simple. Our Stone Age ancestors ate virtually all of their foods fresh and minimally processed. If you do likewise, your health and performance will soar. Whenever possible, choose your foods in this order: (1) fresh, (2) frozen, (3) canned. When you prepare Stone Age recipes with contemporary foods, bear in mind that you want to make sure the ingredients are free of grains, dairy products, salt, refined sugars, legumes (including peanuts), and yeast-containing foods such as baked goods, pickled foods, vinegar, and fermented foods and beverages. Be sure your food choices contain only permitted oils, and remember to select fresh meat, preferably grass fed. Keep in mind the foundation of the Paleo Diet for Athletes: fresh meats, seafood, and fruits and veggies!

PALEO FOOD REPLACEMENTS

Our modern palettes have become jaded with the never-ending onslaught of salt, starch, sugar, and fat laced everywhere into processed foods. After a few weeks of Paleo dieting, you will notice a wonderful change emerging in your taste buds.

Subtle flavors that you never knew existed will materialize. You won't need to add sugar to your fresh strawberries—they will taste delightfully sweet all by themselves. Avocados will have a luscious, creamy flavor that needs no added salt or anything else. Once you have given up sweet, sticky doughnuts, a fresh nectarine will never have tasted so good. Spices you never knew existed will enliven your steaks and roasts, and you will be able to discern these subtle yet incredible flavors because you will no longer be drowning your taste buds in salt and refined sugars.

Vinegar: Vinegar contains acetic acid in a 5 percent solution and consequently contributes to the net metabolic acidosis that plagues the typical American diet. Additionally, unless the vinegar is distilled, it will contain small quantities of yeast—another non-Paleo food substance that should be avoided. We recommend you replace vinegar in your recipes with either lemon or lime juice.

Salt: One of the toughest modern dietary routines to kick is the salt habit. Salt is added to almost everything. In fact, most of us take in an appalling 10 grams per day! These salt substitutes will not only help you get the salt out but will also enliven your recipes: lemon crystals, lemon pepper devoid of salt, powdered garlic, powdered onion, ground red pepper, chili powder, black pepper, cumin, turmeric, celery seeds, coriander seeds, and any commercially available salt-free spice mixtures.

Sugars: There is absolutely no doubt that our Stone Age ancestors had a sweet tooth. Field studies of hunter-gatherers show that they would endure enormous numbers of bee stings to get hold of honey. During certain times of the year, they would gorge themselves with a pound or more of honey a day. However, they couldn't eat it day in and day out, all year long, because it simply wasn't available. Similarly, other naturally occurring sweets such as dates, figs, or maple sugar would have been available seasonally for only a few short weeks during the entire year. We should follow the hunter-gatherer example and get refined sugars out of our diets. That doesn't mean you have to ban sweets entirely—you can eat all of the fresh fruit that you like (unless you are overweight or have one or more symptoms of metabolic syndrome (type 2 diabetes, high blood pressure, high cholesterol, obesity, and gout)), and you can add certain spices such as vanilla, ginger, mint leaves, cinnamon, and nutmeg to recipes. Also, it is entirely permissible to add fruit purees sweetened with lemon or lime juice to your recipes.

Fat: Replace the "bad" fats (trans fats, margarine, and shortening) with these oils: olive, flaxseed, walnut, macadamia, coconut, and avocado. Remember that flaxseed and walnut oils are delicate and susceptible to breakdown by heat and therefore should be used after, not during, cooking.

Alcohol: Perhaps the most important component of any dietary plan is getting people to stick with it. The best way to make you instantly give up on the Paleo Diet for Athletes—or any diet, for that matter—is to make "Thou Shalt Nots." You will notice from Chapter 9 that there are no—repeat, no—absolute requirements in *The Paleo Diet for Athletes*. We have deliberately incorporated this strategy into our nutritional plan to help you with compliance. If you enjoy an occasional glass of wine with your dinner, have it! Realize that you have a certain number of open meals during the week (as fully outlined in Chapter 11), which allow you to enjoy any food you like. However, bear in mind that the further you deviate from the basic plan, the less likely you are to achieve your health and performance goals. Obviously, alcohol was not part of any hunter-gatherer diet, and we do not recommend regular consumption of alcohol for athletes, either. However, it's perfectly acceptable to use certain alcoholic beverages such as wine to add flavor to marinades and sauces. Much of the alcohol is vaporized during cooking.

RECIPES

Meat Dishes

PORK

Barcelona Pork Loin

⅓ cup chili powder

1 teaspoon dried leaf thyme

1 teaspoon Mexican oregano

⅛ teaspoon cloves

⅛ teaspoon allspice

1–2 tablespoons chicken stock

2 pounds boneless pork loin

½ cup water

Preheat the oven to 350°F. In a small bowl, mix together the chili powder, thyme, oregano, cloves, allspice, and stock to form a paste. Thoroughly rub the paste over all sides of the pork loin. Put the pork loin in a small lidded roasting pan. Add the water to the pan. Cover the pan and place in the oven for 2 hours, until tender. Remove the pork from the oven and let stand, covered, for 30 minutes before slicing.

Serves 4

Barbecued Lemon-Pepper Pork Steaks

1 onion, minced

2 teaspoons thyme

¼ teaspoon ground black pepper

¼ teaspoon ground red pepper

2 cloves garlic, minced

½ cup olive oil

6 pork steaks, each 1" thick

⅓ cup fresh lemon juice

1½ teaspoons grated lemon peel

Warm up your grill. Combine the onion, thyme, and ground peppers in a small bowl. Add the garlic and oil, and thoroughly blend the ingredients with a whisk. Mop the steaks with a paper towel, and then smother with the lemon juice. Brush both sides of the steaks with some of the sauce. Briefly flame the steaks over high heat and sprinkle with the lemon peel. Put the steaks on a cool side of the grill and baste liberally with the remaining sauce. Cook about 10 minutes per side under a closed grill.

Serves 6

Oven-Baked Pecan Pork Chops

1 egg, beaten

2 tablespoons olive oil

1 tablespoon dry sherry or water

Ground ginger and garlic powder

4 lean pork chops

¼ cup finely chopped pecans

Preheat the oven to 350°F. In a shallow bowl, beat together the egg, oil, and sherry. Add ginger and garlic powder to taste. Dip the chops in the mixture, and then coat evenly with the pecans. Arrange the pork chops in a single layer in a glass baking dish coated with additional oil. Bake for 30 minutes, turn, and bake until tender, about 20 minutes longer.

Serves 4

Mexico City 1968 Pork Loin Appetizer

½ pound pork tenderloin

3 tablespoons olive oil

1 small carrot, sliced

1 small onion, sliced

4 bay leaves

2 teaspoons minced garlic

2 large tomatoes, peeled and chopped

1 teaspoon black peppercorns

2 stems fresh rosemary

2 tablespoons lime juice

In a large skillet, brown the pork loin in the oil, and then brown the carrot and onion. Place in a 4- to 6-quart pot lightly coated with olive oil, and add the bay leaves, garlic, tomatoes, peppercorns, and rosemary. Add water to cover, and simmer for 1½ hours, adding the lime juice during the last few minutes.

Remove the pork loin and thinly slice it. Place in a dish and cover with the vegetables and sauce. Discard the bay leaves before serving.

Serves 6

CHICKEN AND POULTRY

Ankara Chicken

4 whole skinless chicken breasts

1 large carrot, cut into 1" pieces

1 large rib celery, cut into 1" pieces

½ onion, sliced

2 bay leaves

6 peppercorns

½ teaspoon cumin

½ pound shelled walnuts

3 cloves garlic

Freshly ground black pepper

2 tablespoons olive oil

1 teaspoon paprika

Place the chicken breasts, carrot, celery, onion, bay leaves, and peppercorns in a large Dutch oven. Add cold water to cover the chicken by 1½". Heat to a boil, and skim off all froth and solids that rise to the top. Reduce heat to low. Simmer gently until the chicken is tender, 20 to 30 minutes. Remove the chicken and allow to cool, then debone it. Set aside the cooking liquid, discarding the bay leaves. In a blender or food processor, combine the cumin, walnuts, garlic, and ground pepper. Blend well, and then pour in 1 cup of the cooking liquid. Continue blending until smooth. Cut the chicken breasts in half crosswise, and shred the meat. Mix with the sauce and add ground pepper as needed. Arrange the meat on a platter. Blend the oil and paprika together, and drizzle over the chicken.

Serves 6

Lebanese Walnut Chicken

1 tablespoon olive oil

½ teaspoon powdered cinnamon

½ teaspoon ground nutmeg

2 or 3 cloves

⅓ pound seedless grapes

1½ cups dry white wine

1 tablespoon lemon juice

2 tablespoons chicken stock

1 tablespoon finely chopped onion

2 tablespoons walnut meal

Freshly ground black pepper

½ teaspoon dried thyme

¼ teaspoon chili powder

2¼ pounds skinless chicken breasts

2 large tomatoes, sliced

1 tablespoon chopped walnuts

Preheat the oven to 375°F. Pour the oil in a skillet over medium heat. Add the cinnamon, nutmeg, and cloves. Sear for a few seconds, then take out the cloves. Add the whole grapes and cook for 2 minutes. Add the wine, lemon juice, and stock, and cook to reduce the mixture by half (roughly 8 minutes). When the sauce has reduced to a syrupy consistency, remove from the heat and let cool. Mix the onion, walnut meal, pepper, thyme, and chili powder together in a bowl, and pat onto each chicken breast. Place the chicken breasts in a flat glass baking dish lightly coated with olive oil, and bake for 35 to 40 minutes, or until done. Place on a bed of sliced tomatoes, pour the sauce over them, and sprinkle with the chopped walnuts.

Serves 2

Chicken à la Madrid

4 large skinless chicken breasts

2 red bell peppers, chopped

1 green bell pepper, chopped

6 plum tomatoes, peeled

2 onions, finely chopped

½ teaspoon crushed Anaheim chilies

1 small sprig fresh rosemary

3 cloves garlic, crushed

1 pint reconstituted lime juice

1 pint boiling water

½ teaspoon cayenne pepper

Freshly ground black pepper

Place all the ingredients into a large saucepan. Bring to a boil, then reduce the heat and simmer for 40 minutes, until the chicken is tender.

Serves 4

Zesty Grilled Turkey Breast

5 cloves garlic, minced

¼ cup lime juice

¼ cup lemon juice

¼ cup olive oil

1 teaspoon paprika

1 teaspoon cumin

1 teaspoon turmeric

½ teaspoon white pepper

1½ pounds turkey breast slices, pounded ¼" thick

1 tablespoon olive oil (for basting)

Mix all sauce ingredients together in a blender. Grill or broil the turkey breasts while brushing with the oil to keep them moist. Grill on each side for about 5 minutes. Top each slice with about 2 to 3 tablespoons of the sauce.

Serves 4

Roasted Cornish Game Hens

3 Cornish hens (1½ pounds each)

½ cup unsweetened applesauce

2 teaspoons lemon juice

¼ teaspoon rubbed sage

¼ teaspoon freshly ground black pepper

¼ teaspoon paprika

¼ teaspoon garlic powder

Preheat the oven to 350°F. Remove the skins from the hens and cut the hens in half lengthwise. Place in a shallow glass roasting pan lightly coated with olive oil. Combine the applesauce and remaining ingredients. Brush half over the hens, and set aside the remaining mixture. Bake for 30 minutes. Baste the hens with the reserved applesauce mixture, and bake for 15 to 30 minutes longer, or until done.

Serves 6

BEEF

Sirloin Tips and Tomato Sauce

1½ pounds tomatoes, peeled

2 tablespoons lemon juice

1 onion, thinly sliced

2 tablespoons olive oil

1½ pounds sirloin tips, cubed

1 teaspoon garlic powder

½ teaspoon cinnamon

Freshly ground black pepper

Puree the tomatoes in a blender along with the lemon juice. In a large skillet, brown the onion in the oil. Add the sirloin and cook until brown, stirring frequently. Add the pureed tomato sauce and spices, and simmer for 1 hour.

Serves 4 to 6

Braised Beef with Walnuts, Prunes, and Peaches

3 pounds lean beef

2 cloves garlic, minced

3 tablespoons chopped fresh parsley

3 tablespoons olive oil

1 medium onion, chopped

3 stems fresh thyme

7 ounces white wine

1 large tomato, chopped

3 ounces walnuts, chopped

10 dried prunes, chopped (nonsulfured; available at health food stores)

10 dried peaches, chopped (nonsulfured; available at health food stores)

Cover the beef with the garlic and parsley. Heat the oil in a large casserole dish and brown the beef. Mix in the onion, thyme, and wine, and cook over medium heat for 10 minutes, stirring frequently. Add the tomato and walnuts. Cover and cook over medium-low heat for 90 minutes. Stir in the prunes and peaches, and cook for 15 minutes longer, covered, until the beef is tender and the sauce is thickened.

Serves 6

Isola Pot Roast

3–4 pounds lean pot roast

2 tablespoons olive oil

Freshly ground black pepper

1 pound tomatoes, peeled

1 cup dry red wine

1 medium onion, chopped

1 cup chopped celery

1 tablespoon minced parsley

2 teaspoons oregano

1 clove garlic, minced

Preheat the oven to 300°F. In a Dutch oven, brown the roast in the oil. Add pepper to taste. Puree the tomatoes in a blender and pour over the meat. Stir in the remaining ingredients. Cover and bake for 3 to 4 hours, checking occasionally. If pan liquid seems low, add a small amount of water while roasting.

Serves 6 to 8

Beef Kebabs

1 pound top sirloin steak

1 small onion, finely chopped

½ cup Pinot Noir red wine

8 cubes (1" × 1") fresh pineapple

8 cherry tomatoes

1 can (8 ounces) salt-free water chestnuts, drained

Cut the steak into ¼"-thick strips. Combine the onion and wine in a bowl with the beef strips. Marinate for 4 hours. Alternately thread beef strips, pineapple cubes, cherry tomatoes, and water chestnuts onto metal skewers. Place kebabs on grill over medium coals. Grill 4 minutes, turning once.

Serves 4

Grilled London Broil

1½ pounds London broil steaks, each 1½" thick

5 large cloves garlic, minced

1 teaspoon powdered onion

¼ cup dry red wine

¼ cup lime juice

Place all the ingredients in a shallow dish and marinate in the refrigerator for at least 4 and up to 24 hours. Remove the steaks from the marinade and grill for 12 to 16 minutes for medium-rare, turning once. Place on a cutting board and, holding a sharp knife at a 45-degree angle, cut the steak across the grain into thin slices.

Serves 2 to 4

ORGAN MEATS

Apricot-Raisin Tongue

1 beef tongue

1 tablespoon garlic powder

3 bay leaves

1 tablespoon marjoram

1 pound dried apricots (nonsulfured; available at health food stores)

1 pound tomatoes, peeled

½ cup lime juice

½ cup lemon juice

¼ teaspoon basil

¼ teaspoon ground red pepper

1 tablespoon mustard powder

½ cup raisins

Put the tongue in a large pot, cover completely with water, and bring to a rapid boil. Replace the water and bring to a second boil. Replace the water again and bring to a slow, easy boil. Add the garlic powder, bay leaves, and marjoram, and cook until done, about 2 hours. Discard the water and bay leaves. Skin the tongue and let it cool. Cut into thin slices. Preheat the oven to 350°F. Place the apricots in a saucepan. Puree the tomatoes in a blender. Add the tomato sauce and the remaining ingredients to the apricots, and bring to a boil. Continue to simmer until the mixture thickens. Layer the sliced tongue in a flat casserole dish and pour the sauce over it. Bake for about 20 minutes.

Serves 4

Basque Beef Heart

½ pound beef heart

½ white onion, chopped

4 peppercorns

2 whole cloves

2 teaspoons garlic powder

1 tablespoon flaxseed oil

1 tablespoon lemon juice

1 cup thinly sliced celery

1 cup chopped red onion

1 cup diced tomatoes

½ teaspoon rosemary

½ teaspoon thyme

Put the beef heart in a large pot filled with cold water and add the white onion, peppercorns, cloves, and garlic powder. Bring to a rolling boil, then reduce the heat, cover, and cook until the beef heart is fork-tender. Cool, then cut off the surface covering of the heart and slice it into cubes. Mix together the remaining ingredients and ladle over the beef cubes prior to serving.

Serves 2

Beef Liver in Lime Sauce

1 pound beef liver, sliced ⅜" thick

1 clove garlic, slivered

½ teaspoon cumin

Freshly ground black pepper

2 tablespoons salt-free tomato sauce

2 tablespoons olive oil

2 tablespoons lime juice

1½ tablespoons pecan nut flour

2 tablespoons water

Broil the liver on both sides until lightly browned but not fully cooked. Cut into 1" squares. Place the liver, garlic, cumin, and pepper to taste in a shallow skillet over low heat. Add the tomato sauce and oil and cover with water. Bring to a boil and simmer. In a bowl, mix the lime juice, nut flour, and water until the mixture is the texture of soft custard. Pour into the center of a pan and stir until smooth. Fold into the cooking liver and simmer 5 minutes longer. Serve hot over steamed fresh vegetables.

Serves 4 to 6

Hungarian Chicken Livers with Mushrooms

1 onion, finely chopped

1 green pepper, finely chopped

7 tablespoons olive oil

½ pound mushrooms, sliced

1½ pounds chicken livers, cut into bite-size pieces

1 tablespoon paprika

1 tablespoon nut flour

½ cup chicken stock

Freshly ground black pepper

4 tablespoons dry red wine

3 tablespoons finely chopped parsley

In a large skillet, cook the onion and green pepper in 5 tablespoons of the oil for 3 to 5 minutes or until soft, stirring frequently. Add the mushrooms and cook for 3 to 5 minutes longer. Put in a bowl and add the remaining 2 tablespoons of oil. Add the chicken livers to the skillet and cook for 5 minutes. Return the vegetables to the skillet. Add the paprika and nut flour and stir until the liver and vegetables are evenly coated. Add the stock and simmer until the livers are cooked to the desired state. Season with pepper and reduce the heat. Pour in the wine and reheat, but do not boil. Serve the chicken livers garnished with parsley.

Serves 6

Rocky Mountain Oysters

2 pounds beef testicles

2 bay leaves

1 tablespoon basil

Freshly ground black pepper

1 cup nut flour

Garlic powder

Turmeric

1 cup red wine

Ground red pepper

Olive oil

With a sharp knife, cut and remove the sturdy membrane that covers each testicle and discard. Place the testicles in a large pot filled with water and add the bay leaves and basil. Bring to a slow boil and simmer until done. Let cool and slice each testicle into ¼"-thick ovals. Sprinkle with black pepper to taste. Mix the nut flour, garlic powder, and turmeric to taste in a bowl. In a separate bowl, season the wine with red pepper to taste. Roll each slice in the dry mixture, then dip into the seasoned wine. Sauté in olive oil until slightly browned or tender. Drain on paper towels.

Serves 4 to 6

GAME MEATS

Rooke's Roast Venison

2 yellow onions, sliced

3 carrots, sliced diagonally

1 rib celery, finely chopped

¼ cup olive oil

3 cups red wine

½ cup lemon juice

¼ cup Grand Marnier

1 quart water

1 branch fresh thyme

1 bay leaf

2 tablespoons black peppercorns

5 pounds venison roast

2 cups beef stock

3 tablespoons flaxseed oil

Freshly ground black pepper

In a medium-size pot, cook the onions, carrots, and celery in the olive oil about 5 minutes, until soft, stirring frequently. Add the wine, lemon juice, Grand Marnier, water, thyme, bay leaf, and peppercorns. Bring to a boil and simmer for 20 minutes. Cool, then pour over the venison and refrigerate for 1 to 2 days, stirring occasionally. Remove the venison from the marinade 2 hours prior to cooking. Preheat the oven to 450°F. Place the venison in a roasting pan and roast for 10 minutes, then reduce the heat to 350°F and roast for ½ to 2 hours longer, until done. In the meantime, bring the marinade to a boil over medium heat and reduce to 2 cups, about 45 minutes. Add the stock and simmer to reduce the marinade until it starts to thicken, about 12 minutes. Turn off the heat, cool the marinade to lukewarm, pour in the flaxseed oil, and season to taste with ground pepper. Discard the bay leaf. Cool the venison, slice into serving portions, and cover with the sauce.

Serves 5 or more

Moose Rump Roast

5 to 6 pounds moose rump roast
Olive oil
1 teaspoon garlic powder
Freshly ground black pepper
1 large onion, sliced
2 tablespoons lemon juice
2 tablespoons lime juice
½ cup red Zinfandel wine
1 cup water
Cumin

Preheat the oven to 325°F. Rub the roast completely with oil. Sprinkle on the garlic powder and pepper to taste. Put the onion into the bottom of a roasting pan. Pour 1 tablespoon each of the lemon and lime juices over the onions. Place the roast on the onion slices. Pour the rest of the juices over the meat. Add the wine and water. Cover the pan tightly with foil and bake for 3½ to 4 hours, adding more water as necessary to keep moist. Add cumin and more pepper to taste.

Serves 8 to 10

Buffalo Steaks with Mushroom Sauce

1½ pounds buffalo steak

3 tablespoons freshly chopped thyme

¼ teaspoon garlic powder

Freshly ground black pepper

2 teaspoons + 4 tablespoons olive oil

2 shallots, chopped

½ pound fresh mushrooms, sliced

1½ cups red wine

1 cup beef stock

1 tablespoon chopped parsley

1 tablespoon chives

1 tablespoon flaxseed oil

Cut the steak into 4 pieces and cover with the thyme, garlic powder, and pepper. Cook on both sides in 2 teaspoons of the olive oil for 2 to 3 minutes, or until the centers are still pink, stirring frequently. Remove to a platter and keep warm. Cook the shallots and mushrooms in the remaining 4 tablespoons olive oil, turning frequently. Add the wine and cook to reduce until only about one-fourth is left. Add the stock and reduce until about one-half is left. Season with more pepper to taste and cool. Add the parsley, chives, and flaxseed oil. Pour over the steaks before serving.

Serves 2 to 3

Tarragon Rabbit

4 rabbit legs (boned)
1 tablespoon olive oil
1 cup dry sherry
1 tablespoon tomato puree
1 teaspoon garlic powder
1 teaspoon onion powder
2 tablespoons dried tarragon
Freshly ground black pepper

In a large pan, cook the rabbit slowly in the oil, stirring frequently, but do not brown. Add the sherry, tomato puree, and garlic and onion powders. Stir in 1 tablespoon of the tarragon and season to taste with pepper. Cover and simmer gently for 30 to 40 minutes. Just before serving, turn off the heat and stir in the remaining tablespoon of tarragon.

Serves 4

Barbecued Ostrich Medallions

8 ounces Cabernet Sauvignon wine

1 red onion, finely chopped

1 Jerusalem artichoke, finely chopped

1 green onion, finely chopped

1 rib celery, finely chopped

2 tablespoons fresh or frozen (thawed) mashed blueberries

2 stems fresh thyme

2 stems fresh basil

Juice and chopped rind of 1 lemon

Juice and chopped rind of 1 lime

1 pound ostrich medallions

Combine all the ingredients except the ostrich into a marinade in a large bowl. Add the ostrich and refrigerate for 12 hours. Remove the medallions and save the marinade. Grill the meat until it is cooked to taste. Reduce the marinade until it turns into a thick sauce. Pour over the ostrich.

Serves 4

Seafood

SHELLFISH

Peloponnesian Shrimp

1 teaspoon garlic, finely chopped

2 tablespoons olive oil

2 cups tomatoes, diced

½ cup dry white wine

¼ cup fresh basil, chopped

1 teaspoon dried oregano

Freshly ground black pepper

1½ pounds shrimp, peeled and deveined

⅛ teaspoon ground red pepper

Briefly cook the garlic in 1 tablespoon of the oil, stirring frequently. Add the tomatoes and cook for about a minute. Add the wine, basil, oregano, and black pepper to taste. Cook over moderate heat for 8 to 10 minutes. Heat the remaining 1 tablespoon of oil in a large skillet and add the shrimp. Cook rapidly, 1 to 2 minutes, or until the shrimp turn pink. Dust with the red pepper. Pour the tomato sauce over the shrimp.

Serves 4

Cancún Zesty Mussels

5 pounds mussels

2 tablespoons olive oil

1 cup water

2 cups white wine

½ teaspoon cumin

½ teaspoon garlic powder

¼ teaspoon ground red pepper

3 to 4 large red onions, cut in rings

Freshly ground black pepper

1 bunch parsley

Lemon slices

Rinse and clean the mussels. In a 1-gallon pot, combine the oil, water, wine, cumin, garlic powder, red pepper, onions, and black pepper to taste. Bring to a boil. Add the drained mussels and return to a boil for 15 to 20 minutes. When all of the mussel shells have opened, they are done. Garnish with parsley and serve with lemon slices.

Serves 2 to 4

Tillamook Steamed Clams

6 ounces clams (if open, tap on shell; if it does not close, discard)
Chopped parsley
Olive oil (for serving)

Under cold running water, scrub the sand from the clams with a stiff brush. Place the clams on a rack in a steamer. Fill with enough water to just cover the bottom of the rack. Bring to a boil, reduce the heat, cover the steamer, and steam the clams until they just open, 5 to 10 minutes. Drain and sprinkle with parsley. Serve in soup bowls with oil on the side. To eat the clams, pull them from their shells by their necks and dip in olive oil.

Serves 1

Omega-3 Stuffed Crab

1 pound shredded crabmeat (6 crabs)
Freshly ground black pepper
Paprika
Turmeric
Flaxseed Oil Mayonnaise (see page 241)
1 clove garlic
Olive oil
Cucumber slices

Combine the crabmeat with the pepper, paprika, and turmeric to taste. Add sufficient Flaxseed Oil Mayonnaise to moisten. Rub six crab shells with the garlic and oil. Pile the crab mixture in the shells. Cover with foil and place in a large baking dish. Bake at 400°F for 20 to 25 minutes, or until done. Garnish with cucumber slices.

Serves 6

Lemon Dill Shrimp

3 cloves garlic, minced

⅓ cup olive oil

1 pound large shrimp, shelled and deveined

2 tablespoons lemon juice

⅓ cup fresh dill, minced

In a large skillet, cook the garlic in the oil until soft, stirring frequently. Stir in the shrimp and cook until just pink. Add the lemon juice and dill and blend well.

Serves 4

FISH

Cordain's Fennel Salmon

3 tablespoons extra-virgin olive oil

1 small bulb fresh fennel, cored and slivered

1½ pounds salmon fillets

1 teaspoon dried dill weed

1 teaspoon dried basil

Preheat the oven to 400°F. Coat the bottom and sides of a glass baking dish with 2 tablespoons of the oil. Spread the fennel over the bottom of the dish. Carefully place the salmon on top of the fennel and drizzle the remaining 1 tablespoon of oil over it. Sprinkle with the dill and basil. Cover with foil and bake for 20 to 25 minutes. Serve with steamed broccoli and sliced raw cucumbers.

Serves 4 to 6

Sauterne Squid

1 pound squid, each about 2" long

Pecan nut flour

1 teaspoon garlic powder

½ cup olive oil

¼ cup Sauterne wine

1 tablespoon lemon juice

2 tomatoes, cut into wedges

Parsley sprigs

Wash the squid completely, remove the ink sack and soft backbone from each head, and strip off the black membrane covering the squid. Coat the squid with the nut flour and sprinkle with the garlic powder. Heat the oil in a heavy skillet and cook the squid until brown, stirring frequently. Turn off the heat. Pour the wine over the squid and add the lemon juice. Let stand for 5 to 10 minutes, then drain. Garnish with tomato wedges and parsley sprigs.

Serves 4

Orange Poached Fish

4 medium fillets of any whitefish

¼ cup dry white wine

6 black peppercorns

1 bay leaf

1 small onion, sliced

1 medium orange, quartered

Dried dill weed

In a large skillet, place the fish in a single layer. Add the wine, peppercorns, bay leaf, onion, and enough water to just cover the fish. Poach over medium heat until tender, then remove the fish from the pan and drain on paper towels. Squeeze the juice from the orange over the fish, and dust with dill before serving.

Serves 4

Little Valley Stuffed Trout

½ teaspoon dried dill weed

2 tablespoons finely chopped fresh parsley

2 tablespoons finely chopped yellow onion

¼ cup slivered almonds

1 pound trout (brook trout if you can get one; rainbow trout will do)

Lemon juice

Freshly ground black pepper

Preheat the oven to 400°F. In a small bowl, mix the dill, parsley, onion, and almonds. Fill the cavity of the trout with this mixture. Place the fish on foil and liberally squeeze lemon juice over the fish. Add pepper to taste. Seal the foil and bake for about 25 minutes, until the fish flakes easily with a fork.

Serves 2 to 4

Reese River Barbecued Catfish with Peach Salsa

4 catfish fillets

½ teaspoon freshly ground black pepper

½ teaspoon garlic powder

1 teaspoon ground red pepper

Peach Salsa (see page 245)

Oil and preheat the grill. Sprinkle the catfish fillets with pepper, garlic powder, and red pepper. Place the grill about 4" from the heat source. Cook for about 5 minutes on each side, or until the fish flakes easily with a fork. Serve with Peach Salsa spooned over the fillets.

Serves 2 to 4

CONDIMENTS

Flaxseed Oil Mayonnaise

1 egg

1 tablespoon lemon juice

¼ teaspoon mustard powder

1 cup flaxseed oil

In a blender, combine the egg, lemon juice, and mustard powder and blend for 3 to 5 seconds. Continue blending and slowly add the oil. Blend until thick. Put into a tightly sealed plastic container and refrigerate. The mayonnaise should keep for 5 to 7 days.

Makes 1½ cups

All-Natural Catsup

4 cups vine-ripened fresh tomatoes, diced

1 small sweet onion, diced

¼ teaspoon crushed garlic

½ sweet red bell pepper, diced

1 whole bay leaf

½ Granny Smith apple, peeled, cored, and diced

½ teaspoon allspice

½ teaspoon ground mace

½ cinnamon stick

1 tablespoon black peppercorns

½ teaspoon celery seed

½ cup lemon juice

⅛ teaspoon cayenne pepper

Into a 4-quart saucepan, place the tomatoes, onion, garlic, pepper, bay leaf, and apple. In a small cloth spice bag, put the allspice, mace, cinnamon stick, peppercorns, and celery seed, and place into the tomato mixture. Bring to a boil, and cook until reduced by half, stirring frequently. Remove spice bag and bay leaf. Puree in a food processor until well blended. Return to the saucepan and add lemon juice and cayenne pepper. Continue cooking until catsup reaches a thick, spreadable consistency. Stir frequently, and watch for sticking and scorching as it thickens. Refrigerate or freeze in a well-sealed container.

Makes about 2 cups

Tartar Sauce

1 cup Flaxseed Oil Mayonnaise (see page 241)

¼ cup finely chopped onion

1 tablespoon lemon juice

½ teaspoon dried dill weed

Mix all the ingredients together. Chill before serving.

Makes 1 cup

Colorado Ranch Dressing

1 cup Flaxseed Oil Mayonnaise (see page 241)
1 cup coconut milk
1 teaspoon dried dill weed
½ teaspoon garlic powder
½ teaspoon dried basil
Freshly ground black pepper

Mix all the ingredients together. Refrigerate at least 1 hour before serving.

Makes 1¾ cups

Russian Flaxseed Salad Dressing

1 cup fresh tomatoes
½ cup flaxseed oil
½ cup lemon juice
1 tablespoon honey
1 teaspoon paprika
1 teaspoon onion powder
½ teaspoon garlic powder

Put all the ingredients into a blender and blend until smooth. Refrigerate.

Makes 1½ cups

Tomato Flaxseed Dressing

⅓ cup tomato puree

½ cup flaxseed oil

⅓ cup lime juice

½ teaspoon garlic powder

½ teaspoon onion powder

1 tablespoon honey

Put all the ingredients into a blender and blend until smooth. Refrigerate.

Makes 1¼ cups

Garden-Fresh Salsa

2 cloves garlic

1 large yellow onion, quartered

1 green bell pepper, quartered and seeded

2 jalapeño peppers, stemmed, seeded, and chopped

6 tomatoes, peeled, seeded, and chopped

1 cup fresh cilantro

Freshly ground black pepper

Mince the garlic in a food processor. Add the onion, bell pepper, and jalapeño peppers, and pulse until barely chopped. Add the tomatoes and cilantro, and process until combined but slightly chunky. Add pepper to taste. Refrigerate before using.

Makes 6 to 8 cups

Peach Salsa

1 cup peeled and finely chopped fresh peaches

¼ cup chopped red onion

¼ cup chopped Anaheim chile peppers

½ tablespoon lime juice

½ tablespoon lemon juice

½ teaspoon honey

Cayenne pepper

Combine all the ingredients in a medium bowl. Cover and chill up to 6 hours.

Makes 1½ cups

Sacramento Guacamole

3 ripe avocados

1 teaspoon fresh lemon juice

1 teaspoon coarsely ground black pepper

1 teaspoon garlic powder

1 jalapeño pepper, stemmed, seeded, and finely diced

Mash the avocados with a fork or potato masher until smooth. Stir in the remaining ingredients until well mixed. Refrigerate if not eaten immediately.

Makes 3 cups

Coronado Barbecue Sauce

2 teaspoons olive oil
¼ cup minced onion
1 tablespoon minced, seeded jalapeño pepper
¼ cup All-Natural Catsup (see page 242)
1 tablespoon honey
¼ teaspoon mustard powder
Dash of ground red pepper
2 cups diced tomatoes
Freshly ground black pepper

Heat the oil in a stainless steel saucepan. Add the onion and jalapeño pepper and cook over moderate heat, stirring, until soft, about 3 minutes. Add the All-Natural Catsup, honey, mustard, and red pepper and bring to a simmer. Add the tomatoes and simmer over low heat, stirring until thickened, about 10 minutes. Puree the sauce in a blender or food processor until smooth. Pass through a strainer and season with black pepper to taste. Serve at room temperature.

Makes 2 cups

VEGETABLE DISHES

Stir-Fried Garlic Asparagus

1 clove garlic, minced

2 tablespoons olive oil

1 pound fresh asparagus spears

1 tablespoon lemon juice

Cook the garlic in the oil until soft, stirring frequently. Add the asparagus spears. Cook until tender, 3 to 5 minutes. Pour the lemon juice over the asparagus.

Serves 4

Spicy Lemon Broccoli

4 cups small broccoli florets

1 tablespoon olive oil

2 teaspoons freshly grated lemon peel

Crushed red pepper

Place a vegetable steamer in a medium saucepan and fill with water to the bottom of the steamer. Place the broccoli in the steamer and bring to a boil. Cover and cook for 2 to 3 minutes. Remove the broccoli. Heat the oil in a skillet over medium heat. Add the lemon peel and crushed red pepper to taste. Cook, stirring frequently, until the peel begins to brown, about 1 minute. Add the broccoli and stir until hot, about 1 minute.

Serves 4

Crunchy Garlic Broccoli

1 tablespoon olive oil

4 cups broccoli florets

2 cloves garlic, run through a press

Heat the oil in a large skillet. Add the broccoli, cover, and cook for 3 minutes, stirring occasionally. Turn the heat to low and cook for 2 minutes, or until just tender. Add the garlic, and cook for 1 minute.

Serves 4

Marinated Broccoli Stalks

2 pounds fresh broccoli

1 tablespoon lemon juice

1 tablespoon olive oil

¼ teaspoon dried dill weed

1 clove garlic, minced

Red cabbage leaves

Detach broccoli florets from the stalks, leaving only the secondary stalks attached to the main stalk. (Reserve florets for another use.) Cut off and discard the tough bottom end of the main stalk. Cut the remaining stalks diagonally into ½" slices. (You should have about 2 cups.) Whisk together the lemon juice, oil, dill, and garlic in a medium bowl. Add the sliced stalks and stir to coat evenly. Cover and refrigerate for 3 hours. Serve on cabbage leaves.

Serves 4

Baked Walnut-Stuffed Carrots

4 large carrots, washed and pared
1 medium onion, chopped
¼ cup chopped walnuts
½ green bell pepper, chopped
3 tablespoons olive oil
Freshly ground black pepper

Boil the carrots for 30 minutes, then cut in half lengthwise. Preheat the oven to 350°F. Hollow out the centers and puree the extracted portions. Combine the onion, walnuts, and bell pepper with 1 tablespoon of the oil. Add ground pepper to taste. Mix in the pureed carrots, and stuff the eight carrot halves with the mixture. Bake in a dish coated with the remaining 2 tablespoons of oil. Bake for about 30 minutes.

Serves 8

Steamed Baby Carrots with Basil

20 small carrots, washed and trimmed
1 tablespoon lemon juice
Dried basil

Put a vegetable steamer in the bottom of a medium saucepan, and fill with water to the bottom of the steamer. Bring to a boil, place the carrots in the steamer, cover, and reduce the heat. Steam until tender, 5 to 10 minutes. Pour the lemon juice over the carrots and sprinkle with basil to taste.

Serves 4

Lemon-Vinaigrette Carrots

1 pound carrots, peeled
½ cup olive oil
⅓ cup lemon juice
1 teaspoon minced garlic
1 teaspoon onion powder
¼ teaspoon freshly ground black pepper

Cut the carrots into very thin diagonal slices. Place in a large skillet, cover with water, and boil until tender, 3 to 5 minutes. Whisk together the remaining ingredients in a small bowl. Drain the carrots and toss with the lemon vinaigrette.

Serves 4

Tomato-Pecan Zucchini

2 zucchini, cut in half lengthwise
1 small red onion, finely chopped
4 tablespoons unsalted tomato sauce
½ teaspoon dried parsley
1 clove garlic, chopped
2 tablespoons pecans, chopped

Preheat the oven to 450°F. Hollow out the zucchini halves. In a saucepan, heat the pulp with the onion, tomato sauce, parsley, garlic, and pecans for 5 minutes. Stuff the zucchini shells with the mixture. Place in a baking dish with a little water on the bottom. Bake for 30 minutes, until the zucchini is soft.

Serves 2

Sautéed Cauliflower and Zucchini

1 head cauliflower

½ cup olive oil

1 teaspoon lime juice

1½ teaspoons cumin

¼ teaspoon freshly ground black pepper

1 teaspoon dried basil

1 teaspoon dried oregano

1 tablespoon chopped yellow onion

3 zucchini, cut into ½" slices

Detach the florets from the cauliflower and place in a large skillet with boiling water. Cook until just tender, about 5 minutes. Pour out the water and remove the florets. Pour the oil into the skillet and stir in the lime juice, cumin, pepper, basil, oregano, and onion. Add the zucchini and cauliflower. Cover and cook over low heat for 10 to 15 minutes, or until the zucchini is tender.

Serves 6

Livorno Eggplant

2 eggplants, peeled and cubed

2 cloves garlic, minced

1 yellow onion, diced

2 tablespoons olive oil

1 teaspoon dried basil

1 teaspoon dried oregano

½ teaspoon cumin

3 medium tomatoes, diced

Preheat the oven to 375°F. Add the eggplant to boiling water and boil for 1 minute. Remove and drain the eggplant. Place the eggplant in a bowl and set aside. Cook the garlic and onion in the olive oil about 5 minutes or until soft, stirring frequently. Add the onion, garlic, basil, oregano, and cumin to the eggplant; blend well. Put the mixture into a well-oiled glass baking dish. Layer with the diced tomatoes and bake uncovered for 25 to 30 minutes.

Serves 4

SALADS

Colorado Coleslaw

2 tablespoons lemon juice

2 Granny Smith apples, thinly sliced

3 cups shredded cabbage

1 rib celery, chopped

1 carrot, grated

1 medium yellow onion, thinly sliced

¼ teaspoon garlic powder

½ cup Flaxseed Oil Mayonnaise (see page 241)

In a large bowl, pour the lemon juice over the apple slices and add the cabbage, celery, carrot, and onion. Mix together the garlic powder and Flaxseed Oil Mayonnaise, and combine with the cabbage mixture.

Serves 4

Basil Tomatoes

4 medium tomatoes, sliced

¼ cup flaxseed oil

1½ tablespoons lemon juice

½ teaspoon onion powder

½ teaspoon dried basil

⅛ teaspoon cayenne pepper

1 clove garlic, minced

Place the tomatoes in a shallow dish. Combine the remaining ingredients and pour the dressing over the tomatoes. Cover and refrigerate before serving.

Serves 4

Omega-3 Spinach Salad

1 pound fresh spinach

2 tablespoons lime juice

¼ cup flaxseed oil

1 tablespoon honey

Freshly ground black pepper

1 avocado, diced

8 ounces pork loin (precooked, cooled, and diced)

2 omega-3 eggs, hard-boiled and chopped

Wash the spinach and dry with paper towels. Mix together the lime juice, oil, honey, and pepper to taste in a large bowl. Fold the avocado cubes into the dressing. Toss the spinach, pork loin, and chopped eggs with the avocado and dressing.

Serves 4

Greek Cucumber-Tomato Salad

1 large cucumber, cut into ½" slices, then quartered

2 medium tomatoes, cut into eighths

¼ red onion, very thinly sliced

½ green bell pepper, very thinly sliced

¼ cup lemon juice

2 tablespoons extra-virgin olive oil

Freshly ground black pepper

Mix the cucumber, tomatoes, onion, and bell pepper in a bowl. Toss with the lemon juice and oil. Add black pepper to taste.

Serves 2

Avocado-Cucumber Salad

1 medium unwaxed cucumber, peeled and very thinly sliced

1 yellow bell pepper, sliced

1 tablespoon fresh lime juice

1 jalapeño pepper, seeded and finely diced

1 teaspoon minced onion

Lettuce

1 avocado, sliced

Fresh parsley

In a bowl, combine the cucumber slices with the bell pepper, lime juice, jalapeño pepper, and onion. Arrange lettuce leaves on six serving plates. Pile the cucumber mixture in the center of each plate. Add avocado slices and garnish with parsley.

Serves 6

Bombay Chicken Salad

2 whole skinless chicken breasts, visible fat removed

1 tablespoon curry

4 tablespoons Flaxseed Oil Mayonnaise (see page 241)

1 tablespoon garam masala spice mixture

4 fresh pineapple slices, diced

1 tablespoon raisins

½ teaspoon freshly grated ginger

1 cucumber, peeled and finely chopped

2 ribs celery, finely chopped

Place the chicken breasts and curry in a pot filled with water. Simmer slowly until completely cooked; drain and cool. Cut the chicken into ½" cubes or smaller. In a medium serving dish, combine the Flaxseed Oil Mayonnaise with the remaining ingredients. Add the chicken and mix well.

Serves 4

Guacamole Salad

4 avocados

2½ tablespoons lime juice

1 clove garlic, minced

1 Anaheim chile pepper with seeds, finely chopped

1 teaspoon onion powder

Butter lettuce leaves

1 tomato, diced

Mash the avocados into a chunky paste and add the lime juice, garlic, chile pepper, and onion powder. Stir well and spoon onto the lettuce leaves. Cover with diced tomato.

Serves 2

Omega-3 Crab Salad

2 cups cooked crabmeat, cooled and flaked

1 cup diced celery

¼ cup chopped red bell pepper

1 teaspoon onion powder

¼ teaspoon freshly ground black pepper

1 tablespoon fresh lemon juice

3 tablespoons Flaxseed Oil Mayonnaise (see page 241)

Mixed salad greens

6 avocado wedges

Mix the crabmeat with the celery, bell pepper, onion powder, black pepper, lemon juice, and Flaxseed Oil Mayonnaise. Serve over mixed greens with avocado.

Serves 2

Salsa Shrimp Salad

2 cups boiled shrimp

½ cup diced celery

1 teaspoon finely chopped onion

3 omega-3 eggs, hard-boiled and chopped

⅓ cup Flaxseed Oil Mayonnaise (see page 241)

¼ cup Garden-Fresh Salsa (see page 244)

3 tablespoons lemon juice

Butter lettuce leaves

Combine the shrimp, celery, onion, and eggs. Mix together the Flaxseed Oil Mayonnaise, Garden-Fresh Salsa, and lemon juice. Toss together all the ingredients and spoon onto lettuce leaves. Chill before serving.

Serves 4

Lean Beef Salad

½ cup All-Natural Catsup (see page 242)

⅓ cup flaxseed oil

¼ cup lemon juice

½ teaspoon ground ginger

3 cups cooked lean beef, cut into strips

2 tomatoes, cut into wedges

1 green bell pepper, cut into strips

1 cup fresh mushrooms, sliced

1 cup sliced celery

½ cup green or sweet onion, thinly sliced

4 cups salad greens (romaine lettuce, Chinese cabbage, spinach)

Mix the All-Natural Catsup, oil, lemon juice, and ginger together to make a marinade. Combine the beef, tomatoes, bell pepper, mushrooms, celery, and onion and cover with the marinade. Chill for 2 hours. Put the salad greens into a serving bowl. Drain the marinade from the beef and vegetable mixture; reserve the marinade. Spoon the beef and vegetables onto the greens and toss. Serve with the extra marinade for dressing.

Serves 4

SOUPS

Acapulco Avocado Soup

2 avocados, diced

1 tablespoon chopped green onions

1 jalapeño pepper, seeded and finely chopped

1 tablespoon extra-virgin olive oil

2 cups chicken stock

Freshly ground black pepper

Ground cumin

1 sprig cilantro

1 tomato, diced

Place the avocados in a blender or food processor and puree until smooth. Cook the onions and jalapeño pepper in the oil until tender, stirring frequently. In a large bowl, combine the avocado with the stock and the onions and jalapeño pepper, mixing until smooth. Add black pepper and cumin to taste. Chill for 60 minutes prior to serving. Garnish with cilantro and diced tomato.

Serves 4

Broccoli Soup

1 large onion, chopped

3 cloves garlic, chopped

1 tablespoon olive oil

1½ pounds broccoli florets

3 cups chicken stock

¼ teaspoon ground nutmeg

Freshly ground black pepper

In a large saucepan, cook the onion and garlic in the oil until tender, stirring frequently. Add the broccoli and stock and bring to a boil. Reduce the heat and simmer 10 to 15 minutes, until the broccoli is tender. Put the mixture in a blender and puree until smooth, return it to the saucepan, and heat slowly. Season with the nutmeg and pepper to taste.

Serves 4 to 6

Karachi Carrot Soup

1 butternut squash, cut in half, seeds removed

1 onion, diced

3 cloves garlic, minced

2 tablespoons olive oil

4 cups water

1 pound carrots, peeled and diced

1½" fresh ginger, peeled and thinly sliced

Pinch of ground cinnamon

Freshly ground black pepper

1 sprig parsley

Preheat the oven to 375°F. Place the squash, cut side down, onto a greased baking sheet. Bake for 35 to 40 minutes, or until softened. Cool, then spoon the flesh out of the skin. Cook the onion and garlic in a large saucepan with the oil until soft but not browned, stirring frequently. Pour in the water and add the squash flesh, carrots, and ginger. Bring to a boil and cook for at least 20 minutes, or until the carrots and ginger are tender. Put the mixture in a blender and puree. Return the soup to the saucepan and reheat. Add the cinnamon, season to taste with pepper, and garnish with parsley.

Serves 4

Fresh Tomato-Basil Soup

2 large yellow onions, diced

¼ cup extra-virgin olive oil

2 pounds fresh tomatoes, peeled

1 tablespoon finely grated orange peel

1 tablespoon lemon juice

Freshly ground black pepper

Fresh basil leaves

In a large saucepan, cook the onions in the oil until translucent, stirring frequently. Put the tomatoes in a blender and puree. Add the orange peel, lemon juice, and pureed tomatoes to the saucepan, and cook over medium-low heat, stirring occasionally, for 15 to 20 minutes. Season to taste with pepper and garnish with basil.

Serves 4 to 6

Lean Chicken-Veggie Soup

2 large skinless chicken breasts

½ teaspoon thyme

½ teaspoon marjoram

1 bunch celery, chopped

1 medium head cabbage, chopped

1 large green bell pepper, chopped

1 zucchini, chopped

6 onions, chopped

8 tomatoes, chopped

1 tablespoon onion powder

2 cloves garlic, minced

8 whole peppercorns

1 bay leaf

In a large pot filled with water, simmer the chicken breasts with the thyme and marjoram for 15 to 20 minutes, or until the chicken is fully cooked. Remove the chicken and debone. Chop the chicken into ½" or smaller cubes, discard the bones, and put the chicken back into the pot. Add the remaining ingredients. Bring to a boil, then reduce the heat and simmer for 1½ to 2 hours, until the vegetables are tender and the flavors are well blended. Discard the bay leaf before serving.

Serves 12

FRUITS AND DESSERTS

Granny's Applesauce

8 Granny Smith apples, peeled, cored, and cut into eighths

½ cup water

2 tablespoons lemon juice

1 tablespoon grated lemon peel

Combine the apples and water in a large saucepan and cook over low heat until the apples are tender. Add the lemon juice and cook until the apples are easily mashed with a fork. Remove from the heat and add the lemon peel. Mash with the tines of a fork or a potato masher, leaving a bit of coarse texture. Serve warm.

Serves 4

Baked Cinnamon-Apple Rings

4 Rome baking apples

½ teaspoon powdered cloves

½ teaspoon cinnamon

1 tablespoon honey

½ cup water

Preheat the oven to 400°F. Core the apples and slice into ½" rings. Place into a shallow baking dish lightly greased or coated with cooking spray. Mix the remaining ingredients and pour over the apples. Bake for 15 minutes, or until tender.

Serves 4

Baked Bananas

4 bananas

¼ cup olive oil

Juice and grated rind of 2 lemons

1 tablespoon vanilla

1 teaspoon cinnamon

Preheat the oven to 350°F. Cut the bananas in half lengthwise and place cut side down in a baking dish greased with the oil. Drizzle the bananas with the lemon juice and vanilla and sprinkle with the grated lemon rind and cinnamon. Bake for 15 to 20 minutes.

Serves 4

Cantaloupe-Pineapple Ambrosia

2 cantaloupes

1 pineapple

1 large Granny Smith apple

1 cup raisins

1 cup fresh shredded coconut

1 cup chopped walnuts

Juice of 1 orange

Remove the skins, seeds, and cores from the cantaloupes, pineapple, and apple and cut the fruit into small chunks. In a large salad bowl, mix the fruit with the raisins, coconut, and walnuts and sprinkle with the orange juice.

Serves 4

Walnut-Crusted Strawberries

Fresh strawberries, sliced lengthwise
Honey
Lemon juice
Finely diced walnuts

Wash the strawberries, remove the stems, and cut in thin lengthwise sections. Mix together equal parts honey and lemon juice. Dip the strawberries into the mixture. Arrange on a serving tray and sprinkle with the walnuts.

Servings vary with quantity

STAGE IV RECOVERY RECIPES

The following recipes are intended only for Stage IV recovery and are based on potatoes, sweet potatoes, and yams. Many of these include small amounts of salt as recovery therapy.

Electrolytes are the salts sodium, chloride, potassium, calcium, and magnesium, which occur naturally either within the body's cells or in the extracellular fluids surrounding them. Dissolved in the body fluids as ions, they conduct electric currents and are therefore critical for muscle contraction and relaxation and also for maintaining fluid levels. The body loses a small portion of these salts during exercise, primarily through sweat. The loss is typically not critical in events shorter than 4 hours or in cool-weather events, when the sweat rate is low. But after longer events and exercise in extreme heat, replacement is of greater significance, especially for sodium and possibly for potassium.

There is no doubt that you are losing sodium during extensive exercise. The white blotches on your skin and clothes are visible signs of this. The problem with this is that the excessive loss of sodium during exercise can result in hyponatremia—levels of sodium so low that your health and well-being are at risk. The key to preventing hyponatremia is balancing fluid and sodium intake during long exercise sessions.

In the postexercise recovery period, replacing lost electrolytes will help speed recovery. Most of the electrolytes are found in abundance in natural foods, which makes their replacement fairly easy. Drinking any juices or eating fruits will easily replace nearly all of the electrolytes lost—except sodium, which is also the one most likely to need replenishment. This electrolyte must be added to postexercise recovery drinks and food by adding a bit of table salt. Once you are beyond Stages III and IV, salt should be restricted in your diet.

Marinated Mushrooms

1 pound button mushrooms

¼ cup olive oil

Juice of 1 lemon

2 tablespoons Johannisberg Riesling or other quality Riesling wine

3 cloves garlic, mashed

½ teaspoon mustard powder

¼ teaspoon paprika

Pinch of red pepper flakes

1 tablespoon chopped fresh oregano

1 tablespoon chopped fresh basil

1 tablespoon chopped fresh parsley

Salt

Freshly ground black pepper

In a large glass bowl, toss the mushrooms with all the other ingredients except salt and pepper and marinate for at least 20 minutes. Cook the mushrooms in a dry skillet over high heat for 3 to 5 minutes, until just tender, stirring frequently. Season with salt and pepper to taste. Serve over baked Idaho potatoes, sweet potatoes, or yams. Can be made ahead and refrigerated for quick use.

Serves 4

Herbed New Potatoes

8 small new red potatoes

2 tablespoons olive oil

½ tablespoon chopped fresh parsley

½ tablespoon chopped fresh basil

Salt

Freshly ground pepper

Boil the potatoes until tender, about 12 minutes. Drain and place on a plate or in a bowl. Drizzle with the oil and toss with the herbs and salt and pepper to taste. Make ahead and microwave for quick use.

Serves 2

Herb-Pepper-Almond Potato Toppers

4 tablespoons olive oil

2 cups whole almonds

4 teaspoons herb-pepper seasoning (or make your own mixture of parsley, lemon pepper, black pepper, and garlic powder)

Preheat the oven to 325°F. Spread the oil on a jelly roll pan or flat baking sheet. Stir the nuts and seasonings together and place on the baking sheet. Bake for 20 minutes, stirring occasionally. Remove with a slotted spoon and drain on a paper towel. Sprinkle on potatoes or salad.

Serves 8

Mexican Pecan Potato Toppers

4 tablespoons olive oil

4 cups pecan halves

1 tablespoon chili powder

2 teaspoons ground cumin

Dash of salt

Preheat the oven to 325°F. Spread the oil on a jelly roll pan or flat baking sheet. Stir the nuts and seasonings together and place on the baking sheet. Bake for 20 minutes, stirring occasionally. Remove with a slotted spoon and drain on a paper towel. Sprinkle on potatoes or salad.

Serves 16

Horseradish-Garlic Sauce

2 egg yolks

1 tablespoon white wine

¼ teaspoon salt

1 teaspoon honey

½ teaspoon freshly ground black pepper

⅔ cup olive oil

3 tablespoons prepared horseradish, or to taste

3 cloves garlic, smashed

Place the egg yolks, wine, salt, honey, and pepper in a food processor or blender and mix lightly. With the machine running, add the oil in a thin stream to thoroughly mix. Add half the horseradish and half the garlic, taste, and adjust the seasonings to your liking. Chill and serve as a topping for potatoes, vegetables, or meat. Keeps for 1 week in the refrigerator.

Makes 1 cup

Braised Onion Sauce

1½ pounds sweet onions (about 6 medium), sliced
½ cup olive oil
1 tablespoon honey
¼ cup Madeira wine
Freshly ground nutmeg

Cook the onions in the oil until they're soft and transparent, stirring frequently. Drizzle in the honey, reduce the heat, and simmer slowly for 1 hour. Stir in the wine and cook briefly. Serve as is or puree for a smooth sauce. Sprinkle with nutmeg before serving. Great on potatoes or as a side vegetable.

Makes 4 cups

Fresh Tomato Sauce

1 medium onion, sliced
4 tablespoons olive oil
2½ pounds tomatoes, peeled, seeded, and chopped (or equivalent amount of canned unsalted tomatoes)
½ teaspoon salt
1 tablespoon fresh basil (or 1 teaspoon dried)

Cook the onion in the oil until soft and transparent, stirring frequently. Add the tomatoes and seasonings. Simmer gently for 10 minutes. Pour over potatoes or yams.

Variation: Sauté ½ pound thinly sliced mushrooms with the onion.

Makes 4 cups

Almond-Avocado Spread

1 large ripe avocado, seeded, peeled, and mashed

1 tablespoon lime juice

¼ teaspoon chili powder

Pinch of salt

¼ cup toasted chopped almonds

2 tablespoons diced green chile pepper (Anaheim or other mild variety)

Mix together the avocado, lime juice, chili powder, and salt. Stir in the almonds and pepper. Cover with plastic wrap and refrigerate for 4 hours. Put on baked potatoes, sweet potatoes, or yams.

Makes 1½ cups

Tomato-Ginger Sauce

1½ cups chopped onion

4 thin slices fresh ginger, cut diagonally about 2" long

1 tablespoon olive oil

¼ teaspoon salt (optional)

½ teaspoon ground cumin

½ teaspoon turmeric

⅓ teaspoon allspice

½ teaspoon ground fennel

1 tablespoon minced garlic

½ cup water

1½ pounds crushed tomatoes (if canned, use unsalted tomatoes)

Cook the onion and ginger in the oil, stirring frequently. Add the spices and garlic, and simmer for 5 minutes. Stir in the water and tomatoes. Cook over medium heat for 10 minutes. Spoon over baked potatoes, sweet potatoes, or yams.

Makes 4 cups

Spiced Orange Sauce

3 tablespoons olive oil

3 cups chopped onions

3 tablespoons allspice

¼ teaspoon salt

1½ teaspoons minced garlic

Juice of 3 oranges

1 cup pitted, chopped plums, prunes, or other dried fruit

Heat the oil in a large, heavy saucepan. Add the onions, allspice, and salt, and cook over medium heat, stirring frequently, for 5 minutes. Stir in the garlic and orange juice. Simmer for 5 minutes longer. Add the fruit and simmer for another 5 minutes. Serve hot over potatoes or yams.

Makes 4 cups

REFERENCES

INTRODUCTION

Bar-Yosef, O. The Natufian culture in the Levant, threshold to the origins of agriculture. *Evolutionary Anthropology* 6, no. 5 (1998): 159–77.

Blurton-Jones, N. G., L. C. Smith, J. F. O'Connell, K. Hawkes, and C. L. Kamuzora. Demography of the Hadza, an increasing and high density population of Savanna foragers. *American Journal of Physiological Anthropology* 89 (October 1992): 159–81.

Burke, E. R., and J. R. Berning. *Training Nutrition.* Carmel, IN: Cooper Publishing Group, 1996.

Cabeza de Vaca, N. *Cabeza de Vacas Adventures in the Unknown Interior of America.* New York: Collier Books, 1961.

Caesar, J. G. *Commentaries on the Gallic War, Book VI.* Translated by W. A. McDevitte and W. S. Bohn. New York: Harper & Brothers, 1869.

Carrera-Bastos, P., M. Fontes Villalba, J. H. O'Keefe, S. Lindeberg, and L. Cordain. The western diet and lifestyle and diseases of civilization. *Research Reports in Clinical Cardiology* 2 (March 2011): 215–35.

Cook, J. *A Voyage Towards the South Pole and Round the World.* London: W. Strahan & T. Cadell, 1777.

Cordain, L. Cereal grains: Humanity's double-edged sword. *World Review of Nutrition and Dietetics* 84 (1999): 19–73.

Cordain, L., L. Toohey, M. J. Smith, and M. S. Hickey. Modulation of immune function by dietary lectins in rheumatoid arthritis. *British Journal of Nutrition* 83, no. 3 (March 2000): 207–17.

Cordain, L., S. B. Eaton, A. Sebastian, N. Mann, S. Lindeberg, B. A. Watkins, J. H. O'Keefe, and J. C. Brand-Miller. Origins and evolution of the Western diet: Health implications for the 21st century. *American Journal of Clinical Nutrition* 81, no. 2 (2005): 341–54.

DeVries, A. *Primitive Man and His Food.* Chicago: Chandler Book Company, 1952.

Eaton, S. B., L. Cordain, and S. Lindeberg. Evolutionary health promotion: A consideration of common counterarguments. *Preventive Medicine* 34 (2002): 119–23.

Eaton, S. B., M. Konner, and M. Shostak. Stone agers in the fast lane: Chronic degenerative diseases in evolutionary perspective. *American Journal of Medicine* 84, no. 4 (April 1988): 739–49.

Eaton, S. B., M. Shostak, and M. Konner. *The Paleolithic Prescription.* New York: Harper Row, 1988.

Galloway, J. H. "Sugar." In *The Cambridge World History of Food, Volume 1,* edited by K. F. Kiple and K. C. Ornelas, 437–49. Cambridge: Cambridge University Press, 2000.

Gerrior, S., and L. Bente. Nutrient content of the U.S. food supply, 1909–99: A summary report. U.S. Department of Agriculture, Center for Nutrition Policy and Promotion. Home Economics Report No. 55, 2002.

Hill, K., and A. M. Hurtado. *Ache Life History: The Ecology and Demography of a Foraging People.* New York: Aldine de Gruyter, 1996.

Honeman, W. *American Bicyclist,* 1945.

Jaffee, A. J. "Length of Life: Short and Not So Merry." In *The First Immigrants from Asia: A Population History of the North American Indians,* edited by A. J. Jaffee, 55–66. New York: Plenum Press, 1992.

James, S. R. Hominid use of fire in the lower and middle Pleistocene. *Current Anthropology* 30, no. 1 (1989): 1–26.

Jönsson, T., Y. Granfeldt, B. Ahrén, U. C. Branell, G. Pålsson, A. Hansson, M. Söderström, and S. Lindeberg. Beneficial effects of a Paleolithic diet on cardiovascular risk factors in type 2 diabetes: A randomized cross-over pilot study. *Cardiovascular Diabetology* 8 (July 2009): 35.

Laudonniere, R. G. *Histoire Notable de la Florida.* Gainesville: University of Florida Press, 1975.

Lee, R. B. "The Kung Bushmen of Botswana." In *Hunters and Gatherers Today,* edited by M. G. Bicchieri, 327–35. New York: Holt, Rinehart, and Winston, 1972.

Lindeberg, S., T. Jönsson, Y. Granfeldt, E. Borgstrand, J. Soffman, K. Sjöström, and B. Ahrén. A Palaeolithic diet improves glucose tolerance more than a Mediterranean-like diet in individuals with ischaemic heart disease. *Diabetologia* 50, no. 9 (September 2007): 1795–807.

Mancilha-Carvalho, J. J., R. de Oliveira, and R. J. Esposito. Blood pressure and electrolyte excretion in the Yanomamo Indians, an isolated population. *Journal of Human Hypertension* 3, no. 5 (October 1989): 309–14.

Neel, J. V. "Health and Disease in Unacculturated Amerindian Populations." In *Ciba Foundation Symposium 49—Health and Disease in Tribal Societies,* edited by K. Elliott and J. Whelan, 155–77. The Hague: Elsevier/Excerpta Medica/North-Holland, 1977.

Nieman, D. C. Immunonutrition support for athletes. *Nutrition Reviews* 66, no. 6 (June 2008): 310–20.

O'Keefe, J. H., Jr., and L. Cordain. Cardiovascular disease resulting from a diet and lifestyle at odds with our Paleolithic genome: How to become a 21st-century hunter-gatherer. *Mayo Clinic Proceedings* 79, no. 1 (January 2004): 101–8.

Oliver, W. J., E. L. Cohen, and J. V. Neel. Blood pressure, sodium intake, and sodium related hormones in the Yanomamo Indians, a "no-salt" culture. *Circulation* 52, no. 1 (July 1975): 146–51.

Ramsden, C. E., K. R. Faurot, P. Carrera-Bastos, L. Cordain, M. De Lorgeril, and L. S. Sperling. Dietary fat quality and coronary heart disease prevention: A unified theory based on evolutionary, historical, global, and modern perspectives. *Current Treatment Options in Cardiovascular Medicine* 11, no. 4 (August 2009): 289–301.

Sanderson, P., R. L. Elsom, V. Kirkpatrick, P. C. Calder, J. V. Woodside, E. A. Williams, L. Rink, S. Fairweather-Tait, K. Ivory, M. Cantorna, B. Watzl, and E. M. Stone. UK food standards agency workshop report: Diet and immune function. *British Journal of Nutrition* 103, no. 11 (June 2010): 1684–87.

Savage-Landor, A. H. *Across Unknown South America*. London: Hodder and Stoughton, 1913.

Stefansson, V. Eskimo longevity in northern Alaska. *Science* 127, no. 3288 (1958): 16–19.

US Department of Agriculture, Agricultural Research Service. Data tables: Results from USDA's 1994–96 Continuing Survey of Food Intakes by Individuals and 1994–96 Diet and Health Knowledge Survey. On: 1994–96 Continuing Survey of Food Intakes by Individuals and 1994–96 Diet and Health Knowledge Survey. CD-ROM, NTIS Accession Number PB98-500457, 1997.

US Department of Agriculture, Economic Research Service, 2002. Food consumption (per capita) data system, sugars/sweeteners.

Walsh, N. P., M. Gleeson, R. J. Shephard, J. A. Woods, N. C. Bishop, M. Fleshner, C. Green, B. K. Pedersen, L. Hoffman-Goetz, C. J. Rogers, H. Northoff, A. Abbasi, and P. Simon. Position statement. Part one: Immune function and exercise. *Exercise Immunology Review* 17 (2011): 6–63.

Walsh, N. P., M. Gleeson, D. B. Pyne, D. C. Nieman, F. S. Dhabhar, R. J. Shephard, S. J. Oliver, S. Bermon, and A. Kajeniene. Position statement. Part two: Maintaining immune health. *Exercise Immunology Review* 17 (2011): 64–103.

Wright, K. The origins and development of ground stone assemblages in Late Pleistocene Southwest Asia. *Paleorient* 17, no. 1 (1991): 19–45.

CHAPTER 1

Anthony, J. C., C. H. Lang, S. J. Crozier, T. G. Anthony, D. A. MacLean, S. R. Kimball, and L. S. Jefferson. Contribution of insulin to the translational control of protein synthesis in skeletal muscle by leucine. *American Journal of Physiology–Endocrinology and Metabolism* 282, no. 5 (2002): E1092–101.

Atkins, R. C. *New Diet Revolution*. New York: Avon Books, 1998.

Aude, Y. W., A. S. Agatston, F. Lopez-Jimenez, E. H. Lieberman, M. Almon, M. Hansen, G. Rojas, G. A. Lamas, and C. H. Hennekens. The national cholesterol education program diet vs. a diet lower in carbohydrates and higher in protein and monounsaturated fat: A randomized trial. *Archives of Internal Medicine* 164, no. 19 (October 2004): 2141–46.

Ballmer, P. E., and R. Imoberdorf. Influence of acidosis on protein metabolism. *Nutrition* 11 (1995): 462–68.

Batterham, R. L., H. Heffron, S. Kapoor, J. E. Chivers, K. Chandarana, H. Herzog, C. W. Le Roux, E. L. Thomas, J. D. Bell, and D. J. Withers. Critical role for peptide YY in protein-mediated satiation and body-weight regulation. *Cell Metabolism* 4, no. 3 (September 2006): 223–33.

Beelen, M., R. Koopman, A. P. Gijsen, H. Vandereyt, A. K. Kies, H. Kuipers, W. H. Saris, and L. J. van Loon. Protein coingestion stimulates muscle protein synthesis during resistance-type exercise. *American Journal of Physiology–Endocrinology and Metabolism* 295, no. 1 (July 2008): E70–77.

Beelen, M., L. M. Burke, M. J. Gibala, and L. J. van Loon. Nutritional strategies to promote postexercise recovery. *International Journal of Sport Nutrition and Exercise Metabolism* 20, no. 6 (December 2010): 515–32.

Calder, P. C., and S. Kew. The immune system: a target for functional foods? *British Journal of Nutrition* 88 (2002): S165–76.

Cordain, L. The nutritional characteristics of a contemporary diet based upon Paleolithic food groups. *Journal of American Neutraceutical Association* 5 (2002): 15–24.

Cordain, L., B. A. Watkins, G. L. Florant, M. Kehler, L. Rogers, and Y. Li. Fatty acid analysis of wild ruminant tissues: Evolutionary implications for reducing diet-related chronic disease. *European Journal of Clinical Nutrition* 56 (2002): 181–91.

Due, A., S. Toubro, A. R. Skov, and A. Astrup. Effect of normal-fat diets, either medium or high in protein, on body weight in overweight subjects: A randomised 1-year trial. *International Journal of Obesity and Related Metabolic Disorders* 28, no. 10 (October 2004): 1283–90.

Eades, M. R., and M. D. Eades. *Protein Power.* New York: Bantam Books, 1996.

Farnsworth, E., N. D. Luscombe, M. Noakes, G. Wittert, E. Argyiou, and P. M. Clifton. Effect of a high-protein, energy-restricted diet on body composition, glycemic control, and lipid concentrations in overweight and obese hyperinsulinemic men and women. *American Journal of Clinical Nutrition* 78 (2003): 31–39.

Ferencik, M., and L. Ebringer. Modulatory effects of selenium and zinc on the immune system. *Folia Microbiologica* 48 (2003): 417–26.

Foster, G. D., H. R. Wyatt, J. O. Hill, B. G. McGuckin, C. Brill, B. S. Mohammed, P. O. Szapary, D. J. Rader, J. S. Edman, and S. Klein. A randomized trial of a low-carbohydrate diet for obesity. *New England Journal of Medicine* 348 (2003): 2082–90.

Frassetto, L., R. C. Morris, and A. Sebastian. Potassium bicarbonate reduces urinary nitrogen excretion in postmenopausal women. *Journal of Clinical Endocrinology Metabolism* 82 (1997): 254–59.

Frassetto, L., R. C. Morris Jr., D. E. Sellmeyer, K. Todd, and A. Sebastian. Diet, evolution and aging: The pathophysiologic effects of the post-agricultural inversion of the potassium-to-sodium and base-to-chloride ratios in the human diet. *European Journal of Nutrition* 40 (2001): 200–213.

Hawley, J. A., E. J. Schabort, T. D. Noakes, and S. C. Dennis. Carbohydrate-loading and exercise performance. An update. *Sports Medicine* 24 (1997): 73–81.

Helge, J. W. Adaptation to a fat-rich diet: Effects on endurance performance in humans. *Sports Medicine* 30 (2000): 347–57.

Howarth, K. R., N. A. Moreau, S. M. Phillips, M. J. Gibala. Coingestion of protein with carbohydrate during recovery from endurance exercise stimulates skeletal muscle protein synthesis in humans. *Journal of Applied Physiology* 106, no. 4 (April 2009): 1394–402.

Koopman, R., D. L. Pannemans, A. E. Jeukendrup, A. P. Gijsen, J. M. Senden, D. Halliday, W. H. Saris, L. J. van Loon, and A. J. Wagenmakers. Combined ingestion of protein and carbohydrate improves protein balance during ultra-endurance exercise. *American Journal of Physiology–Endocrinology and Metabolism* 287, no. 4 (October 2004): E712–20.

Kris-Etherton, P. M., D. S. Taylor, S. Yu-Poth, P. Huth, K. Moriarty, V. Fishell, R. L. Hargrove, G. Zhao, and T. D. Etherton. Polyunsaturated fatty acids in the food chain in the United States. *American Journal of Clinical Nutrition* 71 (2000): 179S–88S.

Layman, D. K. Role of leucine in protein metabolism during exercise and recovery. *Canadian Journal of Applied Physiology* 27 (2002): 646–62.

Layman, D. K., R. A. Boileau, D. J. Erickson, J. E. Painter, H. Shiue, C. Sather, and D. D. Christou. A reduced ratio of dietary carbohydrate to protein improves body composition and blood lipid profiles during weight loss in adult women. *Journal of Nutrition* 133, no. 2 (February 2003): 411–17.

Lejeune, M. P., E. M. Kovacs, and M. S. Westerterp-Plantenga. Additional protein intake limits weight regain after weight loss in humans. *British Journal of Nutrition* 93, no. 2 (February 2005): 281–89.

Lemon, P. W., J. M. Berardi, and E. E. Noreen. The role of protein and amino acid supplements in the athlete's diet: Does type or timing of ingestion matter? *Current Sports Medicine Reports* 1 (2002): 214–21.

Levenhagen, D. K., J. D. Gresham, M. G. Carlson, D. J. Maron, M. J. Borel, and P. J. Flakoll. Postexercise nutrient intake timing in humans is critical to recovery of leg glucose and protein homeostasis. *American Journal of Physiology–Endocrinology and Metabolism* 280 (2001): E982–93.

Ludwig, D. S. The glycemic index: Physiological mechanisms relating to obesity, diabetes, and cardiovascular disease. *JAMA* 287 (2002): 2414–23.

Luscombe-Marsh, N. D., M. Noakes, G. A. Wittert, J. B. Keogh, P. Foster, and P. M. Clifton. Carbohydrate-restricted diets high in either monounsaturated fat or protein are equally effective at promoting fat loss and improving blood lipids. *American Journal of Clinical Nutrition* 81, no. 4 (April 2005): 762–72.

May, R. C., J. L. Bailey, W. E. Mitch, T. Masud, and B. K. England. Glucocorticoids and acidosis stimulate protein and amino acid catabolism in vivo. *Kidney International* 49 (1996): 679–83.

McAuley, K. A., C. M. Hopkins, K. J. Smith, R. T. McLay, S. M. Williams, R. W. Taylor, and J. I. Mann. Comparison of high-fat and high-protein diets with a high-carbohydrate diet in insulin-resistant obese women. *Diabetologia* 48, no. 1 (January 2005): 8–16.

Noakes, M., J. B. Keogh, P. R. Foster, and P. M. Clifton. Effect of an energy-restricted, high-protein, low-fat diet relative to a conventional high-carbohydrate, low-fat diet on weight loss, body composition, nutritional status, and markers of cardiovascular health in obese women. *American Journal of Clinical Nutrition* 81, no. 6 (June 2005): 1298–306.

Nuttall, F. Q., and M. C. Gannon. The metabolic response to a high-protein, low-carbohydrate diet in men with type 2 diabetes mellitus. *Metabolism* 55, no. 2 (February 2006): 243–51.

Rasmussen, B. B., K. D. Tipton, S. L. Miller, S. E. Wolf, and R. R. Wolfe. An oral essential amino acid-carbohydrate supplement enhances muscle protein anabolism after resistance exercise. *Journal of Applied Physiology* 88, no. 2 (February 2000): 386–92.

Remer, T. Influence of nutrition on acid-base balance: Metabolic aspects. *European Journal of Nutrition* 40 (2001): 214–20.

Remer, T., and F. Manz. Potential renal acid load of foods and its influence on urine pH. *Journal of the American Dietetic Association* 95 (1995): 791–97.

Rowlands, D. S., K. Rössler, R. M. Thorp, D. F. Graham, B. W. Timmons, S. R. Stannard, and M. A. Tarnopolsky. Effect of dietary protein content during recovery from high-intensity cycling on subsequent performance and markers of stress, inflammation, and muscle damage in well-trained men. *Applied Physiology, Nutrition, and Metabolism* 33, no. 1 (February 2008): 39–51.

Samaha, F. F., N. Iqbal, P. Seshadri, K. L. Chicano, D. A. Daily, J. McGrory, T. Williams, M. Williams, E. J. Gracely, and L. Stern. A low-carbohydrate as compared with a low-fat diet in severe obesity. *New England Journal of Medicine* 348 (2003): 2074–81.

Saunders, M. J. Coingestion of carbohydrate-protein during endurance exercise: Influence on performance and recovery. *International Journal of Sport Nutrition and Exercise Metabolism* 17 (August 2007): S87–103.

Sears, B. *The Zone*. New York: Harper Trade, 1995.

Sebastian, A., L. A. Frassetto, D. E. Sellmeyer, R. L. Merriam, and R. C. Morris Jr. Estimation of the net acid load of the diet of ancestral preagricultural *Homo sapiens* and their hominid ancestors. *American Journal of Clinical Nutrition* 76, no. 6 (December 2002): 1308–16.

Sebastian, A., S. T. Harris, J. H. Ottaway, K. M. Todd, and R. C. Morris Jr. Improved mineral balance and skeletal metabolism in postmenopausal women treated with potassium bicarbonate. *New England Journal of Medicine* 330, no. 25 (June 1994): 1776–81.

Shaw, A., L. Fulton, C. Davis, and M. Hogbin. Using the food guide pyramid: A resource for nutrition educators. US Department of Agriculture. Food, Nutrition, and Consumer Services, Center for Nutrition Policy and Promotion. Washington, DC. http://www.nal. usda.gov/fnic/Fpyr/guide.pdf.

Steward, H. L., M. C. Bethea, S. S. Andrews, and L. A. Balart. *Sugar Busters: Cut Sugar to Trim Fat*. New York: Ballantine Books, 1998.

Taubes, G. What if it's all been a big fat lie? *New York Times Magazine*, July 7, 2002.

Thomson, J. S., A. Ali, and D. S. Rowlands. Leucine-protein supplemented recovery feeding enhances subsequent cycling performance in well-trained men. *Applied Physiology, Nutrition, and Metabolism* 36, no. 2 (April 2011): 242–53.

Tipton, K. D., B. B. Rasmussen, S. L. Miller, S. E. Wolf, S. K. Owens-Stovall, B. E. Petrini, and R. R. Wolfe. Timing of amino acid-carbohydrate ingestion alters anabolic response of muscle to resistance exercise. *American Journal of Physiology–Endocrinology and Metabolism* 281, no. 2 (August 2001): E197–206.

Trinchieri, A., G. Zanetti, A. Curro, and R. Lizzano. Effect of potential renal acid load of foods on calcium metabolism of renal calcium stone formers. *European Urology* 39, suppl. no. 2 (2001): 33–36.

Valentine, R. J., M. J. Saunders, M. K. Todd, and T. G. St. Laurent. Influence of carbohydrate-protein beverage on cycling endurance and indices of muscle disruption. *International Journal of Sport Nutrition and Exercise Metabolism* 18, no. 4 (August 2008): 363–78.

Weigle, D. S., P. A. Breen, C. C. Matthys, H. S. Callahan, K. E. Meeuws, V. R. Burden, and J. Q. Purnell. A high-protein diet induces sustained reductions in appetite, ad libitum caloric intake, and body weight despite compensatory changes in diurnal plasma leptin and ghrelin concentrations. *American Journal of Clinical Nutrition* 82, no. 1 (July 2005): 41–48.

Westerterp-Plantenga, M. S., M. P. Lejeune, I. Nijs, M. van Ooijen, and E. M. Kovacs. High protein intake sustains weight maintenance after body weight loss in humans. *International Journal of Obesity and Related Metabolic Disorders* 28, no. 1 (January 2004): 57–64.

CHAPTER 2

Achten, J., and A. E. Jeukendrup. The effect of pre-exercise carbohydrate feedings on the intensity that elicits maximal fat oxidation. *Journal of Sports Science* 21, no. 12 (2003): 1017–24.

Alghannam, A. F. Carbohydrate-protein ingestion improves subsequent running capacity towards the end of a football-specific intermittent exercise. *Applied Physiology, Nutrition, and Metabolism* 36, no. 5 (2011): 748–57.

Anderson, M. E., C. R. Bruce, S. F. Fraser, N. K. Stepto, R. Klein, W. G. Hopkins, and J. A. Hawley. Improved 2000-meter rowing performance in competitive oarswomen after caffeine ingestion. *International Journal of Sport Nutrition and Exercise Metabolism* 10, no. 4 (2000): 464–75.

Armstrong, L. E., A. C. Pumerantz, M. W. Roti, D. A. Judelson, G. Watson, J. C. Dias, B. Sokmen, D. J. Casa, C. M. Maresh, H. Lieberman, and M. Kellogg. Fluid, electrolyte, and renal indices of hydration during 11 days of controlled caffeine consumption. *International Journal of Sport Nutrition and Exercise Metabolism* 15, no. 3 (2005): 252–65.

Berneis, K., R. Ninnis, D. Haussinger, and U. Keller. Effects of hyper- and hypo-osmolality on whole body protein and glucose kinetics in humans. *American Journal of Physiology* 276 (1999): E188–95.

Berning, J. R., M. M. Leeuders, K. Ratliff, et al. The effects of a high-carbohydrate pre-exercise meal in the consumption of confectionaries of different glycemic indices. *Medicine and Science in Sports and Exercise* 25, no. 5 (1993): S125.

Cox, G. R., B. Desbrow, P. G. Montgomery, M. E. Anderson, C. R. Bruce, T. A. Macrides, D. T. Martin, A. Moquin, A. Roberts, J. A. Hawley, and L. M. Burke. Effect of different protocols of caffeine intake on metabolism and endurance performance. *Journal of Applied Physiology* 93, no. 3 (2002): 990–99.

Graham, T. E. Caffeine and exercise: Metabolism, endurance, and performance. *Sports Medicine* 31, no. 11 (2001): 785–807.

Hargreaves, M., J. A. Hawley, and A. E. Jeukendrup. Pre-exercise carbohydrate and fat ingestion: Effects on metabolism and performance. *Journal of Sports Science* 22, no. 1 (2004): 31–38.

Jenkinson, D. M., and A. J. Harbert. Supplements and sports. *American Family Physician* 78, no. 9 (2008): 1039–46.

Jentjens, R. L., C. Cale, C. Gutch, and A. E. Jeukendrup. Effects of pre-exercise ingestion of differing amounts of carbohydrate on subsequent metabolism and cycling performance. *European Journal of Applied Physiology* 88 (January 2003): 444–52.

Kirwan, J. P., D. O'Gorman, D. Campbell, et al. A low glycemic meal 45 minutes before exercise improves performance. *Medicine and Science in Sports and Exercise* 28, no. 5 (1996): S768.

Kovacs, E. M. R., J. H. C. H. Stegen, and F. Brouns. Effect of caffeinated drinks on substrate metabolism, caffeine excretion, and performance. *Journal of Applied Physiology* 85, no. 2 (1998): 709–15.

Lemon, P. W., and E. E. Noreen. Unpublished paper, 2003.

McArdle, W. D., F. I. Katch, and V. L. Katch. *Exercise Physiology*. Baltimore: Williams & Wilkins, 1996.

Moore, L. J., A. W. Midgley, S. Thurlow, G. Thomas, L. R. McNaughton. Effect of the glycaemic index of a pre-exercise meal on metabolism and cycling time trial performance. *Journal of Science and Medicine in Sport* 13, no. 1 (2010): 182–88.

Moseley, L., G. I. Lancaster, and A. E. Jeukendrup. Effects of timing of pre-exercise ingestion of carbohydrate on subsequent metabolism and cycling performance. *European Journal of Applied Physiology* 88 (January 2003): 453–58.

Paluska, S. A. Caffeine and exercise. *Current Sports Medicine Report* 2, no. 4 (2003): 213–19.

Thomas, D. E., J. R. Brotherhood, and J. C. Brand. Carbohydrate feeding before exercise: Effect of glycemic index. *International Journal of Sports Medicine* 12 (1991): 180–86.

Van Proeyen, K., K. Szlufoik, H. Nielens, M. Ramaekers, and P. Hespel. Beneficial metabolic adaptations due to endurance exercise training in the fasted state. *Journal of Applied Physiology* 110, no. 1 (2010): 236–45.

Van Thuyne, W., and F. T. Delbeke. Distribution of caffeine levels in urine in different sports in relation to doping control before and after the removal of caffeine from the WADA doping list. *International Journal of Sports Medicine* 27, no. 9 (September 2006): 745–50.

White, J. P., J. M. Wilson, K. G. Austin, B. K. Greer, N. St. John, and L. B. Panton. Effect of carbohydrate-protein supplement timing on acute exercise-induced muscle damage. *Journal of the International Society of Sports Nutrition* 19, no. 5 (2008): 5.

Wilmore, J. H., and D. L. Costill. *Physiology of Sport and Exercise*. Champaign, IL: Human Kinetics, 1994.

Wolfe, R. R. Effects of amino acid intake on anabolic processes. *Canadian Journal of Applied Physiology* 26 (December 2001): S220–27.

Wu, C. L., and C. Williams. A low glycemic index meal before exercise improves endurance running capacity in men. *International Journal of Sport Nutrition and Exercise Metabolism* 16, no. 5 (2006): 510–27.

CHAPTER 3

Almond, C. S., E. B. Fortescue, A. Y. Shin, R. Mannix, and D. S. Greenes. Risk factors for hyponatremia among runners in the Boston Marathon. *Academy of Emergency Medicine* 10, no. 5 (2003): 534–35.

Barr, S. I., D. L. Costill, and W. J. Fink. Fluid replacement during prolonged exercise: Effects of water, saline, or no fluid. *Medicine and Science in Sports and Exercise* 23, no. 7 (1991): 811–17.

Below, O., and E. F. Coyle. Fluid and carbohydrate ingestion individually benefit exercise lasting one hour. *Medicine and Science in Sports and Exercise* 27 (1995): 200–210.

Blomstrand, E., F. Celsing, and E. A. Newsholme. Changes in plasma concentrations of aromatic and branched-chain amino acids during sustained exercise in man and their possible role in fatigue. *Acta Physiologica Scandinavica* 133, no. 1 (1988): 115–21.

Blomstrand, E., P. Hassmen, S. Ek, B. Ekblom, and E. A. Newsholme. Influence of ingesting a solution of branched-chain amino acids on perceived exertion during exercise. *Acta Physiologica Scandinavica* 159, no. 1 (1997): 41–49.

Blomstrand, E., P. Hassmen, B. Ekblom, and E. A. Newsholme. Administration of branched-chain amino acids during sustained exercise: Effects on performance and on plasma concentration of some amino acids. *European Journal of Applied Physiology and Occupational Physiology* 63, no. 2 (1991): 83–88.

Blomstrand, E., and E. A. Newsholme. Effect of branched-chain amino acid supplementation on the exercise-induced change in aromatic amino acid concentration in human muscle. *Acta Physiologica Scandinavica* 146, no. 3 (1992): 293–98.

Bossingham, M. J., N. S. Carnell, and W. W. Campbell. Water balance, hydration status, and fat-free mass hydration in younger and older adults. *American Journal of Clinical Nutrition* 81, no. 6 (2005): 1342–50.

Breen, L., K. D. Tipton, and A. E. Jeukendrup. No effect of carbohydrate-protein on cycling performance and indices of recovery. *Medicine and Science in Sports and Exercise* 42, no. 6 (2010): 1140–48.

Brouns, F., W. H. Saris, J. Stroecken, E. Beckers, R. Thijssen, N. J. Rehrer, and F. ten Hoor. Eating, drinking, and cycling. A controlled Tour de France simulation study, Part II. Effect of diet manipulation. *International Journal of Sports Medicine* 10 (May 1989): S41–S48.

Cade, J. R., R. M. Reese, R. M. Privette, N. M. Hommen, J. L. Rogers, and M. J. Fregly. Dietary intervention and training in swimmers. *European Journal of Applied Physiology* 63, no. 3–4 (1991): 210–15.

Convertino, V. A., L. E. Armstrong, E. F. Coyle, G. W. Mack, M. N. Sawka, L. C. Senay Jr., and W. M. Sherman. American College of Sports Medicine position stand: Exercise and fluid replacement. *Medicine and Science in Sports and Exercise* 28, no. 1 (1996): i–vii.

DelCoso, J., E. Estevez, and R. Mora-Rodriguez. Caffeine effects on short-term performance during prolonged exercise in the heat. *Medicine and Science in Sports and Exercise* 40, no. 4 (2008): 744–51.

Dugas, J. P., Y. Oosthuizen, R. Tucker, and T. D. Noakes. Rates of fluid ingestion after pacing but not thermoregulatory responses during prolonged exercise in hot and humid conditions with appropriate convective cooling. *European Journal of Applied Physiology* 105, no. 1 (2009): 69–80.

Ferguson-Stegall, L., E. L. McCleave, Z. Ding, L. M. Kammer, B. Wang, P. G. Doerner, Y. Liu, and J. L. Ivy. The effect of a low carbohydrate beverage with added protein on cycling endurance performance in trained athletes. *Journal of Strength and Conditioning Research* 24, no. 10 (2010): 2577–86.

Fritzsche, R. G., T. W. Switzer, B. J. Hodgkinson, S. H. Lee, J. C. Martin, and E. F. Coyle. Water and carbohydrate ingestion during prolonged exercise increase maximal neuromuscular power. *Journal of Applied Physiology* 88, no. 2 (2000): 730–37.

Fudge, B. W., C. Easton, D. Kingsmore, F. K. Kiplamai, V. O. Onywera, K. R. Westerterp, B. Kayser, T. D. Noakes, and Y. P. Pitsiladis. Elite Kenyan endurance runners are hydrated day-to-day with ad libitum fluid intake. *Medicine and Science in Sports and Exercise* 40, no. 6 (2008): 1171–79.

Gladden, L. B. Lactate metabolism: A new paradigm for the third millennium. *Journal of Physiology* 558 (July 2004): 5–30.

Goulet, E. D. B. Effect of exercise-induced dehydration on time-trial exercise performance: A meta-analysis. *British Journal of Sports Medicine* 45, no. 14 (2011): 1149–56.

Hawley, J. A., B. Sanders, S. C. Dennis, and T. D. Noakes. Effect of ingesting varying concentrations of sodium on fluid balance during exercise. *Medicine and Science in Sports and Exercise* 28, no. 5 (1996): S350.

Hew-Butler, T. D., K. Sharwood, M. Collins, D. Speedy, and T. D. Noakes. Sodium supplementation is not required to maintain serum sodium concentrations during an Ironman Triathlon. *British Journal of Sports Medicine* 40, no. 3 (2006): 255–59.

Hiller, W. D. Dehydration and hyponatremia during triathlons. *Medicine and Science in Sports and Exercise* 21 (October 1989): S219–21.

Hiller, W. D., M. L. O'Toole, E. E. Fortess, R. H. Laird, P. C. Imbert, and T. D. Sisk. Medical and physiological considerations in triathlons. *American Journal of Sports Medicine* 15, no. 2 (1987): 164–67.

Hubbard, R. W., P. C. Szlyk, and L. E. Armstrong. "Influence of Thirst and Fluid Palatability on Fluid Ingestion." In *Perspectives in Exercise Science and Sports Medicine, Volume 3: Fluid Homeostasis During Exercise,* edited by C. V. Gisolfi and D. R. Lamb, 39–96. Indianapolis: Benchmark Press, 1990.

Ivy, J. L., P. T. Res, R. C. Sprague, and M. O. Widzer. Effect of a carbohydrate-protein supplement on endurance performance during exercise of varying intensity. *International Journal of Sport Nutrition and Exercise Metabolism* 13, no. 3 (2003): 388–401.

Jeukendrup, A. E. Carbohydrate supplement: Does it help and how much is too much. *Cycling Performance Digest* 13, no. 6 (2008): 11–12.

Jeukendrup, A. E. Nutrition for endurance sports: Marathon, triathlon, and road cycling. *Journal of Sports Science* 29 (2011): S91–99.

Kratz, A., A. J. Sieger, J. G. Verbalis, M. M. Adner, T. Shirey, E. Lee-Lewandrowski, and K. B. Lewandrowski. Sodium status of collapsed marathon runners. *Archives of Pathology & Laboratory Medicine* 129, no. 2 (2005): 227–30.

Laursen, P. B., R. Suriano, M. J. Quod, H. Lee, C. R. Abbiss, K. Nosaka, D. T. Martin, and D. Bishop. Core temperature and hydration status during an Ironman Triathlon. *British Journal of Sports Medicine* 40, no. 4 (2006): 320–25.

Martínez-Lagunas, V., Z. Ding, J. R. Bernard, B. Wang, and J. L. Ivy. Added protein maintains efficacy of a low-carbohydrate sports drink. *Journal of Strength and Conditioning Research* 24, no. 1 (January 2010): 48–59.

Maughan, R. J., and J. B. Leiper. Limitations to fluid replacement during exercise. *Canadian Journal of Applied Physiology* 24, no. 2 (1999): 173–87.

McCleave, E. L., L. Ferguson-Stegall, Z. Ding, P. G. Doerner III, B. Wang, L. M. Kammer, and J. L. Ivy. A low carbohydrate-protein supplement improves endurance performance in female athletes. *Journal of Strength and Conditioning Research* 25, no. 4 (2011): 879–88.

McConnell, G., K. Kloot, and M. Hargreaves. Effect of timing of carbohydrate ingestion on endurance exercise performance. *Medicine and Science in Sports and Exercise* 28, no. 10 (1996): 1300–1304.

McConnell, G., R. J. Snow, J. Proietto, and M. Hargreaves. Muscle metabolism during prolonged exercise in humans: Influence of carbohydrate availability. *Journal of Applied Physiology* 87, no. 3 (1999): 1083–86.

Merson, S. J., R. J. Maughan, and S. M. Shireffs. Rehydration with drinks differing in sodium concentration and recovery from moderate exercise-induced hypohydration in man. *European Journal of Applied Physiology* 103, no. 5 (2008): 585–94.

Miller, K. C., G. W. Mack, K. L Knight, J. T. Hopkins, D. O. Draper, P. J. Fields, and I. Hunter. Reflex inhibition of electrically induced muscle cramps in hypohydrated humans. *Medicine and Science in Sports and Exercise* 42, no. 5 (2010): 953–61.

Miller, K. C., G. W. Mack, K. L Knight, J. T. Hopkins, D. O. Draper, P. J. Fields, and I. Hunter. Three percent hypohydration does not affect the threshold frequency of electrically-induced cramps. *Medicine and Science in Sports and Exercise* 42, no. 11 (2010): 2056–63.

Miller, S. L., C. M. Maresh, L. E. Armstrong, C. B. Ebbeling, S. Lennon, and N. R. Rodriguez. Metabolic response to provision of mixed protein-carbohydrate supplementation during endurance exercise. *International Journal of Sport Nutrition and Exercise Metabolism* 12, no. 4 (2002): 384–97.

Miller-Stafford, M. L., K. J. Cureton, J. E. Wingo, J. Trilk, G. L. Warren, and M. Buyckx. Hydration during exercise in warm, humid conditions: Effect of a caffeinated sports drink. *International Journal of Sport Nutrition and Exercise Metabolism* 17, no. 2 (2007): 163–77.

Mitchell, H. R., and J. Kirven. Exercise-associated hyponatremia. *Clinical Journal of the American Society of Nephrology* 2, no. 1 (2007): 151–61.

Newsholme, E. A., and E. Blomstrand. The plasma level of some amino acids and physical and mental fatigue. *Experientia* 52, no. 5 (1996): 413–15.

Newsholme, E. A., E. Blomstrand, and B. Ekblom. Physical and mental fatigue: Metabolic mechanisms and importance of plasma amino acids. *British Medical Bulletin* 48, no. 3 (1992): 477–95.

Nielsen, B., J. R. Hales, S. Strange, N. J. Christensen, J. Warberg, and B. Saltin. Human circulatory and thermoregulatory adaptations with heat acclimation and exercise in a hot, dry environment. *Journal of Physiology* 460 (January 1993): 467–85.

Niles, E. S., T. Lachowetz, J. Garfi, W. Sullivan, J. C. Smith, B. P. Leyh, and S. A. Headle. Carbohydrate-protein drink improves time to exhaustion after recovery from endurance exercise. *Journal of Exercise Physiology online* 4, no. 1 (2001): 45–52. faculty.css.edu/tboone2/asep/Niles1Col.doc

Noakes, T. D. Drinking guidelines for exercise: What evidence is there that athletes should drink "as much as tolerable," "to replace the weight lost during exercise" or "ad libitum"? *Journal of Sports Science* 25, no. 7 (2007): 781–96.

Noakes, T. D. Hydration in the marathon: Using thirst to gauge safe fluid replacement. *Sports Medicine* 37, no. 4–5 (2007): 463–66.

Noakes, T. D. Hyponatremia in distance runners: Fluid and sodium balance during exercise. *Current Sports Medicine Report* 1, no. 4 (2002): 197–207.

Noakes, T. D. IMMDA-AIMS advisory statement on guidelines for fluid replacement during marathon running. *New Studies in Athletics: IAAF Technical Quarterly* 17, no. 1 (2003): 7–11.

Noakes, T. D., K. Sharwood, D. Speedy, T. Hew, S. Reid, J. Dugas, C. Almond, P. Wharam, and L. Weschler. Three independent biological mechanisms cause exercise-associated hyponatremia: Evidence from 2,135 weighed competitive athletic performances. *Proceedings of the National Academy of Sciences of the United States of America* 102, no. 51 (2005): 18550–55.

Olsson, K. E., and B. Saltin. Variation in total body water with muscle glycogen changes in man. *Acta Physiologica Scandinavica* 80, no. 1 (1970): 11–18.

Oliver, S. J., S. J. Laing, S. Wilson, J. L. Bilzon, and N. Walsh. Endurance running performance after 48h of restricted fluid and/or energy intake. *Medicine and Science in Sports and Exercise* 39, no. 2 (2007): 316–22.

O'Toole, M. L., P. S. Douglas, R. H. Laird, and D. B. Hiller. Fluid and electrolyte status in athletes receiving medical care at an ultradistance triathlon. *Clinical Journal of Sport Medicine* 5, no. 2 (1995): 116–22.

Papadopoulus, C., J. Doyle, J. Rupp, L. Brandon, D. Benardot, and W. Thompson. The effect of hypohydration on the lactate threshold in a hot and humid environment. *Journal of Sports Medicine and Physical Fitness* 48, no. 3 (2008): 293–99.

Penkman, M. A., C. J. Field, C. M. Sellar, V. J. Harber, and G. J. Bell. Effect of hydration status on high-intensity rowing performance and immune function. *International Journal of Sports Physiology and Performance* 3, no. 4 (2008): 531–46.

Pfeiffer, B., T. Stellingwerff, E. Zaltas, and A. E. Jeukendrup. Carbohydrate oxidation from a carbohydrate gel compared to a drink during exercise. *Medicine and Science in Sports and Exercise* 42, no. 11 (2010): 2038–45.

Pfeiffer, B., T. Stellingwerff, A. B. Hodgson, R. Randell, K. Pöttgen, P. Res, and A. E. Jeukendrup. Nutritional intake and gastrointestinal problems during competitive endurance events. *Medicine and Science in Sports and Exercise* 44, no. 2 (February 2012): 344–51.

Robergs, R. A., F. Ghiasvand, and D. Parker. Biochemistry of exercise-induced metabolic acidosis. *American Journal of Physiology–Regulatory, Integrative and Comparative Physiology* 287 (2004): R502–16.

Romano-Ely, B. C., M. K. Todd, M. J. Saunders, and T. G. St. Laurent. Effect of an isocaloric carbohydrate-protein-antioxidant drink on cycling performance. *Medicine and Science in Sports and Exercise* 38, no. 9 (2006): 1608–16.

Rowlands, D. S., and D. P. Wadsworth. No effect of protein coingestion on exogenous glucose oxidation during exercise. *Medicine and Science in Sports and Exercise* 44, no. 4 (April 2012): 701–8.

Sawka, M. N., L. M. Burke, E. R. Eichner, R. J. Maughan, S. J. Montain, and N. S. Stachenfeld. American College of Sports Medicine position stand. Exercise and fluid replacement. *Medicine and Science in Sports and Exercise* 39, no. 2 (2007): 377–90.

Schena, F., F. Guerrini, P. Tregnaghi, and B. Kayser. Branched-chain amino acid supplementation during trekking at high altitude. The effects on loss of body mass, body composition, and muscle power. *European Journal of Applied Physiology and Occupational Physiology* 65, no. 5 (1992): 394–98.

Speedy, D. B., J. G. Faris, M. Hamlin, P. G. Gallagher, and R. G. Campbell. Hyponatremia and weight changes in an ultradistance triathlon. *Clinical Journal of Sport Medicine* 7, no. 3 (1997): 180–84.

Speedy, D. B., T. D. Noakes, and C. Schneider. Exercise-associated hyponatremia: A review. *Emergency Medicine* 13, no. 1 (2001): 17–27.

Speedy, D. B., I. R. Rogers, T. D. Noakes, J. M. Thompson, J. Guirey, S. Safih, and D. R. Boswell. Diagnosis and prevention of hyponatremia at an ultradistance triathlon. *Clinical Journal of Sport Medicine* 10, no. 1 (2000): 52–58.

Stearns, R. L., H. Emmanuel, J. S. Volek, and D. J. Casa. Effects of ingesting protein in combination with carbohydrate during exercise on endurance performance: A systematic review with meta-analysis. *Journal of Strength and Conditioning Research* 24, no. 8 (2010): 2191–202.

Sulzer, N. U., M. P. Schwellnus, and T. D. Noakes. Serum electrolytes in Ironman triathletes with exercise-associated muscle cramping. *Medicine and Science in Sports and Exercise* 37, no. 7 (2005): 1081–85.

Tucker, R. The anticipatory regulation of performance: The physiological basis for pacing strategies and the development of a perception-based model for exercise performance. *British Journal of Sports Medicine* 43, no. 6 (2009): 392–400.

Utter, A., J. Kang, D. Nieman, and B. Warren. Effect of carbohydrate substrate availability on ratings of perceived exertion during prolonged running. *International Journal of Sport Nutrition* 7, no. 4 (December 1997): 274–85.

Valentine, R. J., M. J. Saunders, M. K. Todd, and T. G. St. Laurent. Influence of carbohydrate-protein beverage on cycling endurance and indices of muscle disruption. *International Journal of Sport Nutrition and Exercise Metabolism* 18, no. 4 (2008): 363–78.

Van Nieuwenhoven, M. A., R. M. Brummer, and F. Brouns. Gastrointestinal function during exercise: Comparison of water, sports drink, and sports drink with caffeine. *Journal of Applied Physiology* 89, no. 3 (2000): 1079–85.

Van Nieuwenhoven, M. A., F. Brouns, and E. M. Kovacs. The effect of two sports drinks and water on GI complaints and performance during an 18-km run. *International Journal of Sports Medicine* 24, no. 4 (2005): 281–85.

Wagenmakers, A. J., A. E. Jeukendrup, and W. H. Saris. Carbohydrate feedings improve 1 hour time trial cycling performance. *Medicine and Science in Sports and Exercise* 28, no. 5 (1996): S221.

Wendt, D., L. J. van Loon, and W. D. Lichtenbelt. Thermoregulation during exercise in the heat: Strategies for maintaining health and performance. *Sports Medicine* 37, no. 8 (2007): 669–82.

Wharam, P. C., D. B. Speedy, T. D. Noakes, J. M. Thompson, S. A. Reid, and L. M. Holtzhausen. NSAID use increases the risk of developing hyponatremia during an Ironman triathlon. *Medicine and Science in Sports and Exercise* 38, no. 4 (2006): 618–22.

Winger, J. M., J. P. Dugas, and L. R. Dugas. Beliefs about hydration and physiology drive drinking behaviors in runners. *British Journal of Sports Medicine* 45, no. 8 (2011): 646–49.

Yamamoto, T., and E. A. Newsholme. Diminished central fatigue by inhibition of the L-system transporter for the uptake of tryptophan. *Brain Research Bulletin* 52, no. 1 (2000): 35–38.

Yaspelkis, B. B., III, J. G. Patterson, P. A. Anderla, Z. Ding, and J. L. Ivy. Carbohydrate supplementation spares muscle glycogen during variable-intensity exercise. *Journal of Applied Physiology* 75, no. 4 (1993): 1477–85.

Yeo, S. E., R. L. Jentjens, G. A. Wallis, and A. E. Jeukendrup. Caffeine increases exogenous carbohydrate oxidation during exercise. *Journal of Applied Physiology* 99, no. 3 (2005): 844–50.

CHAPTER 4

Anthony, J. G., T. G. Anthony, S. R. Kimball, and L. S. Jefferson. Signaling pathways involved in translational control of protein synthesis in skeletal muscle by leucine. *Journal of Nutrition* 131, no. 3 (2001): 856S–60S.

Armstrong, L. E., R. W. Hubbard, B. H. Jones, and J. Daniels. Preparing Alberto Salazar for the heat of the 1984 Olympic marathon. *Physiology and Sports Medicine* 14, no. 3 (1986): 73–81.

Bassit, R. A., L. A. Sawada, R. F. P. Bacurau, F. Navarro, E. Martins Jr., R. V. T. Santos, E. C. Caperuto, P. Rogeri, and L. F. Costa Rosa. Branched-chain amino acid supplementation and the immune response of long-distance athletes. *Nutrition* 18, no. 5 (2002): 376–79.

Berardi, J. M., T. B. Price, E. E. Noreen, and P. W. Lemon. Postexercise muscle glycogen recovery enhanced with a carbohydrate-protein supplement. *Medicine and Science in Sports and Exercise* 38, no. 6 (2006): 1106–13.

Breen, L., A. Philip, O. C. Witard, S. R. Jackman, A. Selby, K. Smith, K. Baar, and K. D. Tipton. The influence of carbohydrate-protein co-ingestion following endurance exercise on myofibrillar and mitochondrial protein synthesis. *Journal of Physiology* 589 (August 2011): 4011–25.

Brouns, F., E. M. Kovacs, and J. M. Senden. The effect of different rehydration drinks on post-exercise electrolyte excretion in trained athletes. *International Journal of Sports Medicine* 19, no. 1 (1998): 56–60.

Brouns, F., W. Saris, and H. Schneider. Rationale for upper limits of electrolyte replacement during exercise. *International Journal of Sport Nutrition* 2, no. 3 (1992): 229–38.

Burke, L. M. Nutrition for postexercise recovery. *Australian Journal of Science and Medicine in Sport* 29, no. 1 (1997): 3–10.

Burke, L. M. Nutritional needs for exercise in heat. *Comparative Biochemical Physiology and Molecular Integrated Physiology* 128, no. 4 (2001): 735–48.

Burke, L. M., G. R. Collier, and M. Hargreaves. Muscle glycogen storage after prolonged exercise: Effect of the glycemic index of carbohydrate feedings. *Journal of Applied Physiology* 75, no. 2 (1993): 1019–23.

Burke, L. M., and R. S. Read. Dietary supplements in sport. *Sports Medicine* 15, no. 1 (1993): 43–65.

Campbell, B., R. B. Kreider, T. Ziegenfuss, P. La Bounty, M. Roberts, D. Burke, J. Landis, H. Lopez, and J. Antonio. International Society of Sport Nutrition position stand: Protein and exercise. *Journal of the International Society of Sport Nutrition* 26, no. 4 (2007): 8.

Cao, J. J., L. K. Johnson, and J. R. Hunt. A diet high in meat protein and potential renal acid load absorption increases fractional calcium absorption and urinary calcium excretion without affecting markers of bone resorption or formation in postmenopausal women. *Journal of Nutrition* 141, no. 3 (2011): 391–97.

Caso, G., and P. J. Garlick. Control of muscle protein kinetics by acid-base balance. *Current Opinion in Clinical Nutrition and Metabolic Care* 8, no. 1 (2005): 73–76.

Cockburn, E., E. Stevenson, P. R. Hayes, P. Robson-Ansley, and G. Howatson. Effect of a milk-based carbohydrate-protein supplement timing on the attenuation of exercise-induced muscle damage. *Applied Physiology, Nutrition, and Metabolism* 35, no. 3 (2010): 270–77.

Etheridge, T., A. Philp, and P. W. Watt. A single protein meal increases recovery of muscle function following an acute eccentric exercise bout. *Applied Physiology, Nutrition, and Metabolism* 33, no. 3 (2008): 483–88.

Ferguson-Stegall, L., E. L. McCleave, Z. Ding, P. G. Doerner III, B. Wang, Y. H. Liao, L. Kammer, Y. Liu, J. Hwang, B. M. Dessard, and J. L. Ivy. Postexercise carbohydrate-protein supplementation improves subsequent exercise performance and intracellular signaling for protein synthesis. *Journal of Strength and Conditioning Research* 25, no. 5 (2011): 1210–24.

Friedman, E., and P. W. Lemon. Effect of chronic endurance exercise on retention of dietary protein. *International Journal of Sports Medicine* 10, no. 2 (1989): 118–23.

Ivy, J. L. Dietary strategies to promote glycogen synthesis after exercise. *Canadian Journal of Applied Physiology* 26 (2001): S236–45.

Ivy, J. L, H. W. Goforth Jr., B. M. Damon, T. R. McCauley, E. C. Parsons, and T. B. Price. Early postexercise muscle glycogen recovery is enhanced with a carbohydrate-protein supplement. *Journal of Applied Physiology* 93, no. 4 (2002): 1337–44.

Ivy, J. L., A. L. Katz, and C. L. Cutler. Muscle glycogen synthesis after exercise: Effect of time of carbohydrate ingestion. *Journal of Applied Physiology* 64, no. 4 (1988): 1480–85.

Layman, D. K. Role of leucine in protein metabolism during exercise and recovery. *Canadian Journal of Applied Physiology* 27, no. 6 (2002): 646–63.

Lemon, P. W. Effects of exercise on dietary protein requirements. *International Journal of Sport Nutrition* 8, no. 4 (1998): 426–47.

Lemon, P. W., D. G. Dolny, and K. E. Yarasheski. Moderate physical activity can increase dietary protein needs. *Canadian Journal of Applied Physiology* 22, no. 5 (1997): 494–503.

Levenhagen, D. K., C. Carr, M. G. Carlson, D. J. Maron, M. J. Borel, and P. J. Flakoll. Postexercise protein intake enhances whole-body and leg protein accretion in humans. *Medicine and Science in Sports and Exercise* 34, no. 5 (2002): 828–37.

Levenhagen, D. K., J. D. Gresham, M. G. Carlson, D. J. Maron, M. J. Borel, and P. J. Flakoll. Postexercise nutrient intake timing in humans is critical to recovery of leg glucose and protein homeostasis. *American Journal of Physiology–Endocrinology and Metabolism* 280, no. 6 (2001): E982–93.

Maughan, R. J., and T. D. Noakes. Fluid replacement and exercise stress. A brief review of studies on fluid replacement and some guidelines for the athlete. *Sports Medicine* 12, no. 1 (1991): 16–31.

Maughan, R. J., and S. M. Shirreffs. Recovery from prolonged exercise: Restoration of water and electrolyte balance. *Journal of Sports Science* 15, no. 3 (1997): 297–303.

Mayer, K., S. Meyer, M. Reinholz-Muhly, U. Maus, M. Merfels, J. Lohmeyer, F. Grimminger, and W. Seeger. Short-time infusion of fish oil–based lipid emulsions, approved for parenteral nutrition, reduces monocyte proinflammatory cytokine generation and adhesive interaction with endothelium in humans. *Journal of Immunology* 171, no. 9 (2003): 4837–43.

Meredith, C. N., M. J. Zackin, W. R. Frontera, and W. J. Evans. Dietary protein requirements and body protein metabolism in endurance-trained men. *Journal of Applied Physiology* 66, no. 6 (1989): 2850–56.

Millard-Stafford, M., G. L. Warren, L. M. Thomas, J. A. Doyle, T. Snow, and K. Hitchcock. Recovery from run training: Efficacy of a carbohydrate-protein beverage? *International Journal of Sport Nutrition and Exercise Metabolism* 15, no. 6 (2005): 610–24.

Ohtani, M., M. Sugita, and K. Maruyama. Amino acid mixture improves training efficiency in athletes. *Journal of Nutrition* 136, no. 2 (2006): 538S–43S.

Pendergast, D. R., J. J. Leddy, and J. T. Venkatraman. A perspective on fat intake in athletes. *Journal of American College of Nutrition* 19, no. 3 (2000): 345–50.

Pennings, B., R. Koopman, M. Beelen, J. M. Senden, W. H. Saris, and L. J. van Loon. Exercising before protein intake allows for greater use of protein-derived amino acids for de novo muscle protein synthesis in both young and elderly men. *American Journal of Clinical Nutrition* 93, no. 2 (2011): 322–31.

Remer, T., and F. Manz. Potential renal acid load of foods and its influence on urine pH. *Journal of the American Dietetic Association* 95, no. 7 (1995): 791–97.

Roy, B., K. Luttmer, M. J. Bosman, and M. A. Tarnopolsky. The influence of postexercise macronutrient intake on energy balance and protein metabolism in active females participating in endurance training. *International Journal of Sport Nutrition and Exercise Metabolism* 12, no. 2 (2002): 172–88.

Sanchez-Benito, J. L., and E. Sanchez-Soriano. The excessive intake of macronutrients: Does it influence the sports performances of young cyclists? *Nutrición Hospitalaria* 22, no. 4 (2007): 461–70.

Sherman, W. M. Recovery from endurance exercise. *Medicine and Science in Sports and Exercise* 24, no. 9 (1992): S336–39.

Shirreffs, S. M., A. J. Taylor, J. B. Leiper, and R. J. Maughan. Postexercise rehydration in man: Effects of volume consumed and drink sodium content. *Medicine and Science in Sports and Exercise* 28, no. 10 (1996): 1260–71.

Symons, T. B., M. S. Moore, and R. R. Wolfe. A moderate serving of high-quality protein maximally stimulates skeletal muscle protein synthesis in young and elderly subjects. *Journal of the American Dietetic Association* 109, no. 9 (2009): 1582.

Tarnopolsky, M. A., M. Bosman, J. R. Macdonald, D. Vandeputte, J. Martin, and B. D. Roy. Postexercise protein-carbohydrate and carbohydrate supplements increase muscle glycogen in men and women. *Journal of Applied Physiology* 83, no. 6 (1997): 1877–83.

Tarnopolsky, M. A., J. D. MacDougall, and S. A. Atkinson. Influence of protein intake and training status on nitrogen balance and lean body mass. *Journal of Applied Physiology* 64, no. 1 (1988): 187–93.

Van Loon, L. J., M. Kruijshoop, H. Verhagen, W. H. Saris, and A. J. Wagenmakers. Ingestion of protein hydrolysate and amino acid-carbohydrate mixtures increases postexercise plasma insulin responses in men. *Journal of Nutrition* 130, no. 10 (October 2000): 2508–13.

Zawadzki, K. M., B. B. Yaspelkis III, and J. L. Ivy. Carbohydrate-protein complex increases the rate of muscle glycogen storage after exercise. *Journal of Applied Physiology* 72, no. 5 (1992): 1854–59.

Zhang, N., T. Terao, and S. Nakano. Effect of time of carbohydrate ingestion on muscle glycogen resynthesis after exhaustive exercise in rats. *Tokai Journal of Experimental Clinical Medicine* 19, no. 3–6 (1994): 125–29.

CHAPTER 5

Beaudet, A. L., and R. P. Goin-Kochel. Some, but not complete, reassurance on the safety of folic acid fortification. *American Journal of Clinical Nutrition* 92, no. 6 (December 2010): 1287–88.

Bohn, T., L. Davidsson, T. Walczyk, and R. F. Hurrell. Phytic acid added to white-wheat bread inhibits fractional apparent magnesium absorption in humans. *American Journal of Clinical Nutrition* 79, no. 3 (March 2004): 418–23.

Boulet, S. L., D. Gambrell, M. Shin, et al. Racial/ethnic differences in the birth prevalence of spina bifida—United States, 1995–2005. *MMWR* 57 (2009): 1409–13.

Chajes, V., and P. Bougnoux. Omega-6/omega-3 polyunsaturated fatty acid ratio and cancer. *World Review of Nutrition and Diet* 92 (2003): 133–51.

Chiaffarino, F., G. B. Ascone, R. Bortolus, P. Mastroia-Covo, E. Ricci, S. Cipriani, and F. Parazzini. Effects of folic acid supplementation on pregnancy outcomes: A review of randomized clinical trials. *Minerva Ginecologica* 62, no. 4 (August 2010): 293–301.

Cole, B. F., J. A. Baron, R. S. Sandler, R. W. Haile, et al. Folic acid for the prevention of colorectal adenomas: A randomized clinical trial. *JAMA* 297, no. 21 (June 2007): 2351–59.

Collin, S. M., C. Metcalfe, H. Refsum, S. J. Lewis, G. D. Smith, et al. Associations of folate, vitamin B12, homocysteine, and folate-pathway polymorphisms with prostate-specific antigen velocity in men with localized prostate cancer. *Cancer Epidemiology, Biomarkers & Prevention* 19, no. 11 (November 2010): 2833–38.

Collin, S. M., C. Metcalfe, H. Refsum, S. J. Lewis, et al. Circulating folate, vitamin B12, homocysteine, vitamin B12 transport proteins, and risk of prostate cancer: A case-control study, systematic review, and meta-analysis. *Cancer Epidemiology, Biomarkers & Prevention* 19, no. 6 (June 2010): 1632–42.

Cordain, L. Cereal grains: Humanity's double-edged sword. *World Review of Nutrition and Diet* 84 (1999): 19–73.

Cordain, L. The nutritional characteristics of a contemporary diet based upon Paleolithic food groups. *Journal of the American Nutraceutical Association* 5 (2002): 15–24.

Cordain, L. "Saturated Fat Consumption in Ancestral Human Diets: Implications for Contemporary Intakes." In *Phytochemicals, Nutrient-Gene Interactions,* edited by M. S. Meskin, W. R. Bidlack, and R. K. Randolph, 115–26. Boca Raton, FL: CRC Press, 2006.

Cordain, L., J. C. Brand-Miller, S. B. Eaton, N. Mann, S. H. A. Holt, and J. D. Speth. Plant-animal subsistence ratios and macronutrient energy estimations in worldwide hunter-gatherer diets. *American Journal of Clinical Nutrition* 71, no. 3 (2000): 682–92.

Cordain, L., S. B. Eaton, J. C. Brand-Miller, N. Mann, and K. Hill. The paradoxical nature of hunter-gatherer diets: Meat-based, yet non-atherogenic. *European Journal of Clinical Nutrition* 56 (March 2002): S42–52.

Cordain, L., S. B. Eaton, A. Sebastian, N. Mann, S. Lindeberg, B. A. Watkins, J. H. O'Keefe, and J. C. Brand-Miller. Origins and evolution of the Western diet: Health implications for the 21st century. *American Journal of Clinical Nutrition* 81, no. 2 (February 2005): 341–54.

Eaton, S. B., M. J. Konner, and L. Cordain. Diet-dependent acid load, Paleolithic nutrition, and evolutionary health promotion. *American Journal of Clinical Nutrition* 91, no. 2 (February 2010): 295–97.

Ebbing, M., K. H. Bønaa, O. Nygård, E. Arnesen, P. M. Ueland, et al. Cancer incidence and mortality after treatment with folic acid and vitamin B12. *JAMA* 302, no. 19 (November 2009): 2119–26.

Favier, R. J., and H. E. Koubi. Metabolic and structural adaptations to exercise in chronic intermittent fasted rats. *American Journal of Physiology* 254, no. 6 (June 1988): R877–84.

Figueiredo, J. C., M. V. Grau, R. W. Haile, R. S. Sandler, R. W. Summers, R. S. Bresalier, C. A. Burke, G. E. McKeown-Eyssen, and J. A. Baron. Folic acid and risk of prostate cancer: Results from a randomized clinical trial. *Journal of the National Cancer Institute* 101, no. 6 (March 2009): 432–35.

Foster-Powell, K., S. H. A. Holt, and J. C. Brand-Miller. International table of glycemic index and glycemic load values: 2002. *American Journal of Clinical Nutrition* 76, no. 1 (January 2002): 5–56.

Frassetto, L. A., R. C. Morris Jr., and A. Sebastian. Potassium bicarbonate reduces urinary nitrogen excretion in postmenopausal women. *Journal of Clinical Endocrinology Metabolism* 82, no. 1 (January 1997): 254–59.

Frassetto, L. A., R. C. Morris Jr., D. E. Sellmeyer, and A. Sebastian. Adverse effects of sodium chloride on bone in the aging human population resulting from habitual consumption of typical American diets. *Journal of Nutrition* 138, no. 2 (February 2008): 419S–22S.

Galli, C., and P. C. Calder. Effects of fat and fatty acid intake on inflammatory and immune responses: A critical review. *Annals of Nutrition and Metabolism* 55, no. 1–3 (2009): 123–39.

Gomez-Cabrera, M. C., E. Domenech, M. Romagnoli, A. Arduini, C. Borras, F. V. Pallardo, J. Sastre, and J. Viña. Oral administration of vitamin C decreases muscle mitochondrial biogenesis and hampers training-induced adaptations in endurance performance. *American Journal of Clinical Nutrition* 87, no. 1 (2008): 142–49.

Gotshall, R. W., T. D. Mickleborough, and L. Cordain. Dietary salt restriction improves pulmonary function in exercise-induced asthma. *Medicine and Science in Sports and Exercise* 32, no. 11 (November 2000): 1815–19.

Harrington, M., and K. D. Cashman. High salt intake appears to increase bone resorption in postmenopausal women but high potassium intake ameliorates this adverse effect. *Nutrition Review* 61, no. 5 (May 2003): 179–83.

Holt, S. H. A., J. C. Miller, and P. Petocz. An insulin index of foods: The insulin demand generated by 1000-kJ portions of common foods. *American Journal of Clinical Nutrition* 66, no. 5 (November 1997): 1264–76.

Honein, M. A., L. J. Paulozzi, T. J. Mathews, J. D. Erickson, and L. Y. Wong. Impact of folic acid fortification of the US food supply on the occurrence of neural tube defects. *JAMA* 285, no. 23 (June 2001): 2981–86.

Hoyt, G., M. S. Hickey, and L. Cordain. Dissociation of the glycaemic and insulinaemic responses to whole and skimmed milk. *British Journal of Nutrition* 93, no. 2 (February 2005): 175–77.

Jenkins, D. J., T. M. Wolever, R. H. Taylor, H. Barker, H. Fielden, J. M. Baldwin, A. C. Bowling, H. C. Newman, A. L. Jenkins, and D. V. Goff. Glycemic index of foods: A physiological basis for carbohydrate exchange. *American Journal of Clinical Nutrition* 34, no. 3 (March 1981): 362–66.

Johnson, N. A., S. R. Stannard, and M. W. Thompson. Muscle triglyceride and glycogen in endurance exercise: Implications for performance. *Sports Medicine* 34, no. 3 (2004): 151–64.

Kuipers, R. S., M. F. Luxwolda, D. A. Dijck-Brouwer, S. B. Eaton, M. A. Crawford, L. Cordain, and F. A. Muskiet. Estimated macronutrient and fatty acid intakes from an East African Paleolithic diet. *British Journal of Nutrition* 104, no. 11 (December 2010): 1666–87.

Lambert, E. V., D. P. Speechly, S. C. Dennis, and T. D. Noakes. Enhanced endurance in trained cyclists during moderate intensity exercise following 2 weeks adaptation to a high fat diet. *European Journal of Applied Physiology and Occupational Physiology* 69, no. 4 (1994): 287–93.

Lemon, P. W. Effects of exercise on dietary protein requirements. *International Journal of Sport Nutrition* 8, no. 4 (December 1998): 426–47.

Levine, A. J., J. C. Figueiredo, W. Lee, D. V. Conti, K. Kennedy, D. J. Duggan, J. N. Poynter, et al. A candidate gene study of folate-associated one carbon metabolism genes and colorectal cancer risk. *Cancer Epidemiology, Biomarkers & Prevention* 19, no. 7 (July 2010): 1812–21.

Liljeberg Elmståhl, H., and I. Björck. Milk as a supplement to mixed meals may elevate postprandial insulinaemia. *European Journal of Clinical Nutrition* 55, no. 11 (November 2001): 994–99.

Lin, J., I. M. Lee, N. R. Cook, J. Selhub, J. E. Manson, J. E. Buring, and S. M. Zhang. Plasma folate, vitamin B-6, vitamin B-12, and risk of breast cancer in women. *American Journal of Clinical Nutrition* 87, no. 3 (March 2008): 734–43.

Lindzon, G. M., A. Medline, K. J. Sohn, F. Depeint, R. Croxford, and Y. I. Kim. Effect of folic acid supplementation on the progression of colorectal aberrant crypt foci. *Carcinogenesis* 30, no. 9 (September 2009): 1536–43

Ludwig, D. S. The glycemic index: Physiological mechanisms relating to obesity, diabetes, and cardiovascular disease. *JAMA* 287, no. 18 (May 2002): 2414–23.

Machado Andrade Pde, M., and M. G. Tavares do Carmo. Dietary long-chain omega-3 fatty acids and anti-inflammatory action: Potential application in the field of physical exercise. *Nutrition* 20, no. 2 (February 2004): 243.

Maughan, R. J., J. Fallah, and E. F. Coyle. The effects of fasting on metabolism and performance. *British Journal of Sports Medicine* 44, no. 7 (June 2010): 490–94.

Micha, R., and D. Mozaffarian. Saturated fat and cardiometabolic risk factors, coronary heart disease, stroke, and diabetes: A fresh look at the evidence. *Lipids* 45, no. 10 (October 2010): 893–905.

Mickleborough, T. D. Salt intake, asthma, and exercise-induced bronchoconstriction: A review. *Physician and Sportsmedicine* 38, no. 1 (April 2010): 118–31.

Mickleborough, T., and R. Gotshall. Dietary components with demonstrated effectiveness in decreasing the severity of exercise-induced asthma. *Sports Medicine* 33, no. 9 (2003): 671–81.

Mickleborough, T. D., R. W. Gotshall, L. Cordain, and M. Lindley. Dietary salt alters pulmonary function during exercise in exercise-induced asthmatics. *Journal of Sports Science* 19, no. 11 (November 2001): 865–73.

Mickleborough, T. D., R. W. Gotshall, E. M. Kluka, C. W. Miller, and L. Cordain. Dietary chloride as a possible determinant of the severity of exercise-induced asthma. *European Journal of Applied Physiology* 85, no. 5 (September 2001): 450–56.

Mickleborough, T. D., M. R. Lindley, and S. Ray. Dietary salt, airway inflammation, and diffusion capacity in exercise-induced asthma. *Medicine and Science in Sports and Exercise* 37, no. 6 (June 2005): 904–14.

Mickleborough, T. D., R. L. Murray, A. A. Ionescu, and M. R. Lindley. Fish oil supplementation reduces severity of exercise-induced bronchoconstriction in elite athletes. *American Journal of Respiratory Critical Care Medicine* 168, no. 10 (November 2003): 1181–89.

Mozaffarian, D., A. Aro, and W. C. Willett. Health effects of trans-fatty acids: Experimental and observational evidence. *European Journal of Clinical Nutrition* 63 (May 2009): S5–21.

Mozaffarian, D., and J. H. Wu. Omega-3 fatty acids and cardiovascular disease: Effects on risk factors, molecular pathways, and clinical events. *Journal of the American College of Cardiology* 58, no. 20 (November 2011): 2047–67.

Nieman, D. C., D. A. Henson, S. R. McAnulty, F. Jin, and K. R. Maxwell. n-3 polyunsaturated fatty acids do not alter immune and inflammation measures in endurance athletes. *International Journal of Sport Nutrition and Exercise Metabolism* 19, no. 5 (October 2009): 536–46.

Nilsson, M., M. Stenberg, A. H. Frid, J. J. Holst, and I. M. Björck. Glycemia and insulinemia in healthy subjects after lactose-equivalent meals of milk and other food proteins: The role of plasma amino acids and incretins. *American Journal of Clinical Nutrition* 80, no. 5 (November 2004): 1246–53.

Nilsson, M., J. J. Holst, and I. M. Björck. Metabolic effects of amino acid mixtures and whey protein in healthy subjects: Studies using glucose-equivalent drinks. *American Journal of Clinical Nutrition* 85, no. 4 (April 2007): 996–1004.

O'Shaughnessy, K. M., and F. E. Karet. Salt handling and hypertension. *Journal of Clinical Investigation* 113, no. 8 (April 2004): 1075–81.

Ostman, E. M., H. G. Liljeberg Elmstahl, and I. M. Björck. Inconsistency between glycemic and insulinemic responses to regular and fermented milk products. *American Journal of Clinical Nutrition* 74, no. 1 (July 2001): 96–100.

Parry-Billings, M., R. Budgett, Y. Koutedakis, E. Blomstrand, S. Brooks, C. Williams, P. C. Calder, S. Pilling, R. Baigrie, and E. A. Newsholme. Plasma amino acid concentrations in the overtraining syndrome: Possible effects on the immune system. *Medicine and Science in Sports and Exercise*, 24, no. 12 (December 1992): 1353–58.

Pedersen, J. I. More on trans fatty acids. *British Journal of Nutrition* 85, no. 3 (March 2001): 249–50.

Peoples, G. E., P. L. McLennan, P. R. Howe, and H. Groeller. Fish oil reduces heart rate and oxygen consumption during exercise. *Journal of Cardiovascular Pharmacology* 52, no. 6 (December 2008): 540–47.

Pizzorno, J., L. A. Frassetto, and J. Katzinger. Diet-induced acidosis: Is it real and clinically relevant? *British Journal of Nutrition* 103, no. 8 (April 2010): 1185–94

Ramsden, C. E., K. R. Faurot, P. Carrera-Bastos, L. Cordain, M. De Lorgeril, and L. S. Sperling. Dietary fat quality and coronary heart disease prevention: A unified theory based on evolutionary, historical, global, and modern perspectives. *Current Treatment Options in Cardiovascular Medicine* 11, no. 4 (August 2009): 289–301.

Ristow, M., K. Zarse, A. Oberbach, N. Klöting, M. Birringer, M. Kiehntopf, M. Stumvoll, C. R. Kahn, and M. Blüher. Antioxidants prevent health-promoting effects of physical exercise in humans. *Proceedings of the National Academy of Sciences of the United States of America* 106, no. 21 (2009): 8665–70.

Salmeron, J., A. Ascherio, E. B. Rimm, G. A. Colditz, D. Spiegelman, D. J. Jenkins, M. J. Stampfer, A. L. Wing, and W. C. Willett. Dietary fiber, glycemic load, and risk of NIDDM in men. *Diabetes Care* 20, no. 4 (April 1997): 545–50.

Salmeron, J., J. E. Manson, M. J. Stampfer, G. A. Colditz, A. L. Wing, and W. C. Willett. Dietary fiber, glycemic load, and risk of non-insulin-dependent diabetes mellitus in women. *JAMA* 277, no. 6 (February 1997): 472–77.

Schmitt, B., M. Fluck, J. Decombaz, R. Kreis, C. Boesch, M. Wittwer, F. Graber, M. Vogt, H. Howald, and H. Hoppeler. Transcriptional adaptations of lipid metabolism in tibialis anterior muscle of endurance-trained athletes. *Physiology Genomics* 15, no. 2 (October 2003): 148–57.

Sebastian, A., L. A. Frassetto, D. E. Sellmeyer, R. L. Merriam, and R. C. Morris Jr. Estimation of the net acid load of the diet of ancestral preagricultural *Homo sapiens* and their hominid ancestors. *American Journal of Clinical Nutrition* 76, no. 6 (December 2002): 1308–16.

Sebastian, A., L. A. Frassetto, D. E. Sellmeyer, R. C. Morris Jr. The evolution-informed optimal dietary potassium intake of human beings greatly exceeds current and recommended intakes. *Seminars in Nephrology* 26, no. 6, (November 2006): 447–53.

Simopoulos, A. P. Evolutionary aspects of the dietary omega-6:omega-3 fatty acid ratio: Medical implications. *World Review of Nutrition and Dietetics* 100 (2009): 1–21.

Simopoulos, A. P. The importance of the ratio of omega-6/omega-3 essential fatty acids. *Bio-medical Pharmacotherapy* 56, no. 8 (October 2002): 365–79.

Simopoulos, A. P. Omega-3 fatty acids in inflammation and autoimmune diseases. *Journal of American College Nutrition* 21, no. 6 (December 2002): 495–505.

Siri-Tarino, P. W., Q. Sun, F. B. Hu, and R. M. Krauss. Meta-analysis of prospective cohort studies evaluating the association of saturated fat with cardiovascular disease. *American Journal of Clinical Nutrition* 91, no. 3 (March 2010): 535–46.

Smith, A. D., Y. I. Kim, and H. Refsum. Is folic acid good for everyone? *American Journal of Clinical Nutrition* 87, no. 3 (March 2008): 517–33.

Stannard, S. R., and N. A. Johnson. Insulin resistance and elevated triglyceride in muscle: More important for survival than "thrifty" genes. *Journal of Physiology* 554 (February 2004): 595–607.

Stellingwerff, T., L. L. Spriet, M. J. Watt, N. E. Kimber, M. Hargreaves, J. A. Hawley, and L. M. Burke. Decreased PDH activation and glycogenolysis during exercise following fat adaptation with carbohydrate restoration. *American Journal of Physiology–Endocrinology and Metabolism* 290, no. 2 (February 2006): E380–88.

Stevens, V. L., M. L. McCullough, J. Sun, and S. M. Gapstur. Folate and other one-carbon metabolism-related nutrients and risk of postmenopausal breast cancer in the Cancer Prevention Study II Nutrition Cohort. *American Journal of Clinical Nutrition* 91, no. 6 (June 2010): 1708–15.

Stolzenberg-Solomon, R. Z., S. C. Chang, M. F. Leitzmann, K. A. Johnson, C. Johnson, S. S. Buys, R. N. Hoover, and R. G. Ziegler. Folate intake, alcohol use, and postmenopausal breast cancer risk in the Prostate, Lung, Colorectal, and Ovarian Cancer Screening Trial. *American Journal of Clinical Nutrition* 83, no. 4 (April 2006): 895–904.

Ströhle, A., A. Hahn, and A. Sebastian. Estimation of the diet-dependent net acid load in 229 worldwide historically studied hunter-gatherer societies. *American Journal of Clinical Nutrition* 91, no. 2 (February 2010): 406–12.

Sublette, M. E., S. P. Ellis, A. L. Geant, and J. J. Mann. Meta-analysis of the effects of eicosapentaenoic acid (EPA) in clinical trials in depression. *Journal of Clinical Psychiatry* 72, no. 12 (December 2011): 1577–84.

Tecklenburg-Lund, S., T. D. Mickleborough, L. A. Turner, A. D. Fly, J. M. Stager, and G.S. Montgomery. Randomized controlled trial of fish oil and montelukast and their combination on airway inflammation and hyperpnea-induced bronchoconstriction. *PLoS ONE* 5, no. 10 (October 2010): e13487.

Tecgala, S. M., W. C. Willett, and D. Mozaffarian. Consumption and health effects of trans fatty acids: A review. *Journal of AOAC International* 92, no. 5 (2009): 1250–57.

Ulrich, C. M., and J. D. Potter. Folate and cancer—timing is everything. *JAMA* 297, no. 21 (June 2007): 2408–9

Van der Merwe, N. J., J. F. Thackeray, J. A. Lee-Thorp, and J. Luyt. The carbon isotope ecology and diet of *Australopithecus africanus* at Sterkfontein, South Africa. *Journal of Human Evolution* 44, no. 5 (May 2003): 581–97.

Vermunt, S. H., B. Beaufrere, R. A. Riemersma, J. L. Sebedio, J. M. Chardigny, R. P. Mensink, and TransLinE Investigators. Dietary trans alpha-linolenic acid from deodorised rapeseed oil and plasma lipids and lipoproteins in healthy men: The TransLinE Study. *British Journal of Nutrition* 85, no. 3 (March 2001): 387–92.

Vogt, M., A. Puntschart, H. Howald, B. Mueller, C. Mannhart, L. Gfeller-Tuescher, P. Mullis, and H. Hoppeler. Effects of dietary fat on muscle substrates, metabolism, and performance in athletes. *Medicine and Science in Sports and Exercise* 35, no. 6 (June 2003): 952–60.

Von Schacky, C. Omega-3 fatty acids and cardiovascular disease. *Current Opinion in Clinical Nutrition and Metabolic Care* 7, no. 2 (March 2004): 131–36.

Williams, M. H. Facts and fallacies of purported ergogenic amino acid supplements. *Clinical Journal of Sport Medicine* 18, no. 3 (July 1999): 633–49.

Williams, M. H. *Nutrition for Health, Fitness and Sport.* New York: McGraw Hill, 2002.

Yeo, W. K., A. L. Carey, L. Burke, L. L. Spriet, and J. A. Hawley. Fat adaptation in well-trained athletes: Effects on cell metabolism. *Applied Physiology, Nutrition, and Metabolism* 36, no. 1 (February 2011): 12–22.

Yeo, W. K., S. J. Lessard, Z. P. Chen, A. P. Garnham, L. M. Burke, D. A. Rivas, B. E. Kemp, and J. A. Hawley. Fat adaptation followed by carbohydrate restoration increases AMPK activity in skeletal muscle from trained humans. *Journal of Applied Physiology* 105, no. 5 (November 2008): 1519–26.

Zehnder, M., E. R. Christ, M. Ith, K. J. Acheson, E. Pouteau, R. Kreis, R. Trepp, P. Diem, C. Boesch, and J. Décombaz. Intramyocellular lipid stores increase markedly in athletes after 1.5 days lipid supplementation and are utilized during exercise in proportion to their content. *European Journal of Applied Physiology* 98, no. 4 (November 2006): 341–54.

CHAPTER 6

Achten, J., and A. E. Jeukendrup. The effect of pre-exercise carbohydrate feedings on the intensity that elicits maximal fat oxidation. *Journal of Sports Science* 21, no. 12 (2003): 1017–24.

Batterham, R. L., H. Heffron, S. Kapoor, J. E. Chivers, K. Chandarana, H. Herzog, C. W. Le Roux, E. L. Thomas, J. D. Bell, and D. J. Withers. Critical role for peptide YY in protein-mediated satiation and body-weight regulation. *Cell Metabolism* 4, no. 3 (2006): 223–33.

Boyadjiev, N. Increase in aerobic capacity by submaximal training and high-fat diets. *Folia Medica* 38, no. 1 (1996): 49–59.

Brown, R. C., C. M. Cox, and A. Goulding. High-carbohydrate versus high-fat diets: Effect on body composition in training cyclists. *Medicine and Science in Sports and Exercise* 32, no. 3 (2000): 690–94.

Burke, L. M., and J. A. Hawley. Effects of short-term fat adaptation on prolonged exercise. *Medicine and Science in Sports and Exercise* 34, no. 9 (2002): 1492–98.

Cameron-Smith, D., L. M. Burke, D. J. Angus, R. J. Tunstall, G. R. Cox, A. Bonen, J. A. Hawley, and M. Hargreaves. A short-term, high-fat diet up-regulates lipid metabolism and gene expression in human skeletal muscle. *American Journal of Clinical Nutrition* 77, no. 2 (2003): 313–18.

Cook, C. M., and M. D. Haub. Low-carbohydrate diets and performance. *Current Sports Medicine Reports* 6, no. 4 (2007): 225–29.

Crovetti, R., M. Porrini, A. Santangelo, and G. Testoling. The influence of thermic effect of food on satiety. *European Journal of Clinical Nutrition* 52, no. 7 (1998): 482–88.

Décombaz, J., D. Sartori, M. J. Arnaud, A. L. Thélin, P. Schürch, and H. Howald. Oxidation and metabolic effects of fructose and glucose ingested before exercise. *International Journal of Sports Medicine* 6, no. 5 (1985): 286–88.

Demarle, A. P., A. M. Heugas, J. J. Slawinski, V. M. Tricot, J. P. Koralsztein, and V. L. Billat. Whichever the initial training status, any increase in velocity at lactate threshold appears as a major factor in improved time to exhaustion at the same severe velocity after training. *Archives of Physiology and Biochemistry* 111, no. 2 (2003): 167–76.

Dumesnil, J. G., J. Turgeon, A. Tremblay, P. Poirier, M. Gilbert, L. Gagnon, S. St. Pierre, C. Garneau, I. Lemieux, A. Pascot, J. Bergeron, and J. P. Després. Effect of a low-glycaemic index-low-fat-high protein diet on the atherogenic metabolic risk profile of abdominally obese men. *British Journal of Nutrition* 86, no. 5 (2001): 557–68.

Farnsworth, E., N. D. Luscombe, M. Noakes, G. Wittert, E. Argyiou, and P. M. Clifton. Effect of a high-protein, energy-restricted diet on body composition, glycemic control, and lipid concentrations in overweight and obese hyperinsulinemic men and women. *American Journal of Clinical Nutrition* 78, no. 1 (2003): 31–39.

Farrell, P. A., J. H. Wilmore, E. F. Coyle, J. E. Billing, and D. L. Costill. Plasma lactate accumulation and distance running performance. *Medicine and Science in Sports* 11, no. 4 (1979): 338–44.

Foster, G. D., H. R. Wyatt, J. O. Hill, B. G. McGuckin, C. Brill, B. S. Mohammed, P. O. Szapary, D. J. Rader, J. S. Edman, and S. Klein. A randomized trial of a low-carbohydrate diet for obesity. *New England Journal of Medicine* 348, no. 21 (2003): 2082–90.

Goedecke, J. H., A. St. Clair-Gibson, L. Grobler, M. Collins, T. D. Noakes, and E. V. Lambert. Determinants of the variability in respiratory exchange ratio at rest and during exercise in training athletes. *American Journal of Physiology–Endocrinology and Metabolism* 276, no. 6 (2000): E1325–34.

Helge, J. W., P. W. Watt, E. A. Richter, M. J. Rennie, and B. Kiens. Fat utilization during exercise: Adaptation to a fat-rich diet increases utilization of plasma fatty acids and very low density lipoprotein-triacylglycerol in humans. *Journal of Physiology* 537 (December 2001): 1009–20.

Helge, J. W., P. W. Watt, E. A. Richter, M. J. Rennie, and B. Kiens. Partial restoration of dietary fat induced metabolic adaptation to training by 7 days of carbohydrate diet. *Journal of Applied Physiology* 93, no. 5 (2002): 1797–805.

Helge, J. W., B. Wulff, and B. Kiens. Impact of a fat-rich diet on endurance in man: Role of the dietary period. *Medicine and Science in Sports and Exercise* 30, no. 3 (1998): 456–61.

Hughson, R. L., and J. M. Kowalchuk. Influence of diet on CO_2 production and ventilation in constant-load exercise. *Respiratory Physiology* 46, no. 2 (1981): 149–60.

Jansson, E., and L. Kaijser. Effect of diet on muscle glycogen and blood glucose utilization during a short-term exercise in man. *Acta Physiologica Scandinavica* 115, no. 3 (1982): 341–47.

Jansson, E., and L. Kaijser. Effect of diet on the utilization of blood-borne and intramuscular substrates during exercise in man. *Acta Physiologica Scandinavica* 115, no. 1 (1982): 19–30.

Keim, N. L., T. F. Barbieri, M. D. VanLoan, and B. L. Anderson. Energy expenditure and physical performance in overweight women: Response to training with and without caloric restriction. *Metabolism* 39, no. 6 (1990): 651–58.

Kiens, B., B. Essen-Gustavsson, N. J. Christensen, and B. Saltin. Skeletal muscle utilization during submaximal exercise in man: Effect of endurance training. *Journal of Physiology* 469 (1993): 459–78.

Lambert, E. V., J. A. Hawley, J. Goedecke, T. D. Noakes, and S. C. Dennis. Nutritional strategies for promoting fat utilization and delaying the onset of fatigue during prolonged exercise. *Journal of Sports Science* 15, no. 3 (1997): 315–24.

Lambert, E. V., D. P. Speechly, S. C. Dennis, and T. D. Noakes. Enhanced endurance in trained cyclists during moderate intensity exercise following 2 weeks adaptation to a high-fat diet. *European Journal of Applied Physiology* 69, no. 4 (1994): 287–93.

Marino, F. E., Z. Mbambo, E. Kortekaas, G. Wilson, M. I. Lambert, T. D. Noakes, and S. C. Dennis. Advantages of smaller body mass during distance running in warm, humid environments. *Pflügers Archiv: European Journal of Physiology* 441, no. 2–3 (2000): 359–67.

McCauley, K. A., K. J. Smith, R. W. Taylor, R. T. McLay, S. M. Williams, and J. I. Mann. Long-term effects of popular dietary approaches on weight loss and features of insulin resistance. *International Journal of Obesity* 30, no. 2 (2006): 342–49.

McMurray, R. G., V. Ben-Ezra, W. A. Forsythe, and A. T. Smith. Responses of endurance-trained subjects to caloric deficits induced by diet or exercise. *Medicine and Science in Sports and Exercise* 17, no. 5 (1985): 574–79.

Muoio, D. M., J. J. Leddy, P. J. Horvath, A. B. Awad, and D. R. Pendergast. Effect of dietary fat on metabolic adjustments to maximal VO2 and endurance in runners. *Medicine and Science in Sports and Exercise* 26, no. 1 (1994): 81–88.

Noakes, M., J. B. Keogh, P. R. Foster, and P. M. Clifton. Effect of an energy-restricted, high-protein, low-fat diet relative to a conventional high-carbohydrate, low-fat diet on weight loss, body composition, nutritional status, and markers of cardiovascular health in obese women. *American Journal of Clinical Nutrition* 81, no. 6 (2005): 1298–306.

Pendergast, D. R., P. J. Horvath, J. J. Leddy, and J. T. Venkatraman. The role of dietary fat on performance, metabolism, and health. *American Journal of Sports Medicine* 24, no. 6 (1996): S53–58.

Phinney, S. D., B. R. Bistrian, W. J. Evans, E. Gervino, and G. L. Blackburn. The human metabolic response to chronic ketosis without caloric restriction: Preservation of sub-maximal exercise capability with reduced carbohydrate oxidation. *Metabolism* 32, no. 8 (1983): 769–76.

Piatti, P. M., F. Monti, I. Fermo, L. Baruffaldi, R. Nasser, G. Santambrogio, M. C. Librenti, M. Galli-Kienle, A. E. Pontiroli, and G. Pozza. Hypocaloric, high-protein diet improves glucose oxidation and spares lean body mass: Comparison to hypocaloric high carbohydrate diet. *Metabolism* 43, no. 12 (1994): 1481–87.

Rankin, J. W. Weight loss and gain in athletes. *Current Sports Medicine Report* 1, no. 4 (2002): 208–13.

Simi, B., B. Sempore, M. H. Mayet, and R. J. Favier. Additive effects of training and high-fat diet on energy metabolism during exercise. *Journal of Applied Physiology* 71, no. 1 (1991): 197–203.

Stevens, J. Does dietary fiber affect food intake and body weight? *Journal of the American Dietetic Association* 88, no. 8 (1988): 939–42.

Tappy, L. Thermic effect of food and sympathetic nervous system activity in humans. *Reproduction Nutrition Development* 36, no. 4 (1996): 391–97.

Toubro, S., T. I. Sørensen, C. Hindsberger, N. J. Christensen, and A. Astrup. Twenty-four-hour respiratory quotient: The role of diet and familial resemblance. *Journal of Clinical Endocrinology & Metabolism* 83, no. 8 (1998): 2758–64.

Vandervater, K., and Z. Vickers. Higher-protein foods produce greater sensory-specific satiety. *Physiology & Behavior* 59, no. 3 (1996): 579–83.

Venkatraman, J. T., J. A. Rowland, E. Denardin, P. J. Horvath, and D. Pendergast. Influence of the level of dietary lipid intake and maximal exercise on the immune status in runners. *Medicine and Science in Sports and Exercise* 29, no. 3 (1997): 333–44.

Westerterp-Plantenga, M. S., N. Luscombe-Marsh, M. P. G. M. LeJenne, K. Diepvens, A. Nieuwenhuizen, M. P. K. J. Engelen, N. E. P. Deutz, D. Azzout-Marniche, D. Tome, and

K. R. Westerterp. Dietary protein, metabolism, and body-weight regulation: Dose-response effects. *International Journal of Obesity* 30 (2006): S16–23.

CHAPTER 7

Bailey, S. P., J. M. Davis, and E. N. Ahlborn. Neuroendocrine and substrate responses to altered brain 5-HT activity during prolonged exercise to fatigue. *Journal of Applied Physiology* 74, no. 6 (1993): 3006–12.

Balaban, E. P., J. V. Cox, P. Snell, R. H. Vaughan, and E. P. Frenkel. The frequency of anemia and iron deficiency in the runner. *Medicine and Science in Sports and Exercise* 21, no. 6 (1989): 643–48.

Bendich, A., and R. K. Chandra. *Micronutrients and Immune Functions*. New York: New York Academy of Sciences, 1990.

Cade, J. R., R. H. Reese, R. M. Privette, N. M. Hommen, J. L. Rogers, and M. J. Fregly. Dietary intervention and training in swimmers. *European Journal of Applied Physiology and Occupational Physiology* 63 (1991): 210–15.

Chandra, R. K. Nutrition and immunity: Lessons from the past and new insights into the future. *American Journal of Clinical Nutrition* 53 (1990): 1087–101.

Cheuvront, S. N., R. I. Carter, and M. N. Sawka. Fluid balance and endurance exercise performance. *Current Sports Medicine Report* 2 (2003): 202–8.

Clement, D. B., D. R. Lloyd-Smith, J. G. Macintyre, G. O. Matheson, R. Brock, and M. Dupont. Iron status in Winter Olympic sports. *Journal of Sports Science* 5, no. 3 (1987): 261–71.

Costill, D. L., E. Coyle, G. Dalsky, W. Evans, W. Fink, and D. Hoopes. Effects of elevated plasma FFA and insulin on muscle glycogen usage during exercise. *Journal of Applied Physiology* 43, no. 4 (1977): 695–99.

Costill, D. L., M. G. Flynn, J. A. Kirwan, J. B. Houmard, J. B. Mitchell, R. Thomas, and S. H. Park. Effects of repeated days of intensified training on muscle glycogen and swimming performance. *Medicine and Science in Sports and Exercise* 20 (1988): 249–54.

Cunningham-Rundles, S. *Nutrient Modulation of the Immune Response*. New York: Marcel Dekker, 1993.

Davis, J. M., and S. P. Bailey. Possible mechanisms of central nervous system fatigue during exercise. *Medicine and Science in Sports and Exercise* 29, no. 1 (1997): 45–57.

Deuster, P. A., S. B. Kyle, P. B. Moser, R. A. Vigersky, A. Singh, and E. B. Schoomaker. Nutritional intakes and status of highly trained amenorrheic and eumenorrheic women runners. *Fertility and Sterility* 46, no. 4 (1986): 636–43.

Deuster, P. A., S. B. Kyle, P. B. Moser, R. A. Vigersky, A. Singh, and E. B. Schoomaker. Nutritional survey of highly trained women runners. *American Journal of Clinical Nutrition* 44, no. 6 (1986): 954–62.

Dressendorfer, R. H., and R. Sockolov. Hypozincemia in runners. *Physiology and Sports Medicine* 8 (1980): 97–100.

Dyck, D. J., C. T. Putman, G. J. Heigenhauser, E. Hultman, and L. L. Spriet. Regulation of fat-carbohydrate interaction in skeletal muscle during intense aerobic cycling. *American Journal of Physiology* 265, no. 6 (1993): E852–59.

Falk, B., R. Burstein, and J. Rosenblum. Effects of caffeine ingestion on body fluid balance and thermoregulation during exercise. *Canadian Journal of Physiology and Pharmacology* 68, no. 7 (1990): 889–92.

Flakoll, P. J., T. Judy, K. Flinn, C. Carr, and S. Flinn. Postexercise protein supplementation improves health and muscle soreness during basic military training in marine recruits. *Journal of Applied Physiology* 96, no. 3 (2004): 951–56.

Fry, R. W., A. R. Morton, and D. Keast. Overtraining in athletes: An update. *Sports Medicine* 12, no. 1 (1991): 32–65.

Fudge, B. W., C. Easton, D. Kingsmore, F. K. Kiplamai, V. O. Onywera, K. R. Westerterp, B. Kayser, T. D. Noakes, and Y. P. Pitsiladis. Elite Kenyan endurance runners are hydrated day-to-day with ad libitum fluid intake. *Medicine and Science in Sports and Exercise* 40, no. 6 (2008): 1171–79.

Gershwin, M. E., R. S. Beach, and L. S. Hurley. *Nutrition and Immunity.* Orlando: Academic Press, 1985.

Hawley, J. A., and W. G. Hopkins. Aerobic glycolytic and aerobic lipolytic power systems. A new paradigm with implications for endurance and ultraendurance events. *Sports Medicine* 19, no. 4 (1995): 240–50.

Ivy, J. L., H. W. Goforth Jr., B. M. Damon, T. R. McCauley, E. C. Parsons, and T. B. J. Price. Early postexercise muscle glycogen recovery is enhanced with a carbohydrate-protein supplement. *Applied Physiology* 93, no. 4 (2002): 1337–44.

Ivy, J. L., P. T. Res, R. C. Sprague, and M. O. Widzer. Effect of a carbohydrate-protein supplement on endurance performance during exercise of varying intensity. *International Journal of Sport Nutrition and Exercise Metabolism* 13, no. 3 (2003): 382–95.

Kirwan, J. P., D. L. Costill, J. B. Mitchell, J. B. Houmard, M. G. Flynn, W. J. Fink, and J. D. Beltz. Carbohydrate balance in competitive runners during successive days of intense training. *Journal of Applied Physiology* 65, no. 6 (1988): 2601–6.

Kovacs, E. M., J. M. Senden, and F. Brouns. Urine color, osmolality, and specific electrical conductance are not accurate measures of hydration status during postexercise rehydration. *Journal of Sports Medicine and Physical Fitness* 39, no. 1 (1999): 47–53.

Lambert, E. V., and J. H. Goedecke. The role of dietary macronutrients in optimizing endurance performance. *Current Sports Medicine Report* 2, no. 4 (2003): 194–201.

Lambert, E. V., D. P. Speechly, S. C. Dennis, and T. D. Noakes. Enhanced endurance in trained cyclists during moderate-intensity exercise following two weeks adaptation to a high-fat diet. *European Journal of Applied Physiology* 69, no. 4 (1994): 287–93.

Lapachet, R. A., W. C. Miller, and D. A. Arnall. Body fat and exercise endurance in trained rats adapted to a high-fat and/or high-carbohydrate diet. *Journal of Applied Physiology* 80, no. 4 (1996): 1173–79.

Marcora, S. M., W. Staiano, and V. Manning. Mental fatigue impairs physical performance in humans. *Journal of Applied Physiology* 106, no. 3 (2009): 857–64.

Marcora, S. M., and W. Staiano. The limit to exercise tolerance in humans: Mind over muscle? *European Journal of Applied Physiology* 109, no. 4 (2010): 763–70.

Muoio, D. M., J. J. Leddy, P. J. Horvath, A. B. Awad, and D. R. Pendergast. Effect of dietary fat on metabolic adjustments to maximal VO_2 and endurance in runners. *Medicine and Science in Sports and Exercise* 26, no. 1 (1994): 81–88.

Noakes, T. D. Time to move beyond a brainless exercise physiology: The evidence for complex regulation of human exercise performance. *Applied Physiology, Nutrition, and Metabolism* 36, no. 1 (2011): 23–25.

Noakes, T. D., A. St. Clair, and E. V. Lambert. From catastrophe to complexity: A novel model of integrative central neural regulation of effort and fatigue during exercise in humans. *British Journal of Sports Medicine* 38, no. 4 (2004): 511–14.

Noakes, T. D., and A. St. Clair. Logical limitations to the "catastrophe" models of fatigue during exercise in humans. *British Journal of Sports Medicine* 38, no. 5 (2004): 648–49.

Noakes, T. D., et al. Effects of a low-carbohydrate, high-fat diet prior to carbohydrate loading on endurance cycling performance. *Clinical Science* 87 (1994): S32–33.

Nose, H., G. W. Mack, X. R. Shi, and E. R. Nadel. Role of osmolality and plasma volume during rehydration in humans. *Journal of Applied Physiology* 65, no. 1 (1988): 325–31.

Oliver, S. J., S. J. Laing, S. Wilson, J. L. Bilzon, and N. Walsh. Endurance running performance after 48h of restricted fluid and/or energy intake. *Medicine and Science in Sports and Exercise* 39, no. 2 (2007): 316–22.

Phinney, S. D., B. R. Bistrian, W. J. Evans, E. Gervino, and G. L. Blackburn. The human metabolic response to chronic ketosis without caloric restriction: Preservation of submaximal exercise capability with reduced carbohydrate oxidation. *Metabolism* 32, no. 8 (1983): 769–76.

Sawka, M. N., S. J. Montain, and W. A. Latzka. Hydration effects on thermoregulation and performance in the heat. *Comparative Biochemistry and Physiology Part A: Molecular & Integrative Physiology* 128, no. 4 (2001): 679–690.

Shephard, R. J., and P. N. Shek. Immunological hazards from nutritional imbalance in athletes. *Exercise Immunology Review* 4 (1998): 22–48.

Sherman, W. M., J. A. Doyle, D. R. Lamb, and R. H. Strauss. Dietary carbohydrate, muscle glycogen, and exercise performance during 7 days of training. *American Journal of Clinical Nutrition* 57 (January 1993): 27–31.

Sherman, W. M., and G. S. Wimer. Insufficient dietary carbohydrate during training: Does it impair athletic performance? *International Journal of Sport Nutrition* 1, no. 1 (1991): 28–44.

Shirreffs, S. M., and R. J. Maughan. Rehydration and recovery of fluid balance after exercise. *Exercise and Sport Sciences Reviews* 28, no. 1 (2000): 27–32.

Slater, G. J., A. J. Rice, K. Sharpe, R. Tanner, D. Jenkins, C. J. Gore, and A. G. Hahn. Impact of acute weight loss and/or thermal stress on rowing ergometer performance. *Medicine and Science in Sports and Exercise* 37, no. 8 (2005): 1387–94.

Snyder, A. C., H. Kuipers, B. Cheng, R. Servais, and E. Fransen. Overtraining following intensified training with normal muscle glycogen. *Medicine and Science in Sports and Exercise* 27, no. 7 (1995): 1063–70.

Steinacker, J. M., W. Lormes, M. Lehmann, and D. Altenburg. Training of rowers before world championships. *Medicine and Science in Sports and Exercise* 30, no. 7 (1998): 1158–63.

Tucker, R. The anticipatory regulation of performance: The physiological basis for pacing strategies and the development of a perception-based model for exercise performance. *British Journal of Sports Medicine* 43, no. 6 (2009): 392–400.

Van Erp-Baart, A. M., W. M. Saris, R. A. Binkhorst, J. A. Vos, and J. W. Elvers. Nationwide survey on nutritional habits in elite athletes. Part II. Mineral and vitamin intake. *International Journal of Sports Medicine* 10 (May 1989): S11–16.

Vogt, M., A. Puntschart, H. Howald, B. Mueller, C. H. Mannhart, L. Gfeller-Tuescher, P. Mullis, and H. Hoppeler. Effects of dietary fat on muscle substrates, metabolism, and performance in athletes. *Medicine and Science in Sports and Exercise* 35, no. 6 (2003): 952–60.

Weiss, H. E. Anamnestic, clinical and laboratory data of 1300 athletes in a basic medical check with respect to the incidence and prophylaxis of infectious diseases. *International Journal of Sports Medicine* 6 (1994): 360.

Wilson, W. M., and R. J. Maughan. Evidence for a possible role of 5-hydroxytryptamine in the genesis of fatigue in man: Administration of paroxetine, a 5-HT re-uptake inhibitor, reduces the capacity to perform prolonged exercise. *Experimental Physiology* 77, no. 6 (1992): 921–24.

Wong, S. H., C. Williams, M. Simpson, and T. Ogaki. Influence of fluid intake pattern on short-term recovery from prolonged, submaximal running and subsequent exercise capacity. *Journal of Sports Science* 16, no. 2 (1998): 143–52.

Zawadzki, K. M., B. B. Yaspelkis III, and J. L. Ivy. Carbohydrate-protein complex increases the rate of muscle glycogen storage after exercise. *Journal of Applied Physiology* 72, no. 5 (1992): 1854–59.

CHAPTER 8

Aiello, L. C., and P. Wheeler. The expensive tissue hypothesis: The brain and the digestive system in human and primate evolution. *Current Anthropology* 36, no. 2 (1995): 199–221.

Allam, A. H., R. C. Thompson, L. S. Wann, M. I. Miyamoto, A. el-Halim Nur El-Din, G. A. El-Maksoud, M. Al-Tohamy Soliman, I. Badr, H. A. El-Rahman Amer, M. L. Sutherland, J. D. Sutherland, and G. S. Thomas. Atherosclerosis in ancient Egyptian mummies: The Horus study. *JACC Cardiovascular Imaging* 4, no. 4 (April 2011): 315–27.

Atkins, R. C., D. Ornish, and T. Wadden. Low-carb, low-fat diet gurus face off. Interview by Joan Stephenson. *JAMA* 289, no. 14 (April 2003): 1767–68, 1773.

Beltrame, M. O., M. H. Fugassa, and N. H. Sardella. First paleoparasitological results from late Holocene in Patagonian coprolites. *Journal of Parasitology* 96, no. 3 (June 2010): 648–51.

Blumenschine, R. J., and J. A. Cavallo. Scavenging and human evolution. *Scientific American* 267 (1992): 90–96.

Bocherens, H., D. G. Drucker, D. Billiou, M. Patou-Mathis, and B. Vandermeersch. Isotopic evidence for diet and subsistence pattern of the Saint-Césaire I Neanderthal: Review and use of a multi-source mixing model. *Journal of Human Evolution* 49, no. 1 (July 2005): 71–87.

Bourbou, C., B. T. Fuller, S. J. Garvie-Lok, and M. P. Richards. Reconstructing the diets of Greek Byzantine populations (6th–15th centuries A.D.) using carbon and nitrogen stable isotope ratios. *American Journal of Physical Anthropology* 146, no. 4 (December 2011): 569–81.

Britton, K., V. Grimes, L. Niven, T. E. Steele, S. McPherron, M. Soressi, T. E. Kelly, J. Jaubert, J. J. Hublin, and M. P. Richards. Strontium isotope evidence for migration in late Pleistocene Rangifer: Implications for Neanderthal hunting strategies at the Middle Palaeolithic site of Jonzac, France. *Journal of Human Evolution* 61, no. 2 (August 2011): 176–85.

Brown, F., J. Harris, R. Leakey, and A. Walker. Early *Homo erectus* skeleton from west Lake Turkana, Kenya. *Nature* 316 (August 1985): 788–92.

Bunn, H. T., and E. M. Kroll. Systematic butchery by plio/pleistocene hominids at Oldulvai Gorge, Tanzania. *Current Anthropology* 27, no. 5 (1986): 431–52.

Burdge, G. C., A. E. Jones, and S. A. Wootton. Eicosapentaenoic and docosapentaenoic acids are the principal products of alpha-linolenic acid metabolism in young men. *British Journal of Nutrition* 88, no. 4 (October 2002): 355–63.

Burdge, G. C., and S.A. Wootton. Conversion of alpha-linolenic acid to eicosapentaenoic, do-cosapentaenoic and docosahexaenoic acids in young women. *British Journal of Nutrition* 88, no. 4 (October 2002): 411–20.

Carrera-Bastos, P., M. Fontes Villalba, J. H. O'Keefe, S. Lindeberg, and L. Cordain. The Western diet and lifestyle and diseases of civilization. *Research Reports in Clinical Cardiology* 2 (March 2011): 15–35.

Chesney, R. W., R. A. Helms, M. Christensen, A. M. Budreau, X. Han, and J. A. Sturman. The role of taurine in infant nutrition. *Advanced Experimental Medical Biology* 442 (1998): 463–76.

Cordain, L. "Saturated Fat Consumption in Ancestral Human Diets: Implications for Contemporary Intakes." In *Phytochemicals: Nutrient-Gene Interactions*, edited by M. S. Meskin, W. R. Bidlack, and R. K. Randolph, 115–26. Boca Raton, FL: CRC Press, 2006.

Cordain, L., J. C. Brand-Miller, S. B. Eaton, N. Mann, S. H. A. Holt, and J. D. Speth. Plant to animal subsistence ratios and macronutrient energy estimations in worldwide hunter-gatherer diets. *American Journal of Clinical Nutrition* 71, no. 3 (2000): 682–92.

Cordain, L., S. B. Eaton, J. C. Brand-Miller, N. Mann, and K. Hill. The paradoxical nature of hunter-gatherer diets: Meat-based, yet non-atherogenic. *European Journal of Clinical Nutrition* 56 (March 2002): S42–52.

Cordain, L., S. B. Eaton, A. Sebastian, N. Mann, S. Lindeberg, B. A. Watkins, J. H. O'Keefe, and J. C. Brand-Miller. Origins and evolution of the Western diet: Health implications for the 21st century. *American Journal of Clinical Nutrition* 81, no. 2 (February 2005): 341–54.

Cordain, L., B. A. Watkins, and N. J. Mann. Fatty acid composition and energy density of foods available to African hominids: Evolutionary implications for human brain development. *World Review of Nutrition and Dietetics* 90 (2001): 144–61.

De Heinzelin, J., J. D. Clark, T. White, W. Hart, P. Renne, G. WoldeGabriel, Y. Beyene, and E. Vrba. Environment and behavior of 2.5-million-year-old Bouri hominids. *Science* 284, no. 5414 (April 1999): 625–29.

Driskell, J. A. *Sports Nutrition.* New York: CRC Press, 2000.

Drucker, D. G., and D. Henry-Gambier. Determination of the dietary habits of a Magdalenian woman from Saint-Germain-la-Rivière in southwestern France using stable isotopes. *Journal of Human Evolution* 49, no. 1 (July 2005): 19–35.

Eaton, S. B., B. I. Strassman, R. M. Nesse, J. V. Neel, P. W. Ewald, G. C. Williams, A. B. Weder, S. B. Eaton III, S. Lindeberg, M. J. Konner, I. Mysterud, and L. Cordain. Evolutionary health promotion. *Preventive Medicine* 34, no. 2 (2002): 109–18.

Emken, R. A., R. O. Adlof, W. K. Rohwedder, and R. M. Gulley. "Comparison of Linolenic and Linoleic Acid Metabolism in Man: Influence of Dietary Linoleic Acid." In *Essential Fatty Acids and Eicosanoids: Invited Papers from the Third International Conference*, edited by A. Sinclair and R. Gibson, 23–25. Champaign, IL: AOCS Press, 1992.

Ermini, L., C. Olivieri, E. Rizzi, G. Corti, R. Bonnal, P. Soares, S. Luciani, I. Marota, G. De Bellis, M. B. Richards, and F. Rollo. Complete mitochondrial genome sequence of the Tyrolean Iceman. *Current Biology* 18, no. 21 (November 2008): 1687–93.

French, L., and S. Kendall. Does a high-fiber diet prevent colon cancer in at-risk patients? *Journal of Family Practice* 52, no. 11 (November 2003): 892–93.

Fuller, B. T., N. Márquez-Grant, and M. P. Richards. Investigation of diachronic dietary patterns on the islands of Ibiza and Formentera, Spain: Evidence from carbon and nitrogen stable isotope ratio analysis. *American Journal of Physical Anthropology* 143, no. 4 (December 2010): 512–22.

Gilbert, M. T., D. L. Jenkins, A. Götherstrom, N. Naveran, J. J. Sanchez, M. Hofreiter, P. F. Thomsen, J. Binladen, T. F. Higham, R. M. Yohe II, R. Parr, L. S. Cummings, and E. Willerslev. DNA from pre-Clovis human coprolites in Oregon, North America. *Science* 320, no. 5877 (May 2008): 786–89.

Gray, J. P. A corrected ethnographic atlas. *World Cultures Journal* 10, no. 1 (1999): 24–85.

Hawkes, K., K. Hill, and J. F. O'Connell. Why hunters gather: Optimal foraging and the Ache of eastern Paraguay. *American Ethnologist* 9 (May 1982): 379–98.

Hohmann, G., and B. Fruth. New records on prey capture and meat eating by bonobos at Lui Kotale, Salonga National Park, Democratic Republic of Congo. *Folia Primatologica* 79, no. 2 (2008): 103–10.

Hu, Y., H. Shang, H. Tong, O. Nehlich, W. Liu, C. Zhao, J. Yu, C. Wang, E. Trinkaus, and M. P. Richards. Stable isotope dietary analysis of the Tianyuan 1 early modern human. *Proceedings of the National Academy of Sciences* 106, no. 27 (July 2009): 10971–74.

Hu, F. B., M. J. Stampfer, E. B. Rimm, J. E. Manson, A. Ascherio, G. A. Colditz, B. A. Rosner, D. Spiegelman, F. E. Speizer, F. M. Sacks, C. H. Hennekens, and W. C. Willett. A prospective study of egg consumption and risk of cardiovascular disease in men and women. *JAMA* 281, no. 15 (1999): 1387–94.

Jay, M., B. T. Fuller, M. P. Richards, C. J. Knüsel, and S. S. King. Iron Age breastfeeding practices in Britain: Isotopic evidence from Wetwang Slack, East Yorkshire. *American Journal of Physical Anthropology* 136, no. 3 (July 2008): 327–37.

Katan, M. B. Trans fatty acids and plasma lipoproteins. *Nutrition Review* 58, no. 6 (2000): 188–91.

Knopf, K., J. A. Sturman, M. Armstrong, and K. C. Hayes. Taurine: An essential nutrient for the cat. *Journal of Nutrition* 108, no. 5 (1978): 773–78.

Kuhn, S. L., and M. C. Stiner. "The Antiquity of Hunter-Gatherers." In *Hunter-Gatherers, an Interdisciplinary Perspective,* edited by C. Panter-Brick, R. H. Layton, and P. Rowley-Conwy, 99–129. Cambridge: Cambridge University Press, 2001.

Kuipers, R. S., M. F. Luxwolda, D. A. Dijck-Brouwer, S. B. Eaton, M. A. Crawford, L. Cordain, and F. A. Muskiet. Estimated macronutrient and fatty acid intakes from an East African Paleolithic diet. *British Journal of Nutrition* 104, no. 11 (December 2010): 1666–87.

Laidlaw, S. A., T. D. Shultz, J. T. Cecchino, and J. D. Kopple. Plasma and urine taurine levels in vegans. *American Journal of Clinical Nutrition* 47 (April 1988): 660–63.

Lee, R. B. "What Hunters Do for a Living, or How to Make Out on Scarce Resources." In *Man the Hunter,* edited by R. B. Lee and I. DeVore, 30–48. Chicago: Aldine, 1968.

Lee-Thorp, J., J. F. Thackeray, and N. van der Merwe. The hunters and the hunted revisited. *Journal of Human Evolution* 39, no. 6 (December 2000): 565–76.

Leonard, W. R., and M. L. Robertson. Evolutionary perspectives on human nutrition: The influence of brain and body size on diet and metabolism. *American Journal of Human Biology* 6, no. 1 (1994): 77–88.

Leonard, W. R., M. L. Robertson, J. J. Snodgrass, and C. W. Kuzawa. Metabolic correlates of hominid brain evolution. *Comparative Biochemistry and Physiology Part A: Molecular & Integrative Physiology* 136, no. 1 (September 2003): 5–15.

Leonard, W. R., J. J. Snodgrass, and M. L. Robertson. Effects of brain evolution on human nutrition and metabolism. *Annual Review of Nutrition* 27 (August 2007): 311–27.

Lieb, C. W. The effects on human beings of a twelve months' exclusive meat diet. *JAMA* 93 (July 1929): 20–22.

Lin, D. S., and W. E. Connor. Fecal steroids of the coprolite of a Greenland Eskimo mummy, AD 1475: A clue to dietary sterol intake. *American Journal of Clinical Nutrition* 74, no. 1 (July 2001): 44–49.

MacDonald, M. L., Q. R. Rogers, and J. G. Morris. Nutrition of the domestic cat, a mammalian carnivore. *Annual Review of Nutrition* 4 (1984): 521–62.

McArdle, W. D., F. I. Katch, and V. L. Katch. *Sports and Exercise Nutrition.* New York: Lippincott Williams & Wilkins, 1999.

Movius, H. L. A wooden spear of third interglacial age from lower Saxony. *Southwest Journal of Anthropology* 6, no. 2 (1950): 139–42.

Müller, W., H. Fricke, A. N. Halliday, M. T. McCulloch, and J. A. Wartho. Origin and migration of the Alpine Iceman. *Science* 302, no. 5646 (October 2003): 862–66.

Murdock, G. P. Ethnographic atlas: A summary. *Ethnology* 6, no. 2 (1967): 109–236.

Nishikimi, M., and K. Yagi. Molecular basis for the deficiency in humans of gulonolactone oxidase, a key enzyme for ascorbic acid biosynthesis. *American Journal of Clinical Nutrition* 54, no. 6 (1991): 1203S–8S.

Niven, L. From carcass to cave: Large mammal exploitation during the Aurignacian at Vogelherd, Germany. *Journal of Human Evolution* 53, no. 4 (October 2007): 362–82.

Noli, D., and G. Avery. Protein poisoning and coastal subsistence. *Journal of Archaeological Science* 15, no. 4 (1988): 395–401.

Pawlosky, R., A. Barnes, and N. Salem. Essential fatty acid metabolism in the feline: Relationship between liver and brain production of long-chain polyunsaturated fatty acids. *Journal of Lipid Research* 35, no. 11 (1994): 2032–40.

Pitts, G. C., and T. R. Bullard. "Some Interspecific Aspects of Body Composition in Mammals." In *Body Composition in Animals and Man,* 45–70. Washington, DC: National Academy of Sciences, 1968.

Richards, M. P., and R. M. Hedges. Focus: Gough's Cave and Sun Hole Cave human stable isotope values indicate a high animal protein diet in the British Upper Palaeolithic. *Journal of Archaeology Science* 27, no. 1 (2000): 1–3.

Richards, M. P., R. Jacobi, J. Cook, P. B. Pettitt, and C. B. Stringer. Isotope evidence for the intensive use of marine foods by Late Upper Palaeolithic humans. *Journal of Human Evolution* 49, no. 3 (September 2005): 390–94.

Richards, M. P., P. B. Pettitt, E. Trinkaus, F. H. Smith, M. Paunovic, and I. Karavanic. Neanderthal diet at Vindija and Neanderthal predation: The evidence from stable isotopes. *Proceedings of the National Academy of Sciences* 97, no. 13 (2000): 7663–66.

Richards, M. P., R. J. Schulting, and R. E. Hedges. Archaeology: Sharp shift in diet at onset of Neolithic. *Nature* 425, no. 6956 (September 2003): 366.

Richards, M. P., G. Taylor, T. Steele, S. P. McPherron, M. Soressi, J. Jaubert, J. Orschiedt, J. B. Mallye, W. Rendu, and J. J. Hublin. Isotopic dietary analysis of a Neanderthal and associated fauna from the site of Jonzac (Charente-Maritime), France. *Journal of Human Evolution* 55, no. 1 (July 2008): 179–85.

Richards, M. P., and E. Trinkaus. Out of Africa: Modern human origins special feature: Isotopic evidence for the diets of European Neanderthals and early modern humans. *Proceedings of the National Academy of Sciences* 106, no. 38 (September 2009): 16034–39.

Rosser, Z. H., T. Zerjal, M. E. Hurles, M. Adojaan, et al. Y-chromosomal diversity in Europe is clinal and influenced primarily by geography, rather than by language. *American Journal of Human Genetics* 67, no. 6 (2000): 1526–43.

Rudman, D., T. J. DiFulco, J. T. Galambos, R. B. Smith, A. A. Salam, and W. D. Warren. Maximal rates of excretion and synthesis of urea in normal and cirrhotic subjects. *Journal of Clinical Investigation* 52, no. 9 (1973): 2241–49.

Semaw, S., M. J. Rogers, J. Quade, P. R. Renne, R. F. Butler, M. Dominguez-Rodrigo, D. Stout, W. S. Hart, T. Pickering, and S. W. Simpson. 2.6-million-year-old stone tools and associated bones from OGS-6 and OGS-7, Gona, Afar, Ethiopia. *Journal of Human Evolution* 45, no. 2 (2003): 169–77.

Simon, H. B. My husband subscribes to *Harvard Men's Health Watch*, but I read it even more than he does. I hope you can help us resolve a disagreement. He wants to have pizza two to three times a week for his prostate, but I don't think it's a healthy food. Who is right? *Harvard Men's Health Watch* 7, no. 11 (June 2003): 8.

Shipman, P. Scavenging or hunting in early hominids: Theoretical framework and tests. *American Anthropologist* 88, no. 1 (1986): 27–43.

Shipman, P., and J. Rose. Early hominid butchering and carcass-processing behaviors: Approaches to the fossil record. *Journal of Anthropological Archaeology* 2, no. 1 (1983): 57–98.

Speth, J. D. Early hominid hunting and scavenging: The role of meat as an energy source. *Journal of Human Evolution* 18, no. 4 (1989): 329–43.

Speth, J. D., and K. A. Spielmann. Energy source, protein metabolism, and hunter-gatherer subsistence strategies. *Journal of Anthropological Archaeology* 2, no. 1 (1983): 1–31.

Stanford, C. B. The hunting ecology of wild chimpanzees: Implications for the behavioral ecology of Pliocene hominids. *American Anthropologist* 98, no. 1 (1996): 96–113.

Stanford, C. B., J. Wallis, H. Matama, and J. Goodall. Patterns of predation by chimpanzees on red colobus monkeys in Gombe National Park, 1982–1991. *American Journal of Physiological Anthropology* 94, no. 2 (June 1994): 213–28.

Sturman, J. A., G. W. Hepner, A. F. Hofmann, and P. J. Thomas. Metabolism of [35S] taurine in man. *Journal of Nutrition* 105, no. 9 (1975): 1206–14.

Teelen, S. Influence of chimpanzee predation on the red colobus population at Ngogo, Kibale National Park, Uganda. *Primates* 49, no. 1 (January 2008): 41–49.

Thieme, H. Lower Palaeolithic hunting spears from Germany. *Nature* 385, no. 6619 (February 1997): 807–10.

Vercellotti, G., G. Alciati, M. P. Richards, and V. Formicola. The Late Upper Paleolithic skeleton Villabruna 1 (Italy): A source of data on biology and behavior of a 14,000-year-old hunter. *Journal of Anthropological Sciences* 86 (2008): 143–63.

Watts, D. P. Scavenging by chimpanzees at Ngogo and the relevance of chimpanzee scavenging to early hominin behavioral ecology. *Journal of Human Evolution* 54, no. 1 (January 2008): 125–33.

Watts, D. P., K. B. Potts, J. S. Lwanga, and J. C. Mitani. Diet of chimpanzees (Pan troglodytes schweinfurthii) at Ngogo, Kibale National Park, Uganda, 1. Diet composition and diversity. *American Journal of Primatology* 74, no. 2 (2012): 114–29.

Watts, D. P., K. B. Potts, J. S. Lwanga, and J. C. Mitani. Diet of chimpanzees (Pan troglodytes schweinfurthii) at Ngogo, Kibale National Park, Uganda, 2. Temporal variation and fallback foods. *American Journal of Primatology* 74, no. 2 (2012): 130–44.

Whiten, A., K. Schick, and N. Toth. The evolution and cultural transmission of percussive technology: Integrating evidence from palaeoanthropology and primatology. *Journal of Human Evolution* 57, no. 4 (October 2009): 420–35.

Wildman, D. E., M. Uddin, G. Liu, L. I. Grossman, and M. Goodman. Implications of natural selection in shaping 99.4% nonsynonymous DNA identity between humans and chimpanzees: Enlarging genus *Homo*. *Proceedings of the National Academy of Sciences* 100, no. 12 (2003): 7181–88.

Willett, W. C., and M. J. Stampfer. Rebuilding the food pyramid. *Scientific American* 288, no. 1 (January 2003): 64–71.

Winterhalder, B. P. "Optimal Foraging Strategies and Hunter-Gatherer Research in Anthropology: Theories and Models." In *Hunter-Gatherer Foraging Strategies,* edited by B. P. Winterhalder and E. A. Smith, 13–35. Chicago: University of Chicago, 1981.

Wood, B. Hominid revelations from Chad. *Nature* 418, no. 6894 (2002): 133–35.

CHAPTER 9

Astrup, A., J. Dyerberg, P. Elwood, K. Hermansen, F. B. Hu, M. U. Jakobsen, F. J. Kok, R. M. Krauss, J. M. Lecerf, P. Legrand, P. Nestel, U. Risérus, T. Sanders, A. Sinclair, S. Stender, T. Tholstrup, and W. C. Willett. The role of reducing intakes of saturated fat in the prevention of cardiovascular disease: Where does the evidence stand in 2010? *American Journal of Clinical Nutrition* 93, no. 4 (April 2011): 684–88.

Aude, Y. W., A. S. Agatston, F. Lopez-Jimenez, E. H. Lieberman, M. Almon, M. Hansen, G. Rojas, G. A. Lamas, and C. H. Hennekens. The national cholesterol education program diet vs. a diet lower in carbohydrates and higher in protein and monounsaturated fat: A randomized trial. *Archives of Internal Medicine* 164, no. 19 (October 2004): 2141–46.

Brand-Miller, J. C., and S. H. A. Holt. Australian Aboriginal plant foods: A consideration of their nutritional composition and health implications. *Nutrition Research Reviews* 11, no. 1 (1998): 5–23.

Clarke, R., C. Frost, R. Collins, P. Appleby, and R. Peto. Dietary lipids and blood cholesterol: Quantitative meta-analysis of metabolic ward studies. *BMJ* 314, no. 7074 (January 1997): 112–17.

Cordain, L. The nutritional characteristics of a contemporary diet based upon Paleolithic food groups. *Journal of American Neutraceutical Association* 5, no. 3 (2002): 15–24.

Cordain, L. *The Paleo Diet.* New York: John Wiley & Sons, 2002.

Cordain, L. "Saturated Fat Consumption in Ancestral Human Diets: Implications for Contemporary Intakes." In *Phytochemicals: Nutrient-Gene Interactions,* edited by M. S. Meskin, W. R. Bidlack, and R. K. Randolph, 115–26. Boca Raton, FL: CRC Press, 2006.

Cordain, L., J. C. Brand-Miller, S. B. Eaton, N. Mann, S. H. A. Holt, and J. D. Speth. Plant to animal subsistence ratios and macronutrient energy estimations in worldwide hunter-gatherer diets. *American Journal of Clinical Nutrition* 71, no. 3 (2000): 682–92.

Cordain, L., S. B. Eaton, J. C. Brand-Miller, N. Mann, and K. Hill. The paradoxical nature of hunter-gatherer diets: Meat-based, yet non-atherogenic. *European Journal of Clinical Nutrition* 56 (March 2002): S42–52.

Cordain, L., R. W. Gotshall, and S. B. Eaton. Physical activity, energy expenditure and fitness: An evolutionary perspective. *International Journal of Sports Medicine* 19, no. 5 (1998): 328–35.

Cordain, L., B. A. Watkins, G. L. Florant, M. Kehler, L. Rogers, and Y. Li. Fatty acid analysis of wild ruminant tissues: Evolutionary implications for reducing diet-related chronic disease. *European Journal of Clinical Nutrition* 56, no. 3 (2002): 181–91.

De Heinzelin, J., J. D. Clark, T. White, W. Hart, P. Renne, G. Wolde-Gabriel, Y. Beyene, and E. Vrba. Environment and behavior of 2.5-million-year-old Bouri hominids. *Science* 284, no. 5414 (1999): 625–29.

Dominguez-Rodrigo, M. Meat-eating by early hominids at the FLK 22 Zinjanthropus site, Olduvai Gorge (Tanzania): An experimental approach using cut-mark data. *Journal of Human Evolution* 33, no. 6 (1997): 669–90.

Farnsworth, E., N. D. Luscombe, M. Noakes, G. Wittert, E. Argyiou, and P. M. Clifton. Effect of a high-protein, energy-restricted diet on body composition, glycemic control, and lipid concentrations in overweight and obese hyperinsulinemic men and women. *American Journal of Clinical Nutrition* 78, no. 1 (July 2003): 31–39.

Feskanich, D., W. C. Willett, M. J. Stampfer, and G. A. Colditz. Milk, dietary calcium, and bone fractures in women: A 12-year prospective study. *American Journal of Public Health* 87, no. 6 (1997): 992–97.

Foster-Powell, K., S. H. A. Holt, and J. C. Brand-Miller. International table of glycemic index and glycemic load values: 2002. *American Journal of Clinical Nutrition* 76, no. 1 (2002): 5–56.

Gannon, M. C., F. Q. Nuttall, P. A. Krezowski, C. J. Billington, and S. Parker. The serum insulin and plasma glucose responses to milk and fruit products in type 2 (non-insulin-dependent) diabetic patients. *Diabetologia* 29, no. 11 (November 1986): 784–91.

Gannon, M. C., F. Q. Nuttall, A. Saeed, K. Jordan, and H. Hoover. An increase in dietary protein improves the blood glucose response in persons with type 2 diabetes. *American Journal of Clinical Nutrition* 78, no. 4 (2003): 734–41.

German, J. B., and C. J. Dillard. Saturated fats: What dietary intake? *American Journal of Clinical Nutrition* 80, no. 3 (September 2004): 550–59.

Gerrior, S., and Bente, L. Nutrient content of the US food supply, 1909–99: A summary report. US Department of Agriculture, Center for Nutrition Policy and Promotion. Home Economics Report no. 55, 2002.

Hartroft, W. S. The incidence of coronary artery disease in patients treated with Sippy diet. *American Journal of Clinical Nutrition* 15 (October 1964): 205–10.

Hegsted, D. M., L. M. Ausman, J. A. Johnson, and G. E. Dallal. Dietary fat and serum lipids: An evaluation of the experimental data. *American Journal of Clinical Nutrition* 57, no. 6 (June 1993): 875–83.

Hegsted, D. M., R. B. McGandy, M. L. Myers, and F. J. Stare. Quantitative effects of dietary fat on serum cholesterol in man. *American Journal of Clinical Nutrition* 17 (November 1965): 281–95.

Hoppe, C., C. Mølgaard, A. Vaag, V. Barkholt, and K. F. Michaelsen. High intakes of milk, but not meat increase s-insulin and insulin resistance in 8-year-old boys. *European Journal of Clinical Nutrition* 59, no. 3 (March 2005): 393–98.

Howell, W. H., D. J. McNamara, M. A. Tosca, B. T. Smith, and J. A. Gaines. Plasma lipid and lipoprotein responses to dietary fat and cholesterol: A meta-analysis. *American Journal of Clinical Nutrition* 65, no. 6 (June 1997): 1747–64.

Hoyt, G., M. S. Hickey, and L. Cordain. Dissociation of the glycaemic and insulinaemic responses to whole and skimmed milk. *British Journal of Nutrition* 93, no. 2 (February 2005): 175–77.

Hu, F. B., J. E. Manson, and W. C. Willett. Types of dietary fat and risk of coronary heart disease: A critical review. *Journal of American College of Nutrition* 20, no. 1 (2001): 5–19.

Krauss, R. M., R. H. Eckel, B. Howard, L. J. Appel, S. R. Daniels, R. J. Deckelbaum, et al. AHA Dietary Guidelines: Revision 2000: A statement for healthcare professionals from the Nutrition Committee of the American Heart Association. *Circulation* 102 (2000): 2284–99.

Kris-Etherton, P. M., and S. Yu. Individual fatty acid effects on plasma lipids and lipoproteins: Human studies. *American Journal of Clinical Nutrition* 65 (May 1997): 1628S–44S.

Layman, D. K., R. A. Boileau, D. J. Erickson, J. E. Painter, H. Shiue, C. Sather, and D. D. Christou. A reduced ratio of dietary carbohydrate to protein improves body composition and blood lipid profiles during weight loss in adult women. *Journal of Nutrition* 133, no. 2 (February 2003): 411–17.

Layman, D. K., H. Shiue, C. Sather, D. J. Erickson, and J. Baum. Increased dietary protein modifies glucose and insulin homeostasis in adult women during weight loss. *Journal of Nutrition* 133, no. 2 (2003): 405–10.

Lee, K. W., and G. Y. Lip. The role of omega-3 fatty acids in the secondary prevention of cardiovascular disease. *QJM: Monthly Journal of the Association of Physicians* 96, no. 7 (2003): 465–80.

Luscombe-Marsh, N. D., M. Noakes, G. A. Wittert, J. B. Keogh, P. Foster, and P. M. Clifton. Carbohydrate-restricted diets high in either monounsaturated fat or protein are equally effective at promoting fat loss and improving blood lipids. *American Journal of Clinical Nutrition* 81, no. 4 (April 2005): 762–72.

Mensink, R. P., P. L. Zock, A. D. Kester, and M. B. Katan. Effects of dietary fatty acids and carbohydrates on the ratio of serum total to HDL cholesterol and on serum lipids and apolipoproteins: A meta-analysis of 60 controlled trials. *American Journal of Clinical Nutrition* 77, no. 5 (May 2003): 1146–55.

Micha, R., and D. Mozaffarian. Saturated fat and cardiometabolic risk factors, coronary heart disease, stroke, and diabetes: A fresh look at the evidence. *Lipids* 45, no. 10 (October 2010): 893–905.

Micha, R., S. K. Wallace, and D. Mozaffarian. Red and processed meat consumption and risk of incident coronary heart disease, stroke, and diabetes mellitus: A systematic review and meta-analysis. *Circulation* 121, no. 21 (June 2010): 2271–83.

Moss, M., and D. Freed. The cow and the coronary: Epidemiology, biochemistry and immunology. *International Journal of Cardiology* 87, no. 2–3 (February): 203–16.

Mozaffarian, D., R. Micha, and S. Wallace. Effects on coronary heart disease of increasing polyunsaturated fat in place of saturated fat: A systematic review and meta-analysis of randomized controlled trials. *PLoS Medicine* 7, no. 3 (March 2010): e1000252.

Muscari, A., U. Volta, C. Bonazzi, G. M. Puddu, C. Bozzoli, C. Gerratana, F. B. Bianchi, and P. Puddu. Association of serum IgA antibodies to milk antigens with severe atherosclerosis. *Atherosclerosis* 77, no. 2–3 (1989): 251–56.

Nelson, G. J. Dietary fat, trans fatty acids, and risk of coronary heart disease. *Nutrition Reviews* 56, no. 8 (August 1998): 250–52.

Nelson, G. J., P. C. Schmidt, and D. S. Kelley. Low-fat diets do not lower plasma choles-terol levels in healthy men compared to high-fat diets with similar fatty acid composition at constant caloric intake. *Lipids* 30, no. 11 (1995): 969–76.

O'Dea, K., K. Traianedes, K. Chisholm, H. Leyden, and A. J. Sinclair. Cholesterol-lowering effect of a low-fat diet containing lean beef is reversed by the addition of beef fat. *American Journal of Clinical Nutrition* 52 (1990): 491–94.

Ostman, E. M., H. G. Liljeberg-Elmstahl, and I. M. Bjorck. Inconsistency between gly-cemic and insulinemic responses to regular and fermented milk products. *American Jour-nal of Clinical Nutrition* 74, no. 1 (2001): 96–100.

Perez-Jimenez, F., J. Lopez-Miranda, and P. Mata. Protective effect of dietary monoun-saturated fat on arteriosclerosis: Beyond cholesterol. *Atherosclerosis* 163, no. 2 (2002): 385–98.

Richards, M. P., and R. M. Hedges. Focus: Gough's Cave and Sun Hole Cave human stable isotope values indicate a high animal protein diet in the British Upper Palaeolithic. *Journal of Archaeology Science* 27, no. 1 (2000): 1–3.

Richards, M. P., P. B. Pettitt, E. Trinkaus, F. H. Smith, M. Paunovic, and I. Karavanic. Neanderthal diet at Vindija and Neanderthal predation: The evidence from stable iso-topes. *Proceedings of the National Academy of Sciences* 97, no. 13 (2000): 7663–66.

Rudman, D., T. J. DiFulco, J. T. Galambos, R. B. Smith III, A. A. Salam, and W. D. War-ren. Maximal rates of excretion and synthesis of urea in normal and cirrhotic subjects. *Journal of Clinical Investigation* 52, no. 9 (1973): 2241–49.

Segall, J. J. Dietary lactose as a possible risk factor for ischaemic heart disease: Review of epidemiology. *International Journal of Cardiology* 46, no. 3 (1994): 197–207.

Siri-Tarino, P. W., Q. Sun, F. B. Hu, and R. M. Krauss. Meta-analysis of prospective cohort studies evaluating the association of saturated fat with cardiovascular disease. *American Journal of Clinical Nutrition* 91, no. 3 (March 2010): 535–46

Siri-Tarino, P. W., Q. Sun, F. B. Hu, and R. M. Krauss. Saturated fat, carbohydrate, and cardiovascular disease. *American Journal of Clinical Nutrition* 91, no. 3 (March 2010): 502–9.

Siri-Tarino, P. W., Q. Sun, F. B. Hu, and R. M. Krauss. Saturated fatty acids and risk of coronary heart disease: Modulation by replacement nutrients. *Current Atherosclerosis Reports* 12, no. 6 (November 2010): 384–90.

Weigle, D. S., P. A. Breen, C. C. Matthys, H. S. Callahan, K. E. Meeuws, V. R. Burden, and J. Q. Purnell. A high-protein diet induces sustained reductions in appetite, ad libitum caloric intake, and body weight despite compensatory changes in diurnal plasma leptin and ghrelin concentrations. *American Journal of Clinical Nutrition* 82, no. 1 (July 2005): 41–48.

Wolfe, B. M., and P. M. Giovannetti. Short-term effects of substituting protein for carbo-hydrate in the diets of moderately hypercholesterolemic human subjects. *Metabolism* 40 (1991): 338–43.

Wolfe, B. M., and Piche, L. A. Replacement of carbohydrate by protein in a conventional-fat diet reduces cholesterol and triglyceride concentrations in healthy normolipidemic subjects. *Clinical Investigations of Medicine* 22, no. 4 (1999): 140–48.

CHAPTER 10

Agostini, F., and G. Biolo. Effect of physical activity on glutamine metabolism. *Current Opinion in Clinical Nutrition & Metabolic Care* 13, no. 1 (January 2010): 58–64.

Blomstrand, E., J. Eliasson, H. K. Karlsson, and R. Köhnke. Branched-chain amino acids activate key enzymes in protein synthesis after physical exercise. *Journal of Nutrition* 136 (January 2006): 269S–73S.

Bowerman, W. J., and W. E. Harris. *Jogging.* New York: Grosset and Dunlap, 1967.

Cordain, L., R. W. Gotshall, and S. B. Eaton. Evolutionary aspects of exercise. *World Review of Nutrition and Diet* 81 (1997): 49–60.

Cordain, L., R. W. Gotshall, and S. B. Eaton. Physical activity, energy expenditure and fitness: An evolutionary perspective. *International Journal of Sports Medicine* 19, no. 5 (1998): 328–35.

Counsilman, J. E. *The Science of Swimming.* New York: Prentice Hall, 1968.

Dreyer, H. C., M. J. Drummond, B. Pennings, S. Fujita, E. L. Glynn, D. L. Chinkes, S. Dhanani, E. Volpi, and B. B. Rasmussen. Leucine-enriched essential amino acid and carbohydrate ingestion following resistance exercise enhances mTOR signaling and protein synthesis in human muscle. *American Journal of Physiology–Endocrinology and Metabolism* 294, no. 2 (February 2008): E392–400.

Hill, K., and A. M. Hurtado. *Ache Life History: The Ecology and Demography of a Foraging People.* New York: Aldine de Gruyter, 1996.

Kargotich, S., D. G. Rowbottom, D. Keast, C. Goodman, B. Dawson, and A. R. Morton. Plasma glutamine changes after high-intensity exercise in elite male swimmers. *Research in Sports Medicine* 13, no. 1 (2005): 7–21.

Karlsson, H. K., P. A. Nilsson, J. Nilsson, A. V. Chibalin, J. R. Zierath, and E. Blomstrand. Branched-chain amino acids increase p70S6k phosphorylation in human skeletal muscle after resistance exercise. *American Journal of Physiology–Endocrinology and Metabolism* 287, no. 1 (July 2004): E1–7.

Kim, H. Glutamine as an immunonutrient. *Yonsei Medical Journal* 52, no. 6 (November 2011): 892–97.

Kraemer, W. J., N. A. Ratamess, and D. N. French. Resistance training for health and performance. *Current Sports Medicine Report* 1, no. 3 (June 2002): 165–71.

Lambert, E. V., D. P. Speechly, S. C. Dennis, and T. D. Noakes. Enhanced endurance in trained cyclists during moderate intensity exercise following 2 weeks adaptation to a high fat diet. *European Journal of Applied Physiology and Occupational Physiology* 69, no. 4 (1994): 287–93.

Loy, S. F., J. J. Hoffmann, and G. J. Holland. Benefits and practical use of cross-training in sports. *Sports Medicine* 19, no. 1 (January 1995): 1–8.

Millet, G. P., R. B. Candau, B. Barbier, T. Busso, J. D. Rouillon, and J. C. Chatard. Modelling the transfers of training effects on performance in elite triathletes. *International Journal of Sports Medicine* 23, no. 1 (January 2002): 55–63.

Mocchegiani, E., J. Romeo, M. Malavolta, L. Costarelli, R. Giacconi, L. E. Diaz, and A. Marcos. Zinc: Dietary intake and impact of supplementation on immune function in elderly. *Age* (January 6, 2012). www.springerlink.com/content/y1rh057np4527371.

Pasiakos, S. M., H. L. McClung, J. P. McClung, L. M. Margolis, N. E. Andersen, G. J. Cloutier, M. A. Pikosky, J. C. Rood, R. A. Fielding, and A. J. Young. Leucine-enriched essential amino acid supplementation during moderate steady state exercise enhances postexercise muscle protein synthesis. *American Journal of Clinical Nutrition* 94, no. 3 (September 2011): 809–18.

Rennie, M. J., J. Bohé, K. Smith, H. Wackerhage, and P. Greenhaff. Branched-chain amino acids as fuels and anabolic signals in human muscle. *Journal of Nutrition* 136 (January 2006): 264S–68S.

Sijben, J. W., and P. C. Calder. Differential immunomodulation with long-chain n-3 PUFA in health and chronic disease. *Proceedings of the Nutrition Society* 66, no. 2 (May 2007): 237–59.

Stellingwerff, T., L. L. Spriet, M. J. Watt, N. E. Kimber, M. Hargreaves, J. A. Hawley, and L. M. Burke. Decreased PDH activation and glycogenolysis during exercise following fat adaptation with carbohydrate restoration. *American Journal of Physiology–Endocrinology and Metabolism* 290, no. 2 (February 2006): E380–88.

White, L. J., R. H. Dressendorfer, S. M. Muller, and M. A. Ferguson. Effectiveness of cycle cross-training between competitive seasons in female distance runners. *Journal of Strength Conditioning Research* 17, no. 2 (May 2003): 319–23.

Yeo, W. K., A. L. Carey, L. Burke, L. L. Spriet, and J. A. Hawley. Fat adaptation in well-trained athletes: Effects on cell metabolism. *Applied Physiology, Nutrition, and Metabolism* 36, no. 1 (February 2011): 12–22.

Yeo, W. K., S. J. Lessard, Z. P. Chen, A. P. Garnham, L. M. Burke, D. A. Rivas, B. E. Kemp, and J. A. Hawley. Fat adaptation followed by carbohydrate restoration increases AMPK activity in skeletal muscle from trained humans. *Journal of Applied Physiology* 105, no. 5 (November 2008): 1519–26.

Zehnder, M., E. R. Christ, M. Ith, K. J. Achéson, E. Pouteau, R. Kreis, R. Trepp, P. Diem, C. Boesch, and J. Décombaz. Intramyocellular lipid stores increase markedly in athletes after 1.5 days lipid supplementation and are utilized during exercise in proportion to their content. *European Journal of Applied Physiology* 98, no. 4 (November 2006): 341–54.

CHAPTER 11

Alderson, L. M., K. C. Hayes, and R. J. Nicolosi. Peanut oil reduces diet-induced atherosclerosis in cynomolgus monkeys. *Arteriosclerosis* 6, no. 5 (1986): 465–74.

Alvarez, J. R., and R. Torres-Pinedo. Interactions of soybean lectin, soyasaponins, and glycinin with rabbit jejunal mucosa in vitro. *Pediatric Research* 16, no. 9 (1982): 728–31.

Amarasiri, W. A., and A. S. Dissanayake. Coconut fats. *Ceylon Medical Journal* 51, no. 2 (June 2006): 47–51.

Baker, B. P., C. M. Benbrook, E. Groth III, and K. Lutz-Benbrook. Pesticide residues in conventional, integrated pest management (IPM)-grown and organic foods: Insights from three US data sets. *Food Additives and Contaminants* 19, no. 5 (May 2002): 427–46.

Bamshad, M., T. Kivisild, W. S. Watkins, M. E. Dixon, C. E. Ricker, B. B. Rao, J. M. Naidu, et al. Genetic evidence on the origins of Indian caste populations. *Genome Research* 11, no. 6 (June 2001): 994–1004.

Barraj, L., N. Tran, and P. Mink. A comparison of egg consumption with other modifiable coronary heart disease lifestyle risk factors: A relative risk apportionment study. *Risk Analysis* 29, no. 3 (March 2009): 401–15.

Batterham, R. L., H. Heffron, S. Kapoor, J. E. Chivers, K. Chandarana, H. Herzog, C. W. Le Roux, E. L. Thomas, J. D. Bell, and D. J. Withers. Critical role for peptide YY in protein-mediated satiation and body-weight regulation. *Cell Metabolism* 4, no. 3 (September 2006): 223–33.

Begom, R., and R. B. Singh. Prevalence of coronary artery disease and its risk factors in the urban population of South and North India. *Acta Cardiologica* 50, no. 3 (1995): 227–40.

Bhopal, R., N. Unwin, M. White, J. Yallop, L. Walker, K. G. Alberti, J. Harland, S. Patel, N. Ahmad, C. Turner, B. Watson, D. Kaur, A. Kulkarni, M. Laker, and A. Tavridou. Heterogeneity of coronary heart disease risk factors in Indian, Pakistani, Bangladeshi, and European origin populations: Cross sectional study. *British Medical Journal* 319, no. 7204 (1999): 215–20.

Borg, K. Physiopathological effects of rapeseed oil: A review. *Acta Medica Scandinavica, Supplementum* 585 (1975): 5–13.

Bourne, D., and J. Prescott. A comparison of the nutritional value, sensory qualities, and food safety of organically and conventionally produced foods. *Critical Review of Food Science Nutrition* 42, no. 1 (2002): 1–34.

Boyle, E. M., S. T. Lille, E. Allaire, A. W. Clowes, and E. D. Verrier. Endothelial cell injury in cardiovascular surgery: Atherosclerosis. *Annual of Thoracic Surgery* 63, no. 3 (March 1997): 885–94.

Childs, M. T., C. S. Dorsett, I. B. King, J. G. Ostrander, and W. K. Yamanaka. Effects of shellfish consumption on lipoproteins in normolipidemic men. *American Journal of Clinical Nutrition* 51, no. 6 (June 1990): 1020–27.

Cordain, L., L. Toohey, M. J. Smith, and M. S. Hickey. Modulation of immune function by dietary lectins in rheumatoid arthritis. *British Journal of Nutrition* 83, no. 3 (March 2000): 207–17.

Cordain, L., B. A. Watkins, G. L. Florant, M. Kehler, L. Rogers, and Y. Li. Fatty acid analysis of wild ruminant tissues: Evolutionary implications for reducing diet-related chronic disease. *European Journal of Clinical Nutrition* 56, no. 3 (2002): 181–91.

Cordain, L. The nutritional characteristics of a contemporary diet based upon Paleolithic food groups. *Journal of the American Nutraceutical Association* 5, no. 3 (2002): 15–24.

Crinnion, W. J. Organic foods contain higher levels of certain nutrients, lower levels of pesticides, and may provide health benefits for the consumer. *Alternative Medicine Review* 15, no. 1 (April 2010): 4–12.

Daley, C. A., A. Abbott, P. S. Doyle, G. A. Nader, and S. Larson. A review of fatty acid profiles and antioxidant content in grass-fed and grain-fed beef. *Nutrition Journal* 9 (March 2010): 10.

Dalla-Pellegrina, C., O. Perbellini, M. T. Scupoli, C. Tomelleri, C. Zanetti, G. Zoccatelli, M. Fusi, A. Peruffo, C. Rizzi, and R. Chignola. Effects of wheat germ agglutinin on human gastrointestinal epithelium: Insights from an experimental model of immune/ epithelial cell interaction. *Toxicology and Applied Pharmacology* 237, no. 2 (June 2009): 146–53.

Dangour, A. D., S. K. Dodhia, A. Hayter, E. Allen, K. Lock, and R. Uauy. Nutritional quality of organic foods: A systematic review. *American Journal of Clinical Nutrition* 90, no. 3 (September 2009): 680–85.

Dangour, A. D., K. Lock, A. Hayter, A. Aikenhead, E. Allen, and R. Uauy. Nutrition-related health effects of organic foods: A systematic review. *American Journal of Clinical Nutrition* 92, no. 1 (July 2010): 203–10.

DebMandal, M., and S. Mandal. Coconut (*Cocos nucifera* L.: Arecaceae): In health promotion and disease prevention. *Asian Pacific Journal of Tropical Medicine* 4, no. 3 (March 2011): 241–47.

De Oliveira e Silva, E. R., C. E. Seidman, J. J. Tian, L. C. Hudgins, F. M. Sacks, and J. L. Breslow. Effects of shrimp consumption on plasma lipoproteins. *American Journal of Clinical Nutrition* 64, no. 5 (1996): 712–17.

El-Tawil, A. M. Prevalence of inflammatory bowel diseases in the Western Nations: High consumption of potatoes may be contributing. *International Journal of Colorectal Disease* 23, no. 10 (2008): 1017–18.

Engfeldt, B., and E. Brunius. Morphological effects of rapeseed oil in rats. I. Short-term studies. *Acta Medica Scandinavica, Supplementum* 585 (1975): 15–26.

Engfeldt, B., and E. Brunius. Morphological effects of rapeseed oil in rats. II. Long-term studies. *Acta Medica Scandinavica, Supplementum* 585 (1975): 27–40.

Feranil, A. B., P. L. Duazo, C. W. Kuzawa, and L. S. Adair. Coconut oil is associated with a beneficial lipid profile in pre-menopausal women in the Philippines. *Asia Pacific Journal of Clinical Nutrition* 20, no. 2 (2011): 190–95.

Freed, D. L. Lectins in food: Their importance in health and disease. *Journal of Nutritional & Environmental Medicine* 2, no. 1 (1991): 45–64.

Grant, G. Anti-nutritional effects of soyabean: A review. *Progress in Food and Nutrition Science* 13, no. 3–4 (1989): 317–48.

Gresham, G. A., and A. N. Howard. The independent production of atherosclerosis and thrombosis in the rat. *British Journal of Experimental Pathology* 41, no. 4 (1960): 395–402.

Halton, T. L., and F. B. Hu. The effects of high protein diets on thermogenesis, satiety and weight loss: A critical review. *Journal of the American College of Nutrition* 23, no. 5 (2004): 373–85.

Hellenäs, K. E., A. Nyman, P. Slanina, L. Lööf, and J. Gabrielsson. Determination of potato glycoalkaloids and their aglycone in blood serum by high-performance liquid chromatography. Application to pharmacokinetic studies in humans. *Journal of Chromatography A* 573, no. 1 (1992): 69–78.

Howell, W. H., D. J. McNamara, M. A. Tosca, B. T. Smith, and J. A. Gaines. Plasma lipid and lipoprotein responses to dietary fat and cholesterol: A meta-analysis. *American Journal of Clinical Nutrition* 65, no. 6 (1997): 1747–64.

Hu, F. B., M. J. Stampfer, J. E. Manson, E. B. Rimm, G. A. Colditz, B. A. Rosner, F. E. Speizer, C. H. Hennekens, and W. C. Willett. Frequent nut consumption and risk of coronary heart disease in women: Prospective cohort study. *British Medical Journal* 317, no. 7169 (November 1998): 1341–45.

Hu, F. B., M. F. Stampfer, E. B. Rimm, J. E. Manson, A. Ascherio, G. A. Colditz, B. A. Rosner, D. Spiegelman, F. E. Speizer, F. M. Sacks, C. H. Hennekens, and W. C. Willett. A prospective study of egg consumption and risk of cardiovascular disease in men and women. *JAMA* 281, no. 15 (1999): 1387–94.

Iablokov, V., B. C. Sydora, R. Foshaug, J. Meddings, D. Driedger, T. Churchill, and R. N. Fedorak. Naturally occurring glycoalkaloids in potatoes aggravate intestinal inflammation in two mouse models of inflammatory bowel disease. *Digestive Diseases and Sciences* 55, no. 11 (November 2010): 3078–85.

Intahphuak, S., P. Khonsung, and A. Panthong. Anti-inflammatory, analgesic, and antipyretic activities of virgin coconut oil. *Pharmaceutical Biology* 48, no. 2 (February 2010): 151–57.

Isherwood, C., M. Wong, W. S. Jones, I. G. Davies, and B. A. Griffin. Lack of effect of cold water prawns on plasma cholesterol and lipoproteins in normo-lipidaemic men. *Cellular and Molecular Biology* 56, no. 1 (February 2010): 52–58.

Keukens, E. A., T. de Vrije, L. A. Jansen, H. de Boer, M. Janssen, A. I. de Kroon, W. M. Jongen, and B. de Kruijff. Glycoalkaloids selectively permeabilize cholesterol containing biomembranes. *Biochimica et Biophysica Acta* 1279, no. 2 (March 1996): 243–50.

Keukens, E. A., T. de Vrije, C. van den Boom, P. de Waard, H. H. Plasman, F. Thiel, V. Chupin, W. M. Jongen, and B. de Kruijff. Molecular basis of glycoalkaloid induced membrane disruption. *Biochimica et Biophysica Acta* 1240, no. 2 (December 1995): 216–28.

Kritchevsky, D., L. M. Davidson, I. L. Shapiro, H. K. Kim, M. Kitagawa, S. Malhotra, P. P. Nair, T. B. Clarkson, I. Bersohn, and P. A. Winter. Lipid metabolism and experimental atherosclerosis in baboons: Influence of cholesterol free, semi-synthetic diets. *American Journal of Clinical Nutrition* 27, no. 1 (1974): 29–50.

Kritchevsky, D., L. M. Davidson, M. Weight, N. P. Kriek, and J. P. du Plessis. Influence of native and randomized peanut oil on lipid metabolism and aortic sudanophilia in the vervet monkey. *Atherosclerosis* 42, no. 1 (1982): 53–58.

Kritchevsky, S. B., and D. Kritchevsky. Egg consumption and coronary heart disease: An epidemiologic overview. *Journal of the American College of Nutrition* 19 (October 2000): 549S–55S.

Kritchevsky, D., S. A. Tepper, and D. M. Klurfeld. Lectin may contribute to the atherogenicity of peanut oil. *Lipids* 33, no. 8 (1998): 821–23.

Larsen, T. M., S. M. Dalskov, M. van Baak, S. A. Jebb, A. Papadaki, A. F. Pfeiffer, J. A. Martinez, T. Handjieva-Darlenska, M. Kunešová, M. Pihlsgård, S. Stender, C. Holst, W. H. Saris, and A. Astrup, for the Diet, Obesity, and Genes (Diogenes) Project. Diets with high or low protein content and glycemic index for weight-loss maintenance. *New England Journal of Medicine* 363, no. 22 (November 2010): 2102–13.

Layman, D. K., P. Clifton, M. C. Gannon, R. M. Krauss, and F. Q. Nuttall. Protein in optimal health: Heart disease and type 2 diabetes. *American Journal of Clinical Nutrition* 87, no. 5 (May 2008): 1571S–75S.

Leheska, J. M., L. D. Thompson, J. C. Howe, E. Hentges, J. Boyce, J. C. Brooks, B. Shriver, L. Hoover, and M. F. Miller. Effects of conventional and grass-feeding systems on the nutrient composition of beef. *Journal of Animal Science* 86, no. 12 (December 2008): 3575–85.

Liener, I. E. Implications of antinutritional components in soybean foods. *Critical Reviews in Food Science and Nutrition* 34, no. 1 (1994): 31–67.

Lindeberg, S., and B. Lundh. Apparent absence of stroke and ischaemic heart disease in a traditional Melanesian island: A clinical study in Kitava. *Journal of Internal Medicine* 233, no. 3 (March 1993): 269–75.

Lipoeto, N. I., Z. Agus, F. Oenzil, M. Wahlqvist, and N. Wattanapenpaiboon. Dietary intake and the risk of coronary heart disease among the coconut-consuming Minangkabau in West Sumatra, Indonesia. *Asia Pacific Journal of Clinical Nutrition* 13, no. 4 (2004): 377–84.

Lochner, N., F. Pittner, M. Wirth, and F. Gabor. Wheat germ agglutinin binds to the epidermal growth factor receptor of artificial Caco-2 membranes as detected by silver nanoparticle enhanced fluorescence. *Pharmaceutical Research* 20, no. 5 (May 2003): 833–39.

Magkos, F., F. Arvaniti, and A. Zampelas. Organic food: Buying more safety or just peace of mind? A critical review of the literature. *Critical Reviews in Food Science and Nutrition* 46, no. 1 (2006): 23–56.

Magkos, F., F. Arvaniti, and A. Zampelas. Organic food: Nutritious food or food for thought? A review of the evidence. *International Journal of Food Science Nutrition* 54, no. 5 (2003): 357–71.

Mensinga, T. T., A. J. Sips, C. J. Rompelberg, K. van Twillert, J. Meulenbelt, H. J. van den Top, and H. P. van Egmond. Potato glycoalkaloids and adverse effects in humans: An ascending dose study. *Regulatory Toxicology and Pharmacology* 41, no. 1 (February 2005): 66–72.

Mensinga, T. T., G. J. Speijers, and J. Meulenbelt. Health implications of exposure to environmental nitrogenous compounds. *Toxicology Review* 22, no. 1 (2003): 41–51.

Micha, R., and D. Mozaffarian. Saturated fat and cardiometabolic risk factors, coronary heart disease, stroke, and diabetes: A fresh look at the evidence. *Lipids* 45, no. 10 (October 2010): 893–905.

Micha, R., S. K. Wallace, and D. Mozaffarian. Red and processed meat consumption and risk of incident coronary heart disease, stroke, and diabetes mellitus: A systematic review and meta-analysis. *Circulation* 121, no. 21 (June 2010): 2271–83.

Misra, A., R. Cherukupalli, K. S. Reddy, A. Mohan, and J. S. Bajaj. Hyperinsulinemia and dyslipidemia in non-obese, normotensive offspring of hypertensive parents in northern India. *Blood Pressure* 7, no. 5–6 (November 1998): 286–90.

Naito, Y., H. Yoshida, T. Nagata, A. Tanaka, H. Ono, and N. Ohara. Dietary intake of rapeseed oil or soybean oil as the only fat nutrient in spontaneously hypertensive rats and Wistar Kyoto rats—Blood pressure and pathophysiology. *Toxicology* 146, no. 2–3 (May 2000): 197–208.

Nieman, D. C. Immunonutrition support for athletes. *Nutrition Reviews* 66, no. 6 (June 2008): 310–20.

Ohara, N., Y. Naito, K. Kasama, T. Shindo, H. Yoshida, T. Nagata, and H. Okuyama. Similar changes in clinical and pathological parameters in Wistar Kyoto rats after a 13-week dietary intake of canola oil or a fatty acid composition-based interesterified canola oil mimic. *Food and Chemical Toxicology* 47, no. 1 (January 2009): 157–62.

Ohara, N., Y. Naito, T. Nagata, S. Tachibana, M. Okimoto, and H. Okuyama. Dietary intake of rapeseed oil as the sole fat nutrient in Wistar rats—lack of increase in plasma lipids and renal lesions. *Journal of Toxicological Sciences* 33, no. 5 (December 2008): 641–45.

Ohara, N., Y. Naito, T. Nagata, K. Tatematsu, S. Y. Fuma, S. Tachibana, and H. Okuyama. Exploration for unknown substances in rapeseed oil that shorten survival time of stroke-prone spontaneously hypertensive rats. Effects of super critical gas extraction fractions. *Food and Chemical Toxicology* 44, no. 7 (July 2006): 952–63.

Papadaki, A., M. Linardakis, T. M. Larsen, M. A. van Baak, A. K. Lindroos, A. F. Pfeiffer, J. A. Martinez, T. Handjieva-Darlenska, M. Kunesová, C. Holst, A. Astrup, W. H. Saris, and A. Kafatos, for the DiOGenes Study Group. The effect of protein and glycemic index on children's body composition: The DiOGenes randomized study. *Pediatrics* 126, no. 5 (November 2010): E1143–52.

Patel, B., R. Schutte, P. Sporns, J. Doyle, L. Jewel, and R. N. Fedorak. Potato glycoalkaloids adversely affect intestinal permeability and aggravate inflammatory bowel disease. *Inflammatory Bowel Diseases* 8, no. 5 (2002): 340–46.

Poikonen, S., T. J. Puumalainen, H. Kautiainen, T. Palosuo, T. Reunala, and K. Turjanmaa. Sensitization to turnip rape and oilseed rape in children with atopic dermatitis: a case-control study. *Pediatric Allergy and Immunology* 15, no. 5 (August 2008): 408–11.

Poikonen S, Puumalainen TJ, Kautiainen H, Burri P, Palosuo T, Reunala T, Turjanmaa K. Turnip rape and oilseed rape are new potential food allergens in children with atopic dermatitis. *Allergy* 61, no. 1 (January 2006): 124–7.

Poikonen, S., F. Rancé, T. J. Puumalainen, G. Le Manach, T. Reunala, and K. Turjanmaa. Sensitization and allergy to turnip rape: A comparison between the Finnish and French children with atopic dermatitis. *Acta Paediatrica* 98, no. 2 (February 2009): 310–15.

Ponnampalam, E. N., N. J. Mann, and A. J. Sinclair. Effect of feeding systems on omega-3 fatty acids, conjugated linoleic acid and trans fatty acids in Australian beef cuts: Potential impact on human health. *Asia Pacific Journal of Clinical Nutrition* 15, no. 1 (2006): 21–29.

Prior, I. A., F. Davidson, C. E. Salmond, and Z. Czochanska. Cholesterol, coconuts, and diet on Polynesian atolls: A natural experiment: The Pukapuka and Tokelau island studies. *American Journal of Clinical Nutrition* 34, no. 8 (August 1981): 1552–61.

Pusztai, A., S. W. Ewen, G. Grant, D. S. Brown, J. C. Stewart, W. J. Peumans, E. J. Van Damme, and S. Bardocz. Antinutritive effects of wheat-germ agglutinin and other N-acetyl-glucosamine-specific lectins. *British Journal of Nutrition* 70, no. 1 (July 1993): 313–21.

Qureshi, A. I., F. K. Suri, S. Ahmed, A. Nasar, A. A. Divani, and J. F. Kirmani. Regular egg consumption does not increase the risk of stroke and cardiovascular diseases. *Medical Science Monitor* 13, no. 1 (January 2007): CR1–8.

Ramachandran, A., C. Snehalatha, A. Kapur, V. Vijay, V. Mohan, A. K. Das, P. V. Rao, C. S. Yajnik, K. M. Prasanna-Kumar, and J. D. Nair. High prevalence of diabetes and impaired glucose tolerance in India: National Urban Diabetes Survey. *Diabetologia* 44, no. 9 (September 2001): 1094–101.

Rule, D. C., K. S. Broughton, S. M. Shellito, and G. Maiorano. Comparison of muscle fatty acid profiles and cholesterol concentrations of bison, beef cattle, elk, and chicken. *Journal of Animal Science* 80, no. 5 (May 2002): 1202–11.

Sanderson, P., R. L. Elsom, V. Kirkpatrick, P. C. Calder, J. V. Woodside, E. A. Williams, L. Rink, S. Fairweather-Tait, K. Ivory, M. Cantorna, B. Watzl, and E. M. Stone. UK food standards agency workshop report: Diet and immune function. *British Journal of Nutrition* 103, no. 11 (June 2010): 1684–87.

Sanford, G. L., and S. Harris-Hooker. Stimulation of vascular cell proliferation by beta-galactoside specific lectins. *FASEB Journal* 4 (August 1990): 2912–18.

Scott, R. F., E. S. Morrison, W. A. Thomas, R. Jones, and S. C. Nam. Short-term feeding of unsaturated vs. saturated fat in the production of atherosclerosis and thrombosis in the rat. *Experimental Molecular Pathology* 3 (1964): 421–43.

Scrafford, C. G., N. L. Tran, L. M. Barraj, and P. J. Mink. Egg consumption and CHD and stroke mortality: A prospective study of US adults. *Public Health Nutrition* 14, no. 2 (February 2011): 261–70.

Siri-Tarino, P. W., Q. Sun, F. B. Hu, and R. M. Krauss. Saturated fat, carbohydrate, and cardiovascular disease. *American Journal of Clinical Nutrition* 91, no. 3 (March 2010): 502–9.

Siri-Tarino, P. W., Q. Sun, F. B. Hu, and R. M. Krauss. Saturated fatty acids and risk of coronary heart disease: Modulation by replacement nutrients. *Current Atherosclerosis Reports* 12, no. 6 (November 2010): 384–90.

Siri-Tarino, P. W., Q. Sun, F. B. Hu, and R. M. Krauss. Meta-analysis of prospective cohort studies evaluating the association of saturated fat with cardiovascular disease. *American Journal of Clinical Nutrition* 91, no. 3 (March 2010): 535–46.

Soenen, S., and M. S. Westerterp-Plantenga. Proteins and satiety: Implications for weight management. *Current Opinion in Clinical Nutrition & Metabolic Care* 11, no. 6 (November 2008): 747–51.

Staprans, I., X. M. Pan, J. H. Rapp, and K. R. Feingold. The role of dietary oxidized cholesterol and oxidized fatty acids in the development of atherosclerosis. *Molecular Nutrition & Food Research* 49, no. 11 (November 2005): 1075–82.

Tasiopoulou, S., A. M. Chiodini, F. Vellere, and S. Visentin. Results of the monitoring program of pesticide residues in organic food of plant origin in Lombardy (Italy). *Journal of Environmental Science and Health, Part B* 42, no. 7 (2007): 835–41.

Veldhorst, M., A. Smeets, S. Soenen, A. Hochstenbach-Waelen, R. Hursel, K. Diepvens, M. Lejeune, N. Luscombe-Marsh, and M. Westerterp-Plantenga. Protein-induced satiety: Effects and mechanisms of different proteins. *Physiology & Behavior* 94, no. 2 (May 2008): 300–307.

Vetter, J. Plant cyanogenic glycosides. *Toxicon* 38, no. 1 (2000): 11–36.

Wang, Q., L. G. Yu, B. J. Campbell, J. D. Milton, and J. M. Rhodes. Identification of intact peanut lectin in peripheral venous blood. *Lancet* 352, no. 9143 (December 1998): 1831–32.

Ward, M. H., S. D. Mark, K. P. Cantor, D. D. Weisenburger, A. Correa-Villasenor, and S. H. Zahm. Drinking water nitrate and the risk of non-Hodgkin's lymphoma. *Epidemiology* 7, no. 5 (September 1996): 465–71.

Walsh, N. P., M. Gleeson, D. B. Pyne, D. C. Nieman, F. S. Dhabhar, R. J. Shephard, S. J. Oliver, S. Bermon, and A. Kajeniene. Position statement. Part two: Maintaining immune health. *Exercise Immunology Review* 17 (2011): 64–103.

Walsh, N. P., M. Gleeson, R. J. Shephard, J. A. Woods, N. C. Bishop, M. Fleshner, C. Green, B. K. Pedersen, L. Hoffman-Goetz, C. J. Rogers, H. Northoff, A. Abbasi, and P. Simon. Position statement. Part one: Immune function and exercise. *Exercise Immunology Review* 17 (2011): 6–63.

Williams, C. M. Nutritional quality of organic food: Shades of grey or shades of green? *Proceedings of the Nutrition Society* 61, no. 1 (2002): 19–24.

Wissler, R. W., et al. Aortic lesions and blood lipids in monkeys fed three food fats. *Federation Proceedings* 26 (1967): 371.

Woese, K., D. Lange, C. Boess, and K. W. Bogl. A comparison of organically and conventionally grown foods: Results of a review of the relevant literature. *Journal of Science Food Agriculture* 74, no. 3 (1997): 281–93.

Worthington, V. Effect of agricultural methods on nutritional quality: A comparison of organic with conventional crops. *Alternative Therapies* 4, no. 1 (1998): 58–68.

Worthington, V. Nutritional quality of organic versus conventional fruits, vegetables, and grains. *Journal of Alternative Complementary Medicine* 7, no. 2 (2001): 161–73.

Yuan, J. M., R. K. Ross, Y. T. Gao, and M. C. Yu. Fish and shellfish consumption in relation to death from myocardial infarction among men in Shanghai, China. *American Journal of Epidemiology* 154, no. 9 (November 2001): 809–16.

Zahm, S. H., and M. H. Ward. Pesticides and childhood cancer. *Environmental Health Perspective* 106 (June 1998): 893–908.

CHAPTER 12

Allsop, K. A., and J. B. Miller. Honey revisited: A reappraisal of honey in pre-industrial diets. *British Journal of Nutrition* 75, no. 4 (April 1996): 513–20.

Burke, L. M., and R. S. Read. Dietary supplements in sport. *Sports Medicine* 15, no. 1 (1993): 43–65.

Costill, D. L. Sweating: Its composition and effects on body fluids. *Annals of New York Academy of Science* 301 (1977): 160–74.

Hew-Butler, T., T. D. Noakes, and A. J. Siegel. Practical management of exercise-associated hyponatremic encephalopathy: The sodium paradox of non-osmotic vasopressin secretion. *Clinical Journal of Sport Medicine* 18, no. 4 (July 2008): 350–54.

Knechtle, B., M. Gnädinger, P. Knechtle, R. Imoberdorf, G. Kohler, P. Ballmer, T. Rosemann, and O. Senn. Prevalence of exercise-associated hyponatremia in male ultraendurance athletes. *Clinical Journal of Sport Medicine* 21, no. 3 (May 2011): 226–32.

Mao, I. F., M. L. Chen, and Y. C. Ko. Electrolyte loss in sweat and iodine deficiency in a hot environment. *Archives of Environmental Health* 56, no. 3 (2001): 271–77.

Noakes, T. D. Hyponatremia in distance runners: Fluid and sodium balance during exercise. *Current Sports Medicine Report* 1, no. 4 (2002): 197–207.

O'Toole, M. L., P. S. Douglas, R. H. Laird, and D. B. Hiller. Fluid and electrolyte status in athletes receiving medical care at an ultradistance triathlon. *Clinical Journal of Sport Medicine* 5, no. 2 (1995): 116–22.

Rogers, I. R., G. Hook, K. J. Stuempfle, M. D. Hoffman, and T. Hew-Butler. An intervention study of oral versus intravenous hypertonic saline administration in ultramarathon runners with exercise-associated hyponatremia: A preliminary randomized trial. *Clinical Journal of Sport Medicine* 21, no. 3 (May 2011): 200–203.

Rosner, M. H. Exercise-associated hyponatremia. *Seminars in Nephrology* 29, no. 3 (May 2009): 271–81.

Shirreffs, S. M., and R. J. Maughan. Whole body sweat collection in humans: An improved method with preliminary data on electrolyte content. *Journal of Applied Physiology* 82, no. 1 (1997): 336–41.

Siegel, A. J. Exercise-associated hyponatremia: Role of cytokines. *American Journal of Medicine* 119 (July 2006): S74–78.

Siegel, A. J. Hypertonic (3%) sodium chloride for emergent treatment of exercise-associated hypotonic encephalopathy. *Sports Medicine* 37, no. 4–5 (2007): 459–62.

Speedy, D. B., J. G. Faris, M. Hamlin, P. G. Gallagher, and R. G. Campbell. Hyponatremia and weight changes in an ultradistance triathlon. *Clinical Journal of Sport Medicine* 7, no. 3 (1997): 180–84.

INDEX

evolution and, 184–86
hydration during, 32–33
sodium and, 34–35
weight loss and, 117–18
Exercise-induced asthma (EIA), 92
Exotic meats, 200
Expensive tissue hypothesis, 149

F

Fatigue
BCAA blood level drop and, 133
bonking, 21, 37, 43, 109
central nervous system, 49
overreaching and, 126
as overtraining sign, 122, 123, 136
theories of, 124–25
Fats, dietary. *See also specific kinds*
balancing, 88–93, 170–71, 197–203, 204, 205–7, 208
chemical structure of, 88–89
comparison of animal meats, 199
in eggs, 168
fat burners and, 106–7, 109, 110
in hunter-gatherer diet, 152–53, 170–71
in lean vs. fatty meats, 167
long-chain fatty acids, 158
monounsaturated, 76, 90, 170, 171, 203
as muscle fuel sources, 83–86
in nuts and seeds, 208
oils, 203, 204, 205–7
omega-3s, 10–11, 70, 91–92, 203
omega-6s, 10–11, 70, 76, 90–91, 203
in organ meats, 169–170
overtraining and, 130–31
percentage of calories from, 171, 177
polyunsaturated, 90–92, 170, 171, 203
during race week, 20
replacements, 213
saturated, 89–90, 169, 171, 203
in shellfish, 201
in Stage II, 48, 49–50
in Stage V, 76
to avoid, 76
trans fatty acids, 76, 92–93

utilization relative to RER, 108
weight loss and, 119–120
FFA, 83
Fiber, 20, 24, 96, 147–49, 160–61
Fish, 69, 200–203
Cordain's Fennel Salmon, 238
Little Valley Stuffed Trout, 240
Orange Poached Fish, 239
recommendations, 202
Reese River Barbecued Catfish with Peach Salsa, 240
Sauterne Squid, 239
Fitness
aerobic capacity, 103–4
anaerobic threshold, 104–5
economy and, 105–6
factors contributing to, 102, 103
health vs., viii–ix
of hunter-gatherers, x–xiv
Flaxseed oil
Basil Tomatoes, 253
Bombay Chicken Salad, 255
Colorado Coleslaw, 253
Colorado Ranch Dressing, 243
Flaxseed Oil Mayonnaise, 241
Lean Beef Salad, 258
Omega-3 Crab Salad, 256
as omega-3 source, 203
Omega-3 Spinach Salad, 254
Omega-3 Stuffed Crab, 237
Russian Flaxseed Salad Dressing, 243
Salsa Shrimp Salad, 257
Tartar Sauce, 242
Tomato Flaxseed Dressing, 244
Folic acid fortification, 99–100
Food Pyramid. *See* USDA Food Pyramid/MyPlate
Foods. *See also specific stages*
acid/base values of selected, 59
amino acid content of common, 74
BCAA content of selected, 55
build period choices, 115
electrolytes in, 57
fresh, 193–97
glycemic load and index of, 63, 82
nutrient density of, 66–67, 172, 174
nutritional adequacy of, 177–78
organic, 195–96, 195

O

Oils, 203, <u>204</u>, 205–7
Oleic acid, 90, 93
Olive oil
  Baked Bananas, 264
  Fresh Tomato-Basil Soup, 261
  Horseradish-Garlic Sauce, 269
  Lemon Dill Shrimp, 238
  Lemon-Vinaigrette Carrots, 250
  Marinated Mushrooms, 267
  Rooke's Roast Venison, 230
  Sautéed Cauliflower and Zucchini,
    251
Omega-3 fatty acids
  inflammation reduced by, 70
  in oils, 203
  Omega-3 Crab Salad, 256
  Omega-3 Spinach Salad, 254
  Omega-3 Stuffed Crab, 237
  ratio to omega-6s, 10–11, 70
  structure and effects of, 91–92
Omega-6 fatty acids, 10–11, 70, 76,
    90–91, 203
Orange
  Cantaloupe-Pineapple Ambrosia,
    264
  Fresh Tomato-Basil Soup, 261
  Orange Poached Fish, 239
  Spiced Orange Sauce, 272
Organic meats, 199–200
Organic produce, 195–96, <u>195</u>
Organ meats, 169–170, 198
  Apricot-Raisin Tongue, 225
  Basque Beef Heart, 226
  Beef Liver in Lime Sauce, 227
  Hungarian Chicken Livers with
    Mushrooms, 228
  Rocky Mountain Oysters, 229
Ornish, Dean, 143
Ostrich
  Barbecued Ostrich Medallions, 234
Overdrinking, 30, 36
Overreaching, 126, 127, 128, 129, 136
Overtraining
  diet and, 127–28
  illness and signs of, 126–27
  macronutrients and, 128–134
  micronutrients and, 134–35

  overreaching vs., 126, 127, 136
  preventing, 136–37
  recovery neglected in, 122
  signs of, 122, 123, 126–27, <u>127</u>,
    136
  treatment of, 136
Oxygen and muscle fuel sources, 84

P

Pacing, poor, 30
Paleo Diet for Athletes
  animal and plant food balance, 165
  athletic world and, 7–8
  cheating, 208–9
  counterarguments against, ix–xvi
  development of, 2–4
  eggs in, 168–69
  Food Pyramid/MyPlate compared to,
    10–13, <u>11</u>, <u>12</u>, 170, 177–78
  food replacements for, 211–13
  foods not part of, 8, 167–68, 171–75,
    <u>172–73</u>
  macronutrient balance, 177
  meats in, 165–67, <u>167</u>, 169–171,
    175–77
  modification for recovery, 18
  nutritional adequacy, 177–78
  nutritional characteristics, 8,
    10–13
  performance enhanced by, 5–7
  principles of, 8, 164
  produce for, 160–61, <u>161</u>, <u>162–63</u>,
    164
  race week, 19–20
  sample 1-day menu, <u>9</u>
  sports nutrition trends compared to,
    viii
  stages of, 19
  weight loss and, 118–121
Peaches
  Braised Beef with Walnuts, Prunes,
    and Peaches, 222
  Peach Salsa, 245
  Reese River Barbecued Catfish with
    Peach Salsa, 240
Peak period diet, 112
Peanut oil and peanuts, 205–6

recipes (Stage IV), 266–272
Stage I as preparation for, 22–23, 24
in Stage III, 52–61
in Stage IV, 61–64
in Stage V, 64–76
Red wine
Barbecued Ostrich Medallions, 234
Beef Kebabs, 223
Braised Onion Sauce, 270
Buffalo Steaks with Mushroom Sauce, 232
Grilled London Broil, 224
Isola Pot Roast, 223
Moose Rump Roast, 231
Rocky Mountain Oysters, 229
Rooke's Roast Venison, 230
Respiratory equivalency ratio (RER), 107, 108, 109–10, 120
Rest. See also Overtraining
needed for fitness, 102
stress/rest balance, 123, 136–37
Restaurants, 209–10
Richards, Mike, 153, 165
Road trips, 210
Robinson, Jo, 199
Rudman, Daniel, 176

S

Salmon
Cordain's Fennel Salmon, 238
Salt and sodium
exercise and, 34–35
hyponatremia, 35–37, 46, 48, 266
potassium/sodium balance, 94
replacements, 212
replenishing, 34–35, 56, 266
salt water ingestion, 31
Stage IV recovery recipes, 266
Satiety, 120
Saturated fatty acids (SAT), 89–90, 169, 171, 203
Seafood. See Fish; Shellfish
Seawater poisoning, 31
Shellfish, 201–3, 201
Cancun Zesty Mussels, 236
Lemon Dill Shrimp, 238

Omega-3 Crab Salad, 256
Omega-3 Stuffed Crab, 237
Peloponnesian Shrimp, 235
Salsa Shrimp Salad, 257
Tillamook Steamed Clams, 237
Sherry
Tarragon Rabbit, 233
Shrimp
Lemon Dill Shrimp, 238
Peloponnesian Shrimp, 235
Salsa Shrimp Salad, 257
Sleep, 102
Sodium. See Salt and sodium
Spinach
Omega-3 Spinach Salad, 254
Sports bars, 27
Sports drinks and gels, 34, 38, 39, 42
Squash
Karachi Carrot Soup, 260–61
Squid
Sauterne Squid, 239
Stage I (eating before exercise)
calories consumed in, 22, 23, 28
carbohydrates in, 17, 22, 23–24, 27–28
food choices in, 25–27
hydration in, 22, 25, 27
importance for performance, 20–21
nutritional goals, 21–23
nutritional guidelines, 23–25
protein in, 24–25, 26, 27
10 minutes before start, 27–28
Stage II (eating during exercise)
carbohydrates in, 38–39, 42–43, 47, 48
18+ hour events, 47–50
fats in, 48, 49–50
food tolerance and, 29–32
4- to 12-hour events, 42–43, 46
hydration in, 30, 31, 32–33, 37–38, 39, 42, 46, 48–49
hyponatremia in, 35–37, 46, 48
90-minute to 4-hour events, 38–39
protein in, 43, 46, 48, 49
sodium, 34–35
12- to 18-hour events, 46–47
2- to 90-minute events, 37–38, 42

ABOUT THE AUTHORS

Loren Cordain, PhD, is a professor in the Department of Health & Exercise Science at Colorado State University in Fort Collins, Colorado. His research emphasis is in evolutionary medicine, and he is nationally and internationally recognized for his expertise in the study of Paleolithic (Stone Age) diets and how they relate to the health and well-being of modern humans. He has contributed more than 120 publications to the medical, nutritional, and scientific literature in the past 30 years, and he is the author of these popular diet books: *The Paleo Diet, The Paleo Diet Cookbook, The Paleo Answer,* and *The Dietary Cure for Acne.* He is a member of the American Institute of Nutrition and the American Society for Clinical Nutrition. Dr. Cordain's research is pushing the envelope regarding the role of diet and disease. He has received the Scholarly Excellence award at Colorado State University for his contributions to understanding optimal human nutrition. He has lectured extensively on the Paleolithic nutrition concept worldwide. For more information, visit Dr. Cordain's Web site: www.thepaleodiet.com.

Joe Friel has coached endurance athletes since 1980, including runners, triathletes, duathletes, road cyclists, mountain bikers, swimmers, rowers, Nordic skiers, and endurance horse racers. These men and women ranged from novice to Olympian and included national champions, world-championship competitors, elite age-group athletes, and those who simply wanted to be in better shape, and have included teens, students, senior citizens, business owners, lawyers, doctors, line workers, and professional athletes. He has a master's degree in exercise science and is a recognized authority on training for endurance sports, having written nine other books on the subject and serving as a columnist for two national sports publications for a decade. He is a widely sought-after speaker on the subject of training and consults with national sports governing bodies on the preparation of athletes for world competitions and the Olympics. Friel is also the founder and president of two successful businesses: TrainingBible Coaching, a sports training company with coaches in three countries; and TrainingPeaks.com, a World Wide Web-based business that provides training tools for athletes and coaches. His blog (www.joefrielsblog.com) is one of the most widely read by endurance athletes around the world.